Advance Praise for *The Birth of Modern Neuroscience in Turin*

"This is a long overdue, erudite presentation of the major role of Turin in shaping modern neurosciences, from Luigi Rolando to Rita Levi-Montalcini. It contributes to a growing critical interest in the interactions among European research centers, while giving original insights on the relationship between scientific institutions and the economic and sociocultural environment."

– Laura Bossi, neurologist and science historian, Paris Diderot University

"This is a beautifully written book, presenting the key figures of modern neuroscience from Turin. The authors shed a unique light when discussing these historical giants— providing descriptions of the people and their works that make the book equally exciting to scientists and to lay readers. As a professor at Washington University in St. Louis, I cannot avoid emphasizing the chapter on Rita Levi-Montalcini: One would argue that nothing new could be said about Rita after dozens of books have been written about her, yet another angle to discuss this exceptional character has been explored. Overall, a delightful book!"

– Professor Jonathan Kipnis, Washington University, St. Louis

"This fascinating collection of essays shows how, for a long time, Turin was the hub of European neuroscience, from anatomy to physiology and anthropology, from brain preservation to plasticity, neural growth and regeneration, and from neurology to neuropsychology and psychiatry."

— Emeritus Professor Jan van Gijn, University of Utrecht

The Birth of Modern Neuroscience in Turin

Edited by

Stefano Sandrone *and* Lorenzo Lorusso

OXFORD
UNIVERSITY PRESS

OXFORD
UNIVERSITY PRESS

Oxford University Press is a department of the University of Oxford. It furthers the University's objective of excellence in research, scholarship, and education by publishing worldwide. Oxford is a registered trade mark of Oxford University Press in the UK and certain other countries.

Published in the United States of America by Oxford University Press
198 Madison Avenue, New York, NY 10016, United States of America.

Library of Congress Cataloging-in-Publication Data
Names: Stefano Sandrone and Lorenzo Lorusso editor.
Title: The birth of modern neuroscience in Turin
Description: New York, NY : Oxford University Press, [2022] |
Includes bibliographical references and index. |
Identifiers: LCCN 2021025250 (print) | LCCN 2021025251 (ebook) |
ISBN 9780190907587 (hardback) | ISBN 9780190907600 (epub) |
ISBN 9780190907617 (online)
Subjects: MESH: Neurosciences—history | Neurology—history | Neurologists |
History, 18th Century | Italy
Classification: LCC QP360 (print) | LCC QP360 (ebook) | NLM WL 11 GI8 |
DDC 612.8/2330945121—dc23
LC record available at https://lccn.loc.gov/2021025250
LC ebook record available at https://lccn.loc.gov/2021025251

DOI: 10.1093/med/9780190907587.001.0001

9 8 7 6 5 4 3 2 1

Printed by Integrated Books International, United States of America

To health workers

who fight the COVID-19 pandemic

with courage and self-denial

CONTENTS

PREFACE

This book is a journey in space and time to discover and rediscover famous and lesser known aspects of the birth of modern neuroscience in Turin, from pre-Enlightenment to the 1980s. Historically, Turin has been an attractive and vibrant city for science and medicine. Not just a background to many discoveries, but an integral part of the social and cultural *humus* that favored cross-fertilization of ideas.

In Turin, in the 18th century, the first scientific academies, allowing people to meet and interact over disparate topics, were founded. Carlo Francesco Giuseppe Bellingeri categorized anatomical and clinical features of cranial nerves, Luigi Rolando realized his anatomical drawings, and Aldo Perroncito completed his histological studies. Angelo Mosso performed his pioneering "neuroimaging" experiments, and Cesare Lombroso from Verona penned his controversial theories. The Sicilian Ernesto Lugaro renovated neurology and psychiatry, and the German Federico Kiesow modernized experimental psychology. Camillo Negro recorded the first clinical cases as neurological movies. Giuseppe Levi from Trieste completed his neuroscientific research and mentored three future Nobel Laureates. Among them, Rita Levi-Montalcini, who was banned from the University because of racial laws, emigrated to the United States and discovered the Nerve Growth Factor. Their pioneering contributions, ranging from basic research to transformative aspects, marked an era and shaped the future of neuroscience.

Turin was founded as a Roman colony in 27 BC under the name of *Castra Taurinorum* and, in 1861, it was chosen as the first capital after the unification of Italy. Located in the North of the country, in the Piedmont region, Turin lies by the Po River and is surrounded by the Alps. Its skyline is dominated by the *Mole Antonelliana*, a tower with an iconic aluminium spire, which hosts the National Museum of Cinema. The Egyptian Museum is the largest in the world outside Egypt and in the Turin Opera House Puccini premiered *La Bohème*. Turin is also associated with renowned publishers and football teams, enogastronomic excellence, and famous automobile manufacturers.

By adopting a multidisciplinary approach, we describe Turin's socio economic context and the productive crosstalk between scientific institutions and the cultural environment. Despite the numerous challenges they had to face, neuroscientists from this city or attracted by this city played a fundamental, although sometimes overlooked, role in the history of neuroscience. Within the Turinese streets, forming an unmistakable Roman street grid, modern neuroscience was born.

Stefano Sandrone and Lorenzo Lorusso

ACKNOWLEDGMENTS

We had the idea of writing this book in May 2017, during a Federation of European Neuroscience Societies seminar in Turin. Many of the speakers who gave a talk agreed to write a chapter for the book: we are thankful to them. Unfortunately, we lost two friends and contributors during the writing journey: Carlo Cristini and Davide Schiffer, to whom we dedicate a thought.

A particular acknowledgement to Oxford University Press: Craig Allen Panner, Jordan McAndrew, Helena Joyce, Joseph Reyman Dickrose, and William Allen.

Our thanks to all authors who have collaborated for the realization of this book.

Many thanks to all the archives and publishers, libraries and librarians, museums and universities who gave their authorisation for reproducing figures and quotes included in the book.

CONTRIBUTORS

Alessandro Bargoni
History of Medicine,
Department of Surgical Sciences,
University of Turin, Turin, Italy

Silvio Bellino
Psychiatry Unit, "Rita Levi Montalcini"
Department of Neuroscience,
University of Turin, Turin, Italy

Giovanni Berlucchi
Department of Neurosciences,
Biomedicine and Movement Sciences,
University of Verona and National
Institute of Neuroscience, Italy

Filippo Bogetto
Psychiatry Unit, "Rita Levi Montalcini"
Department of Neuroscience,
University of Turin, Turin, Italy

Andrea Calvo
Neurology Unit, "Rita Levi Montalcini"
Department of Neuroscience,
University of Turin, Turin, Italy

Adriano Chiò
Neurology Unit, "Rita Levi Montalcini"
Department of Neuroscience,
University of Turin, Turin, Italy

Cristina Cilli
University Museum System, University
of Turin, Turin, Italy

Carlo Cristini
General Psychology,
Department of Clinical and
Experimental Sciences, University of
Brescia, Brescia, Italy

Ariane Dröscher
Independent researcher, Bologna, Italy

Marco R. Galloni
Scientific and Technological Archive
of the University of Turin (ASTUT),
University of Turin, Turin, Italy

Giacomo Giacobini
University Museum System,
University of Turin, Turin, Italy

Paul Knepper
College of Social Science,
Department of Justice Studies,
San José State University, San José,
California, United States

Lorenzo Lorusso
Neurology and Stroke Unit,
Department of Neuroscience,
A.S.S.T.- Lecco, Merate, Lecco, Italy

Giacomo Magrini
Literary Criticism and Comparative
Literature, University of Siena, Siena,
Italy

Giancarla Malerba
University Museum System, University
of Turin, Turin, Italy

Germana Pareti
Department of Philosophy and
Educational Sciences,
University of Turin, Italy

Marco Piccolino
National Institute of Neurosciences,
University of Ferrara, Ferrara, Italy

Alessandro Porro
Environmental Health Center,
Department of Clinical and
Community Sciences
University of Milan, Milan, Italy

Stefano Sandrone
Faculty of Medicine, Imperial College
London, London, United Kingdom

Davide Schiffer
Neurology, Department of
Neuroscience,
University of Turin, Turin, Italy

Nichloas J. Wade
Psychology, School of Social Science,
University of Dundee, Scotland, United
Kingdom

Stefano Zago
Neuropsychology Unit,
Department of Neuroscience and
Mental Health, IRCCS Ca' Granda
Ospedale Maggiore Policlinico
Foundation, University of Milan,
Milan, Italy

CHAPTER 1

The Savoy–Piedmont "Renaissance"

From Pre-Enlightenment to the End of the 18th Century

GERMANA PARETI

ACROSS THE ALPS

In the early 18th century, Piedmontese intellectuals and scientists were keen on dialoguing with colleagues and academic institutions across the Alps. They had a truly cosmopolitan approach to research and its dissemination. Physicians were particularly active, and ideas started to circulate. Turin and the Piedmont found themselves within a network connecting the most important European capitals, along with their scientific societies and the universities.

This stimulating environment was further enriched by the growth of civil society: New academies were funded and scientific works were published. These became the pillars of a renewed "cosmopolitan spirit." During the second half of the century, these exchanges among academic institutions and societies, as well as friendships and personal contacts (sometimes even occasional) favored the "process of Europeanization" (and of "deprovincialization") of Piedmontese culture and its medicine. This process was defined and described by Vincenzo Ferrone, an historian of the Enlightenment. As a result, Turin joined the league of other European capitals, such as Paris, Berlin, and Saint Petersburg (Ferrone, 1988). This became especially evident under Victor Amadeus II, when rationalization programs against myths and false beliefs flourished.

At his father's death in 1675, Victor Amadeus II was Duke of Savoy and remained on the throne until 1730. He started championing a deep change, which had consequences on several levels: institutional, political, military, and cultural, to name a few. The Duke of Savoy also reformed the University of Turin, which, from the end of the 17th century to the turn of the century, was declining. On the one side, the Boards, in particular those of physicians, had filled a noticeable institutional void.

On the other side, the Sabaudian nobility had no interest in modernizing the university, and preferred sending their children to more prestigious institutions in Bologna, Pavia, Padua, and Rome. But after having ratified the Treaty of Utrecht (1713–1715), the sovereign finally enacted reforms in the first two decades of the 18th century: the schools of Medicine and Surgery received new energy through the University Statutes.

REFORMING THE UNIVERSITY

Already reformed in 1720 and finalized in a first cycle in 1729, the university statutes, published in Italian and French, aimed at creating five chairs in Medicine: one in Theory, one in Practical Medicine, one in Anatomy, another in Medical Institutions, and the fifth in Botany. These chairs were assisted by a professor of Surgery who would hold his course over a three-year period. All would have to teach "in accordance with the most recent findings by Physicists." The appointment contract mentioned the salaries for professors (Lupano, 2001). They were based on merit and fame, and generally amounted to some 1,300 *lire* per year for the foundation subjects and 800 lire for the minor subjects. But rules were soon broken. Exceptions for the two most prestigious chairs were made: the Chair in Practical Medicine, assigned to Niccolò Cirillo from Naples, with a yearly allowance of 3,000 lire, and the Chair in Theory, with an annual allowance of 2,000 lire.

Recruiting professors was not an easy task. Without "external" candidates, the chairs could have been easily filled by representatives of the local medical community. As a result, the teaching staff would have remained "parochial" (or "provincial," to use the Italian expression). Yet this was partially avoided: Among the prominent physicians who taught in Turin were the French Pierre Simon Rouhault, professor of Surgery, albeit in Turin only until 1732, and the Turinese Giovanni Fantoni (the son of Giambattista, personal physician to Victor Amadeus II), who held the chair in Medical Theory until 1734. Thanks to the teachings of Friar Joseph Roma, from the Order of Minims in Toulouse, the University also was able to provide a solid preparation in experimental physics.

In the second decade of the 18th century, Turin witnessed the publication of an important book. In 1720, Pierre-Simon Rouhault, *Chirurgien du Roi de Sardaigne et des ses armées* [Surgeon to the King of Sardinia and his armies], along with a member of the French Academy of Sciences, published the *Traité des playes de tête* [Treatise on Head Injuries]. This book, which was dedicated to the sovereign, examined the wounds, contusions, fractures, cranial fractures, and concussions affecting the brain and the meninges, "une matière des plus importantes & plus difficiles de la Chirurgie" ["one of the most important and most difficult subjects of Surgery"] (Rouhault, 1720, p. 1), and provided the rules for completing operations using a drill. In the Preface, Rouhault mentioned his lengthy practice in Parisian hospitals as an important "means for securing new *lumieres* (sic)" so that the young surgeons could be successfully trained via anatomy lessons and surgical procedures (Rouhault, 1720, Preface). It is a well-known fact that graduates in medicine initially shrank from the practice of bloodletting and incisions. By founding the Royal Academy of Surgery, Louis XV of France kept separate the two areas of surgery and practical medicine, and surgery was a separate specialization even within the Kingdom of Sardinia.

Rouhault had the distinction of "ennobling" surgery. One year after publishing this book, he succeeded in making the College of Surgeons a part of the University, thereby contributing to the social and intellectual advancement of this profession. Although initially it dealt only with external (or externally produced) injuries, this specialization gradually grew to include the treatment of internal, localized ones, which no longer had to be considered the exclusive domain of a doctor or "anatomist" (Carpanetto, 1998). The Statutes issued by Charles Emanuel III in 1772 would give a more prominent role to Surgery: These constitutions had to provide a detailed indication of the topics to be covered by individual lecturers in Medicine. For instance, Article XVIII in Chapter VI specifies that the Anatomy Professor must teach "the function of [anatomical] parts through experiments on living animals" and provide knowledge not only of the heart and circulation, but also "the action of nerves and the sensitivity of parts."

BETWEEN EUROPEANIZATION AND LOCAL DEBATES

Yet, these were just the first steps toward a wider "Europeanization." Thanks to the generosity of the Savoy nobility, the aforementioned Professor Giovanni Fantoni could travel around Europe and "network" with the chairs of renowned foreign universities, particularly in Paris and Leiden. He was professor of Anatomy (in 1698) and then head professor of Practical Medicine. In *Dissertationes anatomicae* [Anatomical Dissertations] (Augusta Taurinorum, 1701), subsequently merged into *Anatomia corporis humani ad usum theatri accomodata* (1711) [Anatomy of the Human Body Adapted for Anatomical Theater], "a compendious illustration of the complete workings of the human body" (Bonino, 1824), Fantoni revealed his mechanistic view of the human body, wherein structures stemmed from functions through stimuli and movements.

Considerable transformations were happening in the Turinese pre-illuminist context, characterized by empiricism and the achievements of science, which preceded the age of the Enlightenment, advocating the *lights of reason* against superstition and prejudices. Fantoni brought new energy to local medicine via his interactions with Giambattista Morgagni and Antonio Vallisneri, with Giovanni Lancisi (Lombardi, 1828, pp. 118–120; Freschi, 1843), with the physician and historian of medicine Daniel Le Clerc, and with the Genoese and Parisian circles. The fact that the most important Italian and foreign periodicals (including *Giornale de' Letterati d'Italia* ["Journal of the Italian Literary People"], Lipsia's *Acta Eruditorum*, *Philosophical Transactions*, and *Mémoires* of the French Academy of Sciences) mentioned his name witnesses to the circulation of his ideas beyond academic environments.

But in the early decades of the century, a longstanding debate was catalyzing the attention inside and outside the university, namely, the one between the experimental and microscopic anatomy of Malpighi and Morgagni in opposition to the "practical anatomy" sustained by a lesser-known professor of Anatomy, Giovanni Battista Bianchi, a supporter of the enduring empirical-deductive approach to medicine. Although this was a rather "local" controversy that goes beyond the scope of recounting the origins of neuroscience in Turin, it gives an idea of what the dispute must have meant to Morgagni, and signals that it went well beyond the confines of Piedmontese medicine (Morgagni, 1823).

In the footsteps of Aristotelian tradition, physiology had a central role within the context of medical institutions of the time, even though it remained essentially *physica*, that is the "philosophy of nature." It included the most disparate elements, from Neo-Platonism and Paracelsianism to Cartesian mechanism, and from compliance with Avicenna's Canon of Medicine to the animism of Georg-Ernst von Stahl. Within the corpus of medieval medicine, which had brought together the teachings of Galen and Arab tradition in the search for the causes of health and illness, opposing views coexisted. On the one hand, it sustained the essentially alchemical composition of the body's organs and fluids and the influence of astral bodies on diseases, on which physicians intervened through chemical pharmacology based essentially on the three primes or *tria prima*: sulfur, salt, and mercury. This view would, in some respects, be taken up by Stahlian doctrine, according to which the spirit imparted motion, the *motus tonicus*, which in the German physician-philosopher's view was far from being a mechanical process. On the other hand, the view of the body as a machine, which functions by means of pumps, levers, and other biomechanical contraptions, still persisted. Haller's theory departed from Herman Boerhaave's iatromechanical conception, which, at the start of the century, had taken hold in medical schools throughout Europe. Boerhaave considered the body a system of solid parts in which fluids flow following the laws of hydrodynamics, and the *sensorium commune* was the central switch in the "*machina nervosa*" (Koehler, 2007), whereas his pupil Albrecht von Haller distinguished between sensitivity and irritability (the former typical of the stomach and nerves, the latter of muscle fibers in particular) in his work *Elementa physiologiae* [Elements of Physiology] (1757–1766).

PHYSIOLOGY AS "ANIMATED ANATOMY"

Nevertheless, physiology was still considered "animated anatomy," and this approach was maintained even in the physiology lectures held in Piedmont in the first half of the 18th century. Nevertheless, the textbooks adopted by the programs in Medicine were the expression of innovative teaching, steering toward change and embracing a spirit of freedom, free from a censorial spirit that was still present in the faculties of Theology and Law. This environment generated the school of research on the brain and nervous system that rightfully should be called "Piedmontese," and not just "Turinese." There were continual and fruitful exchanges between the Turinese "center" and the province, as well as between academic medicine and physicians in the provinces. Moreover, some of these protagonists did not work in Piedmont alone, but went on to practice in northern Italy and taught in other universities, including Pavia and Padua. For quite a few of these scholars, physics opened the door to studies in medicine, in a period in which Savoyard science also progressed under the impulses of technological progress (and with the development of military and artillery equipment in the Savoyard state), with an impact that was not confined to the Savoyard state.

For example, the Piarist Giovanni Battista Beccaria (1716–1781), one of the fathers of Italian studies on electricity, began his research in the context of Galilean physics. In 1748, he succeeded Joseph Roma in the chair of Experimental Physics. He had embraced the new scientific paradigm represented by the theory of Benjamin Franklin.

Once in Turin, he declared war on the academic sophistries and the Cartesian ideals that had long reigned at the University, and he became the first to introduce the principles of Galileo, of Newton, and of their followers (Bonino, 1824, p. 185).

Beccaria was the author of the two-volume *Dell'elettricismo artificiale e naturale* [On the Artificial and Natural Electricity] (1753) and of numerous subsequent works on magnetism. He could access the University laboratories, which also were frequented by students in medicine and surgery. In addition to this, he could use the instrumentation, thereby successfully surrounding himself with an entourage of promising scholars, many of whom became illuminists. Among these, Giovanni Francesco Cigna, a doctor and chemist from Mondovì, Luigi Lagrange, Tommaso Valperga Caluso, and Giuseppe Angelo Saluzzo from Monesiglio, who in 1757 founded the Society of Science "with the common goal of furthering science and progress" (Reale Accademia delle Scienze di Torino, 1883; Figure 1.1). Founded as a private Turinese society in 1759, it immediately opened its doors to medicine, welcoming, among its first members, the aforementioned Swiss naturalist Albrecht von Haller, but also local physicians, surgeons, and naturalists (in particular, Carlo Allioni, Ambrogio Bertrandi, Michele Antonio Plaza, and Giambattista Gaber). It changed its name to the Royal Academy of Sciences when King Victor Amadeus III granted the society a Royal Charter on July 25, 1783. The "College of Nobles," built in 1679 by the architect Guarino Guarini, became (and remains to this day) its seat. The founding of the Academy set the scene for an open European cultural environment free from prejudice and superstitions and upheld freedom of the press. Unlike universities, it did not aim to provide education, but a "modern" environment permeated by a broad range of scientific interests. Because its aim was not simply the professionalization of students, the Academy focused on the social *utilitas* of knowledge: observations, comparisons, analyses, and experiences were to be shared among all scholars thanks to "a continuous social exchange of information and ideas" (Ferrone, 1998).

AN ELECTRIFYING DEBATE

In the June 1789 opening lecture, the president, Carlo Ludovico Count of Morozzo della Rocca, addressed King Victor Amadeus III to request his patronage and mentioned physiology and its debt to physics, as well as its contribution to anatomy (Morozzo, 1790). Piedmontese scientists were on the same wavelength as their European fellows: In the Galvani Committee recently established within

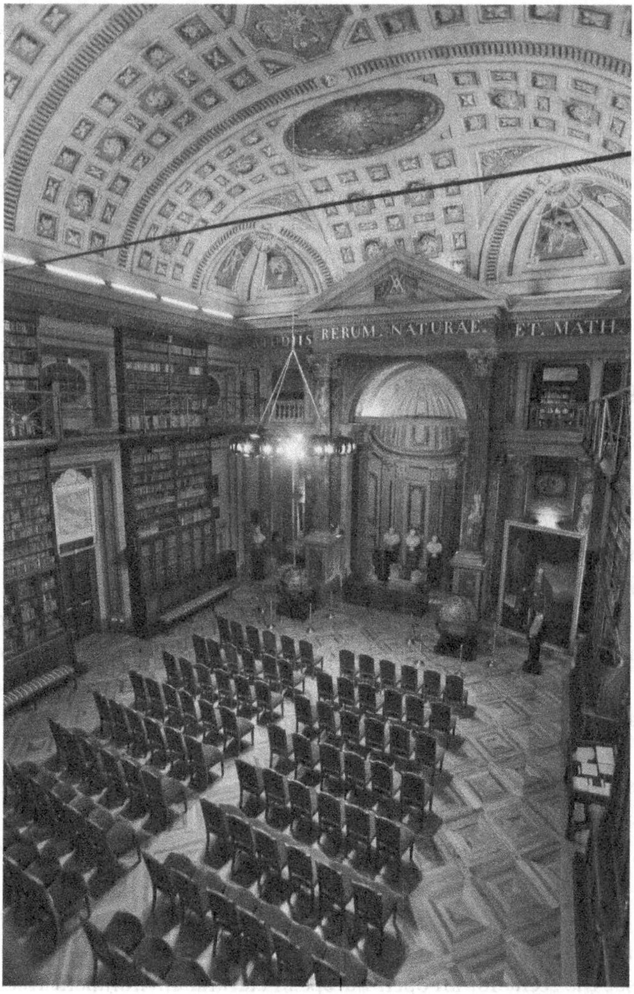

Figure 1.1. *Sala dei Mappamondi (Room of the Globes)*, within the Accademia delle Scienze. This photo was taken by Marco Saroldi in 2014 for Accademia delle Scienze, to whom the rights for publication belong. Thanks to them and to President Massimo Mori for granting the use of it.

the Academy of Sciences, besides completing experiments with batteries on the corpses of those decapitated, hanged, or drowned (Fantonetti, 1838) and discussing methods of dissection, topics of debate included the Hallerian theory of muscular irritability and the controversy between Galvani's "electrobiological" theory and Volta's "electrophysical" hypothesis.

The animating principle of Galvanic fluid, which was also considered a therapeutic stimulant, was similar to the vital principle; academics, physicians, and physiologists did not disdain contributions from experts in electricism to counteract the reductionist, organicistic leanings deriving from Condillac's sensism, and especially from the ideas of French materialists such as Holbach and Helvétius. Although academics such as Beccaria and Cigna aimed to quantify electrical phenomena, there were also charlatans who attributed fanciful properties to the electrical fluid. The debate between strongly opposing views that was polarizing the major European cities quickly overcame Turin.

At the end of the 18th century, controversies were sparked by the careful scrutiny of Brownism, which came to Italy through Giovanni Rasori's reformulation of the doctrine of counterstimulus. Brown's idea was essentially that of *restitutio*, namely of "reintegrating," a deprived organism through stimulation therapy. Medicine merged with philosophy, especially moral philosophy. On the one hand, in the wake of "the healing power of nature" advocated by Rousseau, the idea began to take hold that man does not require remedies, let alone physicians. On the other hand, influenced by Samuel-Auguste Tissot's thesis of "the moral causes of nervous disorders," which, resulting in confusion and weakness "make the heart and mind suffer" (Tissot, 1779)—the medicine of *sensibilité*, based on the union of "physical" and "moral," was emerging. It was a "philosophical" medicine (Maffiodo, 1996), like the one of the Savoyard Amédée Doppet, "docteur en Médecine de la faculté de Turin" and author of *Le Médecin Philosophe.*

Capitalizing on the link between "physical" and "moral," Amédée Doppet demonstrated how to heal by acting on the patient's stirrings of the soul (Doppet, 1787). Another Savoyard physician, Joseph Daquin, author of *Philosophie de la folie* [Philosophy of Madness] (1791) and a friend of Rousseau, was among the first supporters of the "moral" treatment of illnesses, in particular mental illnesses. While Brownism was a strong response to that which has been aptly defined as the "temptation to disengage" of natural medicine inspired by Rousseau, there were increasing attempts to investigate the neurophysiological nature of certain pathologies. More in-depth research was undertaken on the fundamentals of the nervous system to sustain the thesis, more philosophical than scientific, of a correlation between "body" and "spirit." The literature produced by historians of the early modern period highlighted the contiguity of ideas that developed in the field of practical medicine, irrespective of physicians' affiliations to different cultural domains. Rejecting the application of rigid mechanistic classifications, this empirical approach rapidly gained consensus, mostly because of the immediate, basic results obtained.

MAGNETISM, MESMERISM, AND MASONRIES IN THE CAPITAL OF THE OCCULT

The scientific debate was on fire. It involved professionals, part of the public, and even penetrated into the smaller centers, as shown by the work of the lesser known, but well-informed, physicians in the provinces. Emblematic, in this respect, is the figure of Francesco Giuseppe Gardini (1783–1816), who worked between the cities of Alba and Asti. A corresponding member of the Lyon Academy and of the Royal Academy of Science, he was in touch with some of the most important European scientists, including Galvani, Giovanni Battista Beccaria, and Giuseppe A. Eandi (Carpanetto, 2011). Gardini wrote several works on the usefulness of electric fluid, in which ("anticipating Bichat" according to historians), he divided nerves into three spheres, depending on whether they originated from (1) the brain, cerebellum, or medulla oblongata; (2) from the spinal cord; or (3) from their "interweaving" and independent of one's own will. He was such a fervent supporter of Galvanism and of the effects of electric fluid that Galvani himself wrote in a letter to his friend: "*Galvanic fluid should be more aptly called* GARDINISM *rather than* GALVANISM" (Bonino, 1824, p. 298).

In the early 19th century, the "fluid theory" took different forms even in Piedmont, and various schools and movements flourished around the application of this universal principle. Magnetism, mesmerism, hypnosis, and somnambulism (Gallini, 1983), along with physiognomy and rhabdomancy, were new "alternatives" to the official medicine, which continued to reflect mechanistic views. On the wave of a renewed vision of nature (one that was dynamic, vital, and in continuous transformation, as advocated particularly by Diderot and other French illuminists), popular science was gaining momentum. Its success was often linked to the crisis of the physical–mathematical mechanicism, which also reflected on 18th-century medicine in Piedmont (Ferrone, 2000). These movements, albeit liminal and underground as compared to experimentalism, were nurtured by a pantheistic–vitalist vision of man and nature. These movements found fertile terrain in the "humanitarian" approach of healers and magnetisers, which soon would translate into the figure of the physician seen not only as a man of science, but also as a philanthropist.

Despite their popularity, the Academy continued to strongly refuse any form of neo-naturalism, which gained a foothold in Freemasonry. Piedmont thus became a land of conquest for animal magnetism, and this was probably also favored by its liberal tradition. From a therapeutic perspective, this became a cultural phenomenon revolving around the "extraordinary." Francesco Guidi, one of the most prominent magnetizers in Italy during the 19th century, commented:

> In the last ten years Piedmont has been the only part of Italy in which magnetism was well accepted, and given that it is [. . .] a science of progress, I daresay the best progress, necessarily requires freedom, and in Piedmont, in the wake of the freedom of association and of press accorded by the Savoyard constitutional Statute, it was freely studied, experimented and applied by enthusiastic magnetophiles and scholarly physicians-magnetists—among whom doctors Borgna, Coddè, Gatti and Peano excelled. (Guidi, 1863, p. 362)

In 1856, the recently founded Philomagnetic Society counted 66 members, including 15 physicians, and although "the Medical Council of Turin requested that the government issue repressive laws against the magnetizers," an authoritative expert such as Giovanni Stefano Bonacossa, future director of the asylum and founder of the *Clinica delle malattie mentali* [Mental Illness Clinic], urged:

> not to relegate everything that is and has been said about animal magnetism and somnambulism to fairy tales, nor are the magnetic phenomena observed in many individuals just a cunning invention, and one must therefore not refer to those who

practiced magnetism or who believed in it as charlatans, yokels or simpletons. (*Atti*, 1840, p. 376)

The effect was still perceptible in the 19th century in the form of what Georges Gusdorf named, "romantic knowledge," which had developed in opposition to Cartesianism and Illuminism; this profound contradiction would make Turin—already "a singular city [in which] anything could happen"—one of the capitals of the occult in the coming centuries.

REFERENCES

Atti della II riunione degli scienziati italiani tenuta in Torino nel settembre del 1840 (1841). Torino: Cassone e Marzorati.

Bonino GG (1824) *Biografia Medica Piemontese*. II. Torino: Bianco.

Carpanetto D (1998) *Scienza e arte del guarire. Cultura, formazione universitaria e professioni mediche a Torino tra Sei e Settecento*. Torino: Deputazione Subalpina di Storia Patria.

Carpanetto D (2006) Elettricità animale e riforma della medicina in uno scritto autobiografico di Francesco Giuseppe Gardini (1740–1816). *Medicina & Storia* 12: 115–137.

Doppet A (1787) *Le Médecin Philosophe*. Turin: Reycends.

Fantonetti GB (1838) *Effemeridi delle scienze mediche*. X. Milano: Molina.

Ferrone V (1988) *La Reale Accademia delle Scienze di Torino: Le premesse e la fondazione*. In V Ferrone, *La Nuova Atlantide e i Lumi. Scienza e politica nel Piemonte di Vittorio Emanuele* III, pp. 107–157. Torino: Meynier.

Ferrone V (2000) *I profeti dell'Illuminismo. Le metamorfosi della ragione nel tardo Settecento italiano*. Roma-Bari: Laterza.

Freschi F (1843) *Storia della medicina in aggiunta, e continuazione a quella di Curzio Sprengel*. VI. Firenze: Tipografia della Speranza.

Gallini C (1983) *La sonnambula meravigliosa. Magnetismo e ipnotismo nell'Ottocento italiano*. Milano: Feltrinelli.

Guidi F (1863) *Il magnetismo animale considerato secondo le leggi della natura*. Milano: Sanvito.

Koehler PJ (2007) *Neuroscience in the Work of Boerhaave and Haller*. In H Whitaker, CUM Smith, and S Finger (Eds.), *Brain, Mind, and Medicine. Neuroscience in 18th Century*, pp. 213–232. New York: Springer.

Lombardi A (1828) *Storia della letteratura italiana nel secolo XVIII*. II. Modena: Tipografia Camerale.

Lupano A (2001) *Le Regie Costituzioni universitarie del 1772*. In *Costituzioni di Sua Maestà per l'Università di Torino*, pp. iv–xii. Torino: Università degli Studi di Torino.

Maffiodo B (1996) *I borghesi taumaturghi. Medici, cultura scientifica e società in Piemonte fra crisi dell'Antico Regime ed età napoleonica*. Firenze: Olschki.

Morgagni GB (1823) *Delle sedi e cause delle malattie anatomicamente investigate*. I. Milano: Rusconi.

Morozzo (Count) CL (1790) Discours adressé au Roi dans la séance publique du 28 juin 1789. *Mémoires de l'Académie Royale des Sciences de Turin* 4: xx–xxvi.

Reale Accademia delle Scienze di Torino (1883) *Il primo secolo della Reale Accademia delle Scienze di Torino. Notizie storiche e bibliografiche (1783–1883)*. Torino: Stamperia Reale Paravia.

Rouhault PS (1720) *Traité des playes de tête*. Turin: Radix & Mairesse.

Tissot SAD (1779) *Traité des nerfs et de leurs maladies*. II. Paris-Lausanne: Didot.

CHAPTER 2

The Savoy–Piedmont "Renaissance"

Between Materialism and Spiritualism

GERMANA PARETI

VINCENZO MALACARNE'S PIONEERING RESEARCH

More than 50 kilometers away from Turin is the city of Saluzzo, where Vincenzo Malacarne (1743–1816) was born. He was a professor at Padua from 1794 until his death; he first held a chair in Clinical Surgery, and subsequently, when his eyesight worsened, in Principles of Surgery. But let's go back to the beginning of his career. Malacarne started as a student of the surgeon and anatomist Ambrogio Bertrandi (1723–1765), who maintained that anatomy should be considered together with physiology: "the Anatomist [. . .] with knowledge of Mechanics, Physics and Chemistry, gleans the working of life from these" (Bertrandi, 1786, p. 109). Formed by this school, Malacarne was outstanding in human and comparative anatomy: When Bertrandi became ill, he nominated Malacarne to the chair in Practical Surgery (Ruggieri, 1817). Before joining Pavia and Padua, Malacarne had worked intensely in Piedmont. He had been "a tutor in anatomy and surgical foundations" in Turin, and the director of the baths of Acqui from 1775 to 1783. In that year, Victor Amadeus III nominated him "Head Physician of the hospital of the city and citadel," a position he held until 1789, when he was awarded the chair in surgical foundations in Pavia.

Malacarne made an important examination of hydrocephalus in a deceased 17-year-old, and this was an important milestone for his research, because it allowed him to make important observations of the brain, the cerebellum, and the nervous system, as described in the first chapter of the second part of *Osservazioni in Chirurgia* [Observations in Surgery]. This work was conceived between 1764 and 1772, but published only in 1784. Malacarne inferred the existence of a close link between variations in psyche or behavior and cerebral lesions. He observed that a series of disorders had led to the "compression" of the cerebellum (Malacarne, 1784,

p. LXXXIII), "excessively developed bones," dural thickening, robust laminae, and so on, corresponding to "increasing [degrees of] stupidity," weakened limbs, irregular eye movements, agitation starting from the 10th year, voracity, and convulsions leading to death.

Malacarne's interest in the brain increased. At the end of the 1770s, he produced what is considered the first detailed description of the cerebellum (Zanatta et al., 2018), with the introduction of many new anatomical terms, including "tonsil," "pyramid," "lingual," and "uvula," which subsequently came into common use (Clarke & Jacyna, 1987). *Nuova esposizione della vera struttura del cerveletto umano* [New Presentation of the True Structure of the Human Cerebellum], published in Turin in 1776 and comprising 44 cases, was followed in 1780 by *Encefalotomia nuova universale* [New Universal Encephalotomy]. Malacarne's work was largely descriptive: In dissecting the cadavers, he aimed to "very clearly describe the incisions, and operations" (Malacarne, 1780, p. xiv), and the "alterations, the morbid or benign deformities, found in any miniscule portion of the brain" and in the brain of brutes, and so on. He aimed to "change" the name or even give a new name to those parts observed that did not have one, and these names would derive from their shape and structure or their similarity to other known anatomical parts. During his anatomical observations, Malacarne identified a minuscule portion of the lower cerebellar vermis that was slightly prominent (from an evolutionary standpoint the oldest portion of the cerebellum), from which four lobes branched: It became known as "the Malacarne pyramid" or "transverse eminence of Malacarne."

CRETINISM, SCALPELS, AND NEUROANATOMY

Another object of his investigation was the phenomenon of cretinism in the Cuneo and Aosta valleys. He concluded that the disorders found in cretins, imbeciles, lunatics, and half-wits were due to cranial malformations, the excessive width of the foramina of Valsalva, the "distressed" cerebellar masses, an anomalous number of "small lobes" or laminae, the latter always fewer than those of healthy specimens (Malacarne, 1789). According to his son Gaetano, who wrote his father's biography, Malacarne authored a work titled, *Direzione di uno spedale di pazzi e cura delle diverse specie di pazzia* [Direction of a Hospital for Insane People and Treatment of Different Kinds of Insanity], where he examined numerous cases of cretinism. This book, however, was never published or perhaps was lost, but nonetheless it might witness his interest in mental illnesses. In his 1788, *Lettre sur l'état des Crétins* [Note on Cretinism], addressed to Johann Peter Frank, Professor of Clinical Medicine in Pavia, Malacarne described in detail the series of alterations, thickening and/or flattening, narrowing or excessive widening of the cranium, cavities, laminae, and especially, *la masse du cervelet infiniment plus gênée* ["the mass of cerebellum infinitely more constipated"] (Malacarne, 1789, p. 35): a set of factors that could "provide a vast amount of extremely useful information for explaining [. . .] the faculties of organs contained in our body's three main cavities" (Belloni, 1977). The hypothesis of a parallelism between imbecility and hypoplasia of the cerebellum stemmed from this and was a topic of discussion with Charles Bonnet, who instead maintained that *le travail de l'esprit* ["the work of the spirit"], and therefore exercising the intellect, increased the number of lamellae, and not *vice versa*. At the time, scholars such as Bonnet and Haller were searching for the *siège de l'âme* ["seat of the human soul"]. The former especially voiced pessimism regarding our knowledge of brain anatomy and the location of human faculties, thereby stimulating, through his sensistic psychology, Malacarne to perform research on the cerebellum and collect a greater number of case studies.

Notwithstanding his excellent results, Malacarne doubted that neuroanatomy "would discover the tiniest pieces." He engaged in an intense exchange of correspondence with Bonnet, to whom he wrote 53 letters between 1778 and 1789 (the year in which he moved to Pavia). Among these, Letter II is of particular importance. Malacarne replied to the Swiss naturalist that "our scalpels will never find the smallest particles of this admirable machine that is the direct instrument of the soul; nevertheless, we always try to find the differences" (Malacarne, 1791, p. 18). And he stated that he was increasingly convinced that differences affected individuals: Those whose cerebellum has a larger number of laminae, have a "better memory," are wiser and livelier, providing as an example the case of a cerebellum particularly rich in laminae from a commoner married to a custodian, but endowed with great intellectual curiosity. In Letter III he agreed with Bonnet that the continued, intense exercise of mental faculties could stimulate the development of certain portions of the brain. He supported this hypothesis with an example that would become famous in the history of neuroscience:

"Who knows whether different trials on sibling pairs of dogs, goldfinches, parrots and blackbirds etc., nourished with the same food in the same home, who knows, I say, whether similar trials could teach us something interesting [. . .]? One from each pair should receive careful training, the other none at all, and after some years both should be analyzed using an anatomical scalpel" (Malacarne, 1791, p. 32).

FAME AND MISFORTUNE IN EUROPE

By analyzing the cerebellum, Malacarne became famous throughout Europe, to the extent that he was complimented by the French physician and anatomist Félix Vicq d'Azyr ("Monsieur Malacarne spoke of [the cerebellum] with the greatest erudition and knowledge") (G. Malacarne, 1819, p. 69; Vicq d'Azyr, 1786) and by the German physician and anatomist Samuel Thomas Soemmerring, who wondered whether the use of the brain, and especially mental exercise, could change the structure of the brain. Based on observations by Malacarne, the response seemed to be affirmative, "although the scalpel cannot easily demonstrate this" (Soemmerring, 1800, p. 91). His name appears a number of times in *De Partium corporis humani praecipuarum fabrica et functionibus* [On the Structure and Functions of the Primary Parts of the Human Body] by Albrecht von Haller (1778, vol. 8), who expressed his difficulty with "the new terms that Malacarne had been obliged to adopt, given that he described therein things that had never been found before" (G. Malacarne, 1819,

p. 78). His greatest merit was the pioneering contribution to what would be known in the 20th century as "cortical plasticity," as was acknowledged in the late 1960s by Mark R. Rosenzweig and colleagues at the University of California. They described neuroanatomical modifications of the occipital cortex after enriched experiences (Rosenzweig et al., 1968, 1972a and 1972b) and recalled the exchange of views between the two 18th century scientists.

In 1783, Bonnet and Malacarne discussed the possibility of testing experimentally whether mental exercise could induce growth of the brain. Malacarne agreed to test the hypothesis and carefully designed the experimental strategy. He chose as subjects two littermate dogs and pairs of birds, each pair coming from the same clutch of eggs. He gave one animal of each pair extensive training while the other received none. After a few years of this differential treatment, Malacarne sacrificed the animals and compared the brains of each pair (Rosenzweig, 2007). Rosenzweig concluded by citing the review of the experiment's positive results in *Journal de Physique* in 1793 (n° 43, p. 73).

However, the German phrenologist Franz Joseph Gall was probably not among Malacarne's admirers. According to Malacarne, Gall failed to adequately cite him in his works: In 1807 he began to examine the works of his German colleague, without losing occasion to argue against his ideas (Buzzi, 2012, 2015; Martelli et al., 1993). During his study of modifications to endocranial organs, Malacarne became convinced that a link existed between the morphology of the cranium (and brain) and mental disorders: This idea preceded Gall's tenets of phrenology, announced in 1810. Using his *cephalometer*, Malacarne intended not only to "measure" endocranial conformations, but also to demonstrate the precise correspondence of cerebral and cerebellar structures with intellective and moral faculties. According to Father Juan Andrés y Morell, a Catalan Jesuit who was very active in the Piedmontese region in the early 19th century, Malacarne had given "the brain its, so to speak, clear and distinct geography, and its true, genuine history, its philosophical anatomy" (Alfieri, 2014, p. 11). According to Malacarne, the brain consisted of individual apparatuses, each corresponding to a specific intellectual activity, distinct and different from one individual to the other, depending on cranial morphology. Apparently, the Jesuit Andrés did not consider this view as being dangerously materialist. On the contrary, in Malacarne's studies he saw—"almost an essay on *psychotomy* or *phrenotomy*, that is of different organs through which the brain or soul acts upon us in different ways"—indispensable information to improve the intellectual faculties of individuals and cure mental illness, for which anatomical evidence can be found. By sectioning subjects affected by cretinism, Malacarne had identified a cranial anomaly accompanied by hypoplasia of the cerebellum and a reduced number of lamellae. Andrés noted that it would be even more useful to dissect subjects who were "crazy but not born so," having followed the development of the illness. These discoveries would have even benefitted the history of the same Society of Jesus, so that Andrés joked, "How many lamellae was Boscovich missing, and how battered they must have been after his illness, if modifications do indeed occur in them?" (Alfieri, 2014, p. 11).

The individual apparatuses to which the Jesuit refers confirm that Malacarne's conception was essentially a *morphological* one: He aimed to compile an atlas of "topographical anatomy." In his treatise titled *Osservazioni in Chirurgia* [Observations in Surgery], Malacarne illustrated the results of his study on 60 dissected parts of the human brain, determining the weight of the cerebrum and cerebellum, the number of laminae in the two surfaces (upper and lower) of the cerebellum, and comparing findings from subjects affected by cretinism with those from normal subjects. The cerebellum of the former weighed much less (about one ounce) and had far fewer laminae (half to as little as one quarter) than in healthy subjects. While trying to rationalize the organization of cerebral structures, Malacarne also adopted a *mathematical* criterion to define the relationship between faculties and a lack of development due to brain pathologies (Cherici, 2006; Pajon & Cathiard, 2015). The human brain was found to be "superior" to that of animals because of its greater complexity; based on the number of fissures and circumvolutions, it was possible to delineate an evolutionary scale among vertebrates, with the brain structure of man at the apex. Note that through this research approach Malacarne subtracted the development of intellectual faculties from the influence of society and education and returned to a "morphological" rather than "dynamic" view of physiology. Nevertheless, in subsequent studies published in the early 1800s, he postulated a possible parallelism between the arrangement of the "innards" (the lamellar structure) of the cerebrum, cerebellum and spinal cord, and Volta's galvanic column, wondering whether this organization could "perhaps be the main source of the Galvanic Fluid, the actual animator of the animal machine" (Malacarne, 1808). Although the idea indicated a shift from an anatomical-surgical reductionist paradigm to a "more subtle" physiological vision based on animal electricity, it was to remain an unfinished project, because Malacarne died in 1816.

NAPOLEON AND TOURBILLON

The sequence of political and military events across the Alps—the end of the French Revolution, Napoleon's rise to power, his fall and the Restoration—had significant repercussions on the medicine in Piedmont between the 18th and 19th centuries. Even the biographies of Turinese physicians and scientists of that period often reveal the effects of that *tourbillon* of historical events. For example, the anatomist Luigi Rolando, who completed a degree in Turin in 1793 and was a pupil of Gianfrancesco Cigna, had to go to Sardinia, where he followed the Savoy family into exile during the Subalpine Republic established by Bonaparte, to then return to Piedmont in 1814 as a Professor of Anatomy.

Bonaparte's policies had contrasting effects. Although the ideal of a "renewal of order" advocated by Bonaparte suited the generally moderate positions of the academics, Piedmontese physicians took a collective stance against the incorporation of Subalpine medicine in the French university system. At the same time, Napoleon strengthened the central role of hospitals as a place of research and care, as well as the importance of practical medicine, which was a fertile meeting ground for university and academia. But with the Restoration and the return of the Savoys to Turin, much of the experience accumulated during the previous years was lost. Numerous appeals were made to discard obscurantism, partly represented also by a return to spiritualistic and neo-vitalistic positions that were more pronounced in medicine than surgery. The medical environment already had a solid representation within the Academy of Sciences, strengthened by the previous revolutionary and Napoleonic experiences. Despite this, in December 1819, a group of 19 physicians, including university professors (also of physiology, such as Michele Buniva and Lorenzo Martini), signed a petition requesting of the king that they be allowed to periodically meet to discuss medical-scientific topics and publish reports on these sessions.

Following the revolutionary events of 1821, in which many physicians and members of the university took part, the government looked upon the Society (private) of Medicine-Surgery with hostility. Only in 1842, Carlo Alberto, namely Charles Albert, King of Sardinia, gave it official recognition, and in 1846 its status was raised to Royal Academy of Medicine and Surgery. In the climate of tension that had developed in Piedmont, Carlo Alberto managed to overcome the resistance of the Ministry of Police, even though the time had long been right. In fact, in 1832 the members of the Society of Medicine and Surgery had renewed their appeal to the king to subsidize the publication of a journal (*[Giornale delle Scienze Mediche]*, first published four years later).

ROYAL ACADEMY OF MEDICINE AND SURGERY

This institution did not have an easy life, and there were heavy restrictions to avoid having discussions veer toward politics. Despite initial restrictions on political discussions, the establishment of this institution was of great importance for Piedmontese medicine: It promoted new ideas, allowed interactions with the institutions of foreign countries, and had a good representation by academics of diverse disciplines. It also served as a hub during an era when it was difficult to attend international congresses. Among those writing articles (from the first issues of *Giornale*) were distinguished physicians involved in the study of the nervous system. Along with many future presidents of the Academy, the name of Carlo F. Bellingeri, a philosophy student who turned to medicine and was admitted to the College of Medicine in 1818, was included. He dedicated himself to the so-called *res tenebrosa* ("the dark," as he himself defined it) of brain anatomy and physiology, including the clinical examination of encephalitis and neurological pathologies, and to studies in comparative anatomy based on animal dissection, focusing on the pathways and connections of nerve fibers and the spinal cord. Bernardino Bertini and Giovanni Stefano Bonacossa also appeared: Under the guidance of Benedetto Trompeo and Cipriano Bertolini, the latter came to the Royal [Lunatic] Asylum in 1820 and headed it between 1842 and 1874, whereas Bertini, a physician and member of Parliament, proposed the law invoked by his colleague Bonacossa for the care of those who had "lost their intellectual faculties" (Bonacossa, 1846, 1849, 1851; Baral, 2016). In 1838 there were 29 members. The number rose to 40 in 1848 and, in the pages dedicated to its history, the role of the Academy of Medicine in the foundation of the Faculty of Medicine was mentioned. From 1848, Clinical Medicine in Mental Illness was included among the new Chairs.

"Medicine of Passions"

In the meantime, the more or less underground movements that, drawing inspiration from a neo-naturalistic vision, had affirmed themselves in the 18th century continued to exist on the fringes of the institutional positions represented by the "noble" part of scientific culture—the one that had never wavered from Galilean-Newtonian experimentalism. If the close ties between man and nature downscaled the role of official pharmacopeia, the value of expressions of sensibility, as manifested in sentiments, passions, and emotions, were recovered. Moving away from 18th-century sensism, the new "medicine of passions" did not ascribe these conditions to the organs of sense alone but to a more interior "knowledge of the spirit." Deriving from the French tradition and typical of the Romanticism of the start of the century, this approach continued the work of the previous century's "moral medicine," which aimed to educate individuals morally (and therefore socially). The medicine of "disorders of the spirit" also had a following in Savoyard Piedmont, where it became widespread through the influence of Jean-Louis Alibert, a dermatologist and court physician to the kings of France, among the founders of the Academy of Sciences in Paris and a member of the one in Turin, as well as author of *Physiologie des passions* [Physiology of the Passions] (1825), which was subtitled "new doctrine of moral sentiments." Twenty years later, in *Médecine des passions* [Medicine of the Passions] (1841) besides defining a classification for passions and attempting to identify both moral and physical causes, Jean-Baptiste Félix Descuret investigated the relationship between insanity and its effects on accountability. Reaffirming the value of anatomical–pathological investigation in determining the organic causes of insanity and the influence of moral causes, respectively, the two opposing conceptions of mental illness, organicistic and psychological, accused each other of dogmatism and materialism. In the search for a possible middle ground, phrenological doctrine represented a third solution.

Although its emphasis on localization stemmed from a rigid determinism, in Piedmontese medicine, instead, it seemed to steer more toward identifying the *moral* causes of illness. The analysis of craniums, undertaken especially on the organs of assassins and criminals, revealed the influence of "internal organization and external causes" on behavior, an interweaving that could be investigated only through medical appraisal. It was therefore possible to reconcile the opposing views in the thesis according to which one could stimulate the brain in the direction of good by "operating" on the physical causes (*Atti*, 1841). And although even the French psychiatrist Jean-Étienne Dominique Esquirol maintained that Piedmontese psychiatry was lagging behind its French counterpart, things were about to change.

Piedmontese Psychiatry

Establishing itself as a discipline focusing not only on deviant behavior, but also on the social aspects (and legal implications) of insanity, the psychiatry that was emerging in Piedmont was inspired by the idea of a correlation between organic conditions and moral and intellectual states. It also adopted moral treatment as a potential therapy with beneficial effects on organic mechanisms. Incarnated in the figures of the earlier-mentioned Trompeo and Bonacossa, academics with a past "faith in phrenology," the psychiatrist represented an authority with the dual function of physician and director of the hospital. This novel approach to medicine would have revolutionary effects on the management of insane asylums, which became "medical institutions" and resulted in the modernization of treatments, the medicalization of interventions with a view to creating a more humane relationship between doctor and patient, and the introduction of statistical analyses, favored by Trompeo through his hospital statistical register in 1828.

Bonacossa studied in major European cities and believed in the existence of a link between anatomical-pathological conditions and behavioral disorders. In the assembly of Italian scientists held in Turin (Figure 2.1) on September 23, 1840, he entered into a slight dispute with the earlier-mentioned Bellingeri. In identifying the

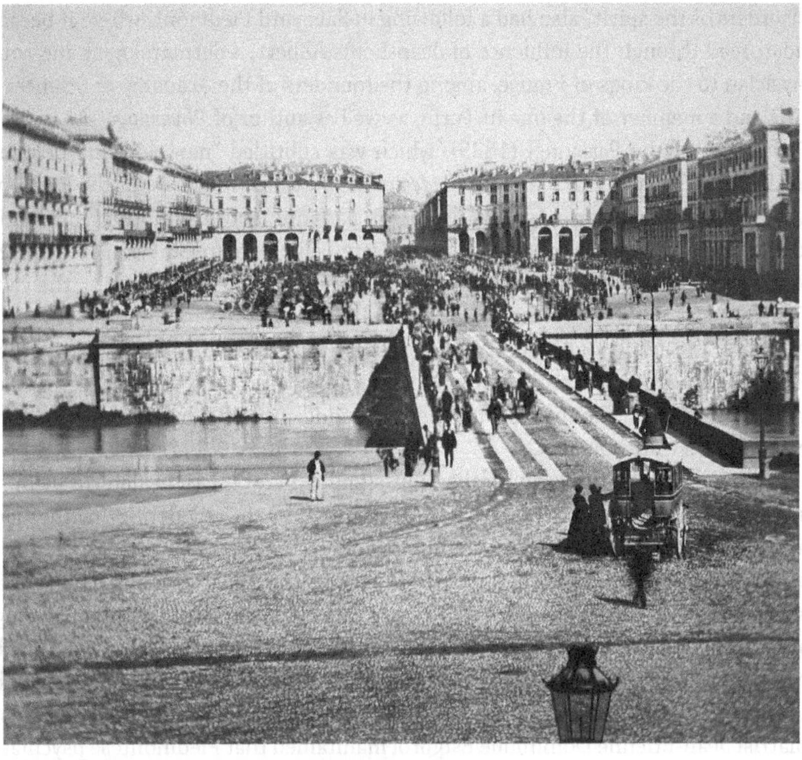

Figure 2.1. Turin in 1860. Courtesy of Marco Galloni.

location of mental lesions, the latter maintained that "the lesions of the senses and intellectual faculties [. . .] indicate that the affection lies solely in the brain's gray matter" (*Atti*, 1841, p. 326), whereas the damage to motor faculties lies in the matter of the spinal cord. Bonacossa, instead, believed there should have been a number of "specific" organs of mental illness, without excluding affections, not only of the cerebral cortex but also of the spinal cord as causes of psychiatric alienation.

Embracing the hypothesis of the organic nature of insanity, suitable medical treatment had to take place in a mental hospital under the guidance of experts in mental disorders. Doing his utmost to have the laws whereby "a madman is still responsible and punishable for his own actions" repealed, Bonacossa appealed to politicians, advocating the importance of establishing a "committee of physicians" to decide on the morbid condition. His appeal was heard by Bernardino Bertini, a doctor and member of parliament who in 1850 proposed a law for "the custody and care of half-wits" (Bonacossa, 1851, pp. 21–22).

DECLINE AND REBIRTH OF VITALISM

Historians who have investigated the status of Piedmontese medicine in the early 19th century agree that local physicians were mostly vitalists, although this philosophical current had influenced Turinese surgery to a lesser extent. In his studies devoted to Piedmontese physicians, general pathologist Mario Umberto Dianzani, who was president of the Medical Academy in Turin between 1998 and 2002, found that provincialism, which also had afflicted the medical sciences, was only overcome in the second half of the 19th century, when Jakob Moleschott was assigned the chair in Physiology and Giulio Bizzozero the one in Pathology.

In reconstructing the history of Turinese physiology, which was constantly wavering between materialism and spiritualism at the end of the century, the words of Turin-born physiologist Angelo Mosso during the opening of the academic year at the University of Turin on November 4, 1895 are emblematic. After mentioning the "resurrection" of 18th-century materialism (by the French La Mettrie, Holbach, and Cabanis), Mosso commented that, in general, "for each action there is a reaction" and that "materialism [thus] fueled mysticism" (Mosso, 1896, p. 31), a movement he took to include Lavater and Mesmer, given that his animal magnetism was a "mysterious fluid" acting at a distance and not contained in humans in equal amounts.

The physiology of Johannes Müller gave renewed life to sensorial studies, although they still concerned the "physiology of the spirit," given that Müller was a vitalist and admirer of Giordano Bruno. Nevertheless, a real change came with his pupils, Hermann van Helmholtz, Emil du Bois-Reymond, Ernst W. von Brücke, and others, who fought against vitalism. While Carl Ludwig reintroduced mechanicism into the study of life manifestations, Moleschott returned to materialism, although veiled with mysticism. Unfortunately, Mosso commented, things were regressing: He did not intend to give up on an explanation involving "only force and matter," but it was evident that to "unravel the secret of life," many were again referring to "a mystical force that acts with discernment and consciousness" (Mosso, 1896, p. 36). It was a resurgence of vitalism, deplored by du Bois, to which Mosso wished to add his own voice. He saw disturbing signs of the influence of neo-vitalism and mysticism even in Italy, and this was particularly discouraging, given that, at that moment, there was no hope of understanding the essence of life and of the soul, the nature of thought and of consciousness, notwithstanding the progress in the understanding of the structure of nerve cells and their chemistry.

These words not only depict the Zeitgeist at the end of the century, but also highlight some among the unresolved questions—no longer merely philosophical, but truly neuroscientific—on the link between mind and body.

REFERENCES

Alfieri F (2014) La Compagnia di Gesù e la medicina nel primo Ottocento. Ipotesi di ricerca. *Mélanges de l'École Française de Rome. Italie et Mediterranée modernes et contemporaines* 126(1): 83–100.

Alibert J-L (1825) *Physiologie des Passions, ou Nouvelle doctrine des sentiments moraux.* 2 vols. Paris: Béchet jeune.

Atti della II riunione degli scienziati italiani tenuta in Torino nel settembre del 1840 (1841). Torino: Cassone e Marzorati.

Baral S (2016) *Le phrénologiste au tribunal. Notes pour une recherche sur le cas italien.* http://criminocorpus.revues.org/3209.

Belloni L (1977) Charles Bonnet et Vincenzo Malacarne sur le cervelet siège de l'âme et sur l'impression basilaire du crâne dans le crétinisme. *Gesnerus* 34: 69–81.

Bertrandi A (1758) *Orazione sopra gli Studj per la Chirurgia* in *Opere* (1786), I. Torino: Reycends.

Bonacossa GS (1846) Dell'importanza della perizia medica nel giudicare sullo stato mentale dell'uomo in alcune questioni del foro civile e criminale. *Atti della Reale Accademia Medico-Chirurgica di Torino* 2: 348–383.

Bonacossa GS (1849) *Osservazioni sulla proposizione di legge del medico collegiato Bernardino Bertini membro della Camera de' Deputati riguardante la custodia e la cura dei mentecatti e considerazioni sullo stato attuale de' pazzi in Piemonte.* Torino: Favale.

Bonacossa GS (1851) *Petizione presentata al Parlamento nazionale il 18 febbraio 1849*, in *Elementi teorico-pratici di patologia mentale.* Torino: Favale.

Buzzi S (2012) Lumen Fortunae Vincentii Malacarnae. In S Messina and P Trivero (Eds.), *Metamorfosi dei Lumi. Le belle lettere e le scienze*, pp. 169–183. Torino: Accademia University Press.

Buzzi S (2015) Un carteggio sepolto nel tempo: alcune lettere di Vincenzo Malacarne da Saluzzo. *Rivista di Storia dell'Università di Torino* 4(2): 1–47.

Cherici C (2006) Vincenzo Malacarne (1744–1816): A researcher in neurophysiology between anatomophysiology and electrical physiology of the human brain. *Comptes Rendus Biologies* 329(5–6): 319–329.

Clarke E, Jacyna LS (1987) *Nineteenth-Century Origins of Neuroscientific Concepts.* Berkeley-Los Angeles-London: University of California Press.

Descuret J-BF (1841) *La médecine des passions ou Les passions considérées dans leurs rapports avec les maladies, les lois et la religion.* Paris: Labé.

Haller A (von) (1778) *De Partium corporis humani praecipuarum fabrica et functionibus. Cerebrum. Nervi.* 8. Bernae at Lausannae: Ex Pérelis Societatum Typographicarum.

Malacarne G (1819) *Memorie storiche intorno alla vita e alle opere di Michele Vincenzo Giacinto Malacarne da Saluzzo . . .* Padova: Tipografia del Seminario.

Malacarne V (1776) *Nuova esposizione della vera struttura del cerveletto umano.* Torino: Briolo.

Malacarne V (1780) *Encefalotomia nuova universale*. Torino: Briolo.
Malacarne V (1784) *Trattato delle osservazioni in chirurgia*, II. Torino: Briolo.
Malacarne V (1789) *Sui gozzi e la stupidità che in alcuni paesi gli accompagna*. Torino: Stamperia Reale.
Malacarne V (1791) *Lettere Anatomico-fisiologiche* in *Neuroencefalotomia*. Pavia: Stamperia del monastero di san Salvadore.
Malacarne V (1808) Conoscendo dalla organizzazione del cervelletto in ispezie, e forse anche da più attento esame del cervello e dalla midolla spinale che queste viscere formano qualche cosa di somigliante alla colonna galvanica del Volta, cercare per mezzi di sperimenti se fossero mai la sorgente principale del fluido galvanico animator materiale della macchina animale. *Giornale della società di incoraggiamento delle scienze e delle arti di Milano* 4: 122–130.
Martelli F, Baratta L, Arieti S (1993) Considerazioni preliminari sull'origine della frenologia: L'opera di Vincenzo Malacarne. *Medicina nei secoli* 5: 405–418.
Mosso A (1896) Materialismo e Misticismo. *Annuario Accademico per l'anno 1895–96*. 20: 23–52.
Pajon P, Cathiard MA (Eds.) (2015) *Les imaginaires du cerveau*. Fernelmont: EME.
Rosenzweig MR (2007) Modification of brain circuits through experience. In F Bermúdez-Rattoni (Ed.), *Neural plasticity and memory: From genes to brain imaging*, Chapter 4, 67–94. Boca Raton, FL: CRC Press/Taylor & Francis.
Rosenzweig MR, Bennett EL (1972a) Cerebral changes in rats exposed individually to an enriched environment. *Journal of Comparative and Physiological Psychology* 80(2): 304–313.
Rosenzweig MR, Bennett EL, Diamond MC (1972b) Brain changes in response to experience. *Scientific American* 226: 22–29.
Rosenzweig MR, Love W, Bennett EL (1968) Effects of a few hours a day of enriched experience on brain chemistry and brain weight. *Physiology and Behavior* 3: 819–825.
Ruggieri C (1817) *Elogio funebre di Vincenzo Malacarne*. Venezia: Andreola.
Soemmerring ST (1800) *Vom Bau des menlischen Koerpers. Hirnlehre und Nervenlehre*. 5. Frankfurt a.M.: Varrentrapp und Werren.
Vicq d'Azyr F (1786) *Traité d'anatomie et de physiologie, avec planches coloriées représentant au naturel les divers organes de l'homme et des animaux*. 2 vols. Paris: Didot l'aîné.
Zanatta A, Cherici C, Bargoni A, Buzzi S, Cani V, Mazzarello P (2018) Vincenzo Malacarne (1744–1816) and the first description of the human cerebellum. *Cerebellum* 17: 461–464. https://doi.org/10.1007/s12311-018-0932-7.

CHAPTER 3

Carlo Francesco Giuseppe Bellingeri

A Forgotten Pioneer of Italian Neurology

LORENZO LORUSSO AND STEFANO ZAGO

I have tried to shed more light on the structure, functions, and diseases of the nervous system; both in my inaugural dissertation, in which I exposed at length my thoughts on the functions of the nerves of the face, that is, of the fifth and seventh pairs of the brain nerves. I have the satisfaction of having in these studies preceded the works of Charles Bell, a Professor in London, because this work of mine was published in the year 1818, and Charles Bell published his writing three years later, that is in 1821. I don't know if the English author has consulted or read this work of mine; I know that I sent a copy to the Royal Society of London, and that it arrived and was presented to the Scientific Committee on January 20, 1820, as published in the volume of the Philosophical Transactions of the Royal Society of London for the year 1820, in whose catalogue of works, donated by the Authors, my dissertation is found with my name and indicated the date.

With these words, written in the preface of his *Ragionamenti, Sperienze ed Osservazioni Patologiche comprovanti l'Antagonismo Nervoso* [Reasonings, Experiences and Pathological Observations Proving the Nervous Antagonism] published in 1833, Carlo Francesco Giuseppe Bellingeri (1785–1848) claimed precedence over the discovery of the distinct functions of the facial nerves and, more precisely, of the fifth and seventh pairs of brain nerves. This was one of the leitmotifs of Bellingeri's work and life, and he often reiterated how this would have given him worldwide fame (Bellingeri, 1834a). A long diatribe followed with Charles Bell (1774–1842), universally recognized, along with the Frenchman, François Magendie (1783–1855), as the true modern discoverer of the functions of the facial nerves (Tomey, Komotar, & Mocco, 2007).

In the 19th and 20th centuries, several works throughout Europe and the United States recognized Bellingeri as a pioneer in the study of cranial nerves (e.g., Walker, 1834; Negri, 1835; *The Edinburgh Medical and Surgical Journal*, 1834; Bostock, 1836; Lewis & Dandy, 1930; Harris, 1952) and research on the spinal cord (Brown-Séquard, 1860). Bellingeri, however, seems to have been "lost" over time.

His name was not even included in any of the most important reviews concerning the history of Italian neurology (e.g., Belloni, 1963; Zanchin & Premuda, 1990; Bentivoglio & Mazzarello, 2009), nor were his descriptions on the cranial nerves (Fine & Darkhabani, 2009; Ng, Rosenfeld, & Di Ieva, 2019). This neglect of Bellingeri was perhaps also due to the theory of "nervous antagonism" he had put forward at the time (Bellingeri, 1825a, 1833a). He discussed the anachronistic idea of neural competition between the cerebral lobes and their function of driving flexion and adduction movements, and the cerebellum and its function involving extension and abduction movements (Bellingeri, 1824, 1833a). Bellingeri tried to corroborate his theory with the observations made by ancient and contemporary authors, and even through his own experiments on animals; this theory, however, failed to gain consensus. Despite the mixed fortunes of his writings, Bellingeri should be counted among the leading Italian scholars of neurology. He advocated the importance of studying the central and the peripheral sensory and motor brain functions, because this could have finally detached medicine from the metaphysical or magical shackles that immobilized the whole medical field in what has been defined as a cul de sac (Silvano, 1987).

He attributed the functions of the intellect and senses to the cortical substance, and the functions of movement to the medulla. He discussed the importance of the sensory organs and their connections with the brain during a presentation at the Royal Academy of Sciences in Turin in 1833, which was focused on the difference between sight and hearing. He published an essay on the cerebral hemispheres, according to a phylogenetic approach in mammals, following the phrenological theories of Franz Gall (Bellingeri, 1838, 1839). With regards to mental illness, Bellingeri followed the footsteps of one of the founding fathers of Italian psychiatry, Vincenzio Chiarugi (1759–1820), who defined mental illness as ". . . a primitive insult of the brain". This was also supported by the founders of the clinics for nervous and mental illnesses in Italy (Mazzarello, 2018). In 1840, Bellingeri read a paper at the *Second Congress of Italian Scientists*, which took place in Turin, on the influence of the cortex on mental functions and malfunctions. He observed that several psychiatric diseases were associated with lesions of the cortical substance of the brain, which, in his opinion, was undergoing an inflammatory process (Leidesdorf, 1865). Bellingeri's scientific work is vast, and he was also a valuable clinician, as documented by several publications on the subject (Banchieri, 1963).

CARLO FRANCESCO GIUSEPPE BELLINGERI: A BIOGRAPHICAL SKETCH

Bellingeri was born in Sant'Agata Fossili, a charming hilly town in the area of Tortona, about one hundred kilometers from Turin. According to his baptismal certificate, he was born on the 15th of October 1785, and not in 1779 or 1787 as misreported by some sources, due to births of the same name (Banchieri, 1963; Balestrasse, 1968; Silvano, 1987). Bellingeri spent his childhood in the castle owned by the ancient Bellingeri family and studied in Tortona. He was then sent to Turin, where he attended courses in philosophy and joined the Faculty of Medicine and Surgery. He graduated with honors on the 31st of December 1811, at the age of 24, with a thesis on clinical pharmacology titled, *Nuovi succedanei alla china—china nella cura delle febbri intermittenti* [New cinchona substitutes in the treatment of intermittent fevers] (Bellingeri, 1811). He then returned to his hometown, where he began to practice as a medical doctor, but two years later he returned to Turin to join the university and focus on research. When Bellingeri arrived in Turin, Vittorio Emanuele I (1759–1824) had already been in exile in Sardinia since 1802, and the political and social effects of the French Revolution were evident throughout the peninsula. The clinical tools of the time were essentially based on physical semiotics (*ratio et observatio*), and in Turin he was able to continue honing his observational skills. Bellingeri was accepted at the Turin Medical College and devoted his inaugural conference (held publicly on May 9th, 1818, as a Doctor Philosophiae et Medicinae) to original methodologies to investigate the distribution of the cranial and spinal nerves (Bellingeri, 1818). The conference was given particular attention and proceedings were published in the same year (see Figure 3.2). Sixteen years later, in 1834, a translation was published in the *Medical Chirurgical Review*.

Bellingeri was also a professor of psychiatry at the Faculty of Medicine at the University of Turin, where he then became Dean. He was also a consultant at the *Spedale Maggiore of the Equestrian Order of SS. Maurizio and Lazzaro*, and a court doctor to the Royal Family. He was later appointed a *Member of the Royal Academy of Sciences of Turin*, the prestigious institution founded in 1783 by Vittorio Amedeo III of Savoy (1726–1796). Bellingeri was also a corresponding member of the *Imperial and Royal Academy of Sciences, Letters and Arts of Padua*, and of the *Royal Academy of Sciences of Siena*. A shy man, but highly esteemed academically (Chiari, 1835; Silvano, 1987), he married Gertrude Vegezzi (1797–1848), with whom he had seven children. He died in Turin on May 15th, 1848, at the age of 53; the cause of his death is unknown. The city of Rome, but not Turin, named a street in his honor.

NEUROANATOMY AND NEUROPHYSIOLOGY WORKS

We can broadly distinguish three main research areas of interest for Bellingeri in the neuroscientific field: (i) neuroanatomy and physiology, with a particular focus on the spinal cord and cranial nerves; (ii) clinical neurology, with his descriptions of neuralgia and infectious diseases, especially encephalitis, and (iii) galvanism and electricity.

Bellingeri, according to the Italian tradition studies considered that the description of the anatomy of a structure should always precede any hypotheses on its independent action. Several renowned Italian scholars explored this area, among them Domenico Cotugno (1736–1822) in Naples, who described the two aqueducts of the vestibule and the cochlea, and Domenico Mistichelli (1675–1725), in Rome, who first described the crossing of the nerve fibers. Others included Felice Fontana (1730–1805) in Florence, who studied the cylindrical, myelin sheath of the brain and the degeneration of the ninth pair of cranial nerves. There were also three leading anatomists working in Pavia, namely Vincenzo Rocchetti (1777–1819), known for spinal cord pathology, Antonio Scarpa (1752–1832), whose name is linked to the vestibular ganglion, the large cardiac nerve, and the nasopalatine nerve, and Bartolomeo Panizza (1785–1867), who studied the cranial nerves and cerebral lobes. As we have already seen in the previous chapters, there were also Michele Vincenzo Giacinto Malacarne (1744–1816) in Saluzzo and Luigi Rolando (1773–1831) in Turin.

Bellingeri's monograph was translated into German by Hermmann Kaulla (Kaulla, 1773). Of particular interest are Bellingeri's studies on the structure of the spinal cord, of which he was one of the pioneers from both an anatomical and a pathophysiological perspective. In 1823, the work, *De Medulla Spinali Nervisque ex ea Prodeuntibus Annotationes Anatomico-Physiologicae* (Figure 3.1, center; Figure 3.2), written in Latin, proposed a subdivision between the gray matter, which is linked to sensory processes, and the white matter, assigned to the functions of motion. He also noted that children, who have maximum sensitivity and weak muscle movements, had more gray than white matter, whereas in adults the situation was reversed, thus favoring motion over sensitivity. Bellingeri concluded that:

> *the nerves that come from the brain and its productions, such as the pyramidal bodies, and the anterior bands of the spinal cord, generally serve the flexion movements, while the nerves that stem from the cerebellum, and its productions, that is, from the posterior bands of the spinal cord, produce the movements of erection and extension.* (Bellingeri, 1823)

Bellingeri sent his observations to Scarpa and received the following reply on December 9th, 1824:

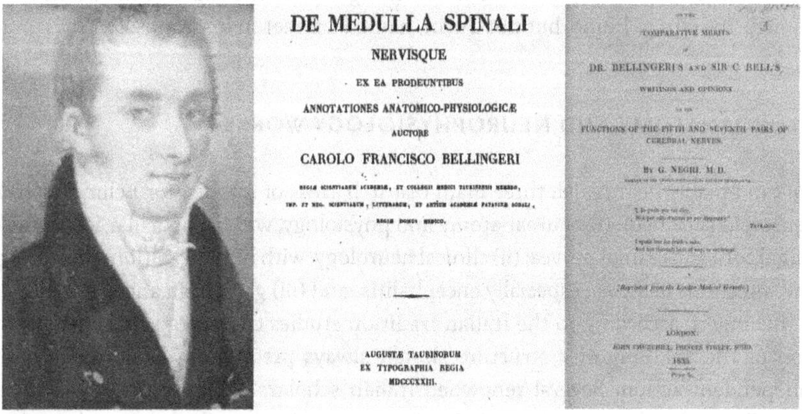

Figure 3.1. Left: Title page of *Il dissertatio inauguralis* held by Bellingeri in 1818, at the *Regio Ateneo di Torino*. Center: Title page of *De Medulla Spinali Nervisque ex ea Prodeuntibus Annotationes Anatomico-Physiologicae,* printed in 1823. Right: Title page of Giovanni Negri's work of 1835 on the roles Bellingeri and Bell played in the discovery of the role of the V and VII cranial nerves. Courtesy of Bellingeri family.

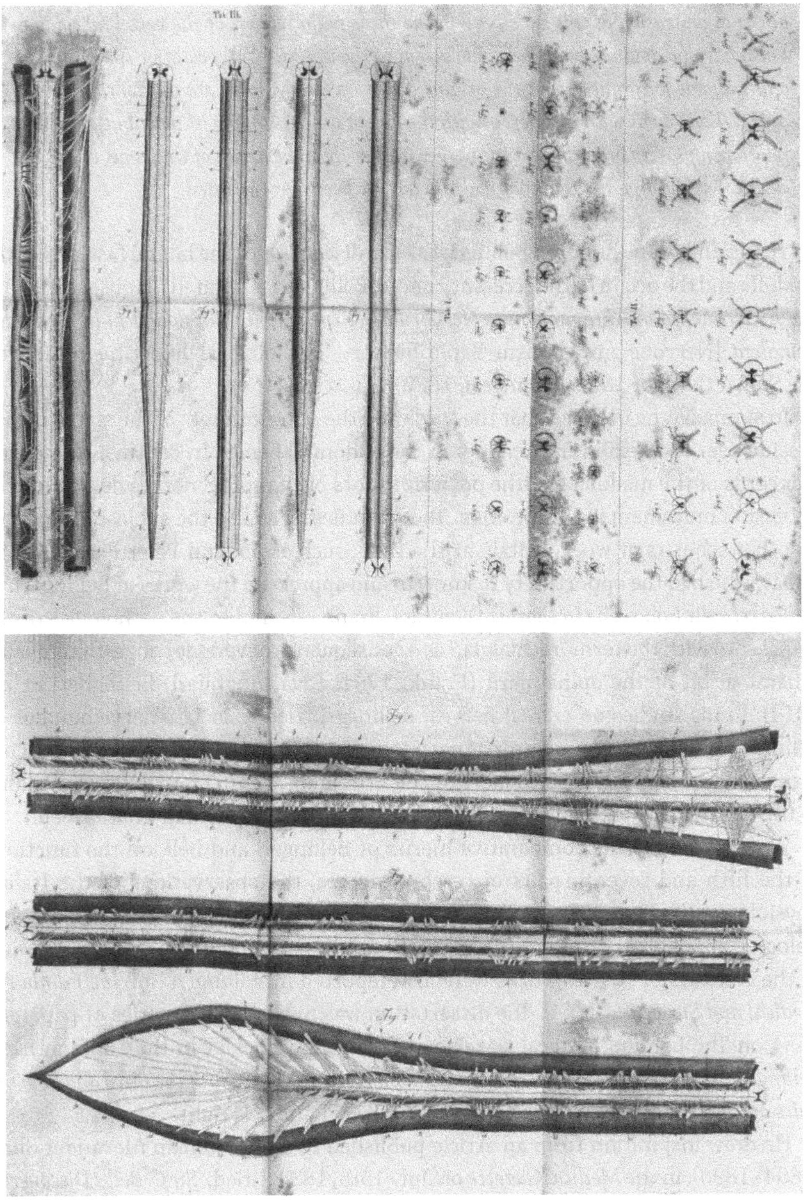

Figure 3.2. Illustrations of the spinal cord, reported in *Medulla Spinali Nervisque ex ea Prodeuntibus Annotationes Anatomico-Physiologicae*" Courtesy of Bellingeri family.

I read with great interest your anatomical notes on the spinal cord which you kindly sent me. After some observations on the corpse, I have no doubts in stating that the purely anatomical part of your booklet is very accurate and true. The existence of the lateral cords, and therefore the distinction of the spinal cord into six fascicles, is in accordance with the truth. Your observations on the location and form of the cinereal substance are exact, and in the organization of this substance in the three main regions of the vertebral column. I also have no doubts about the triple origin of the anterior and posterior spinal nerves, and I take it for granted that the origins of the accessory nerve are all from the lateral cord. When I dealt with this nerve, with the aim of understanding its distribution and its relationships with other important nerves, rather than the origin of the same, it was not clear to me the organization that had still not yet been demonstrated.

Scarpa's admissions honored Bellingeri as the discoverer of the lateral fascicles of the medulla and the origin of the accessory nerve. Bellingeri reiterated his observations in the *Experimenta in Antagonismum Nervorum—Experimenta Physiological in Medullam Spinalem* [Nervous Antagonism Experiments—Physiological Experimentation on the Spinal Cord] of 1826 (Bellingeri, 1826).

In summary, he believed that the cords and the anterior roots of the spinal nerves preside over the flexion movements in the abdominal ends. In contrast, the posterior cords of the medulla and the posterior roots of the spinal nerves determine the extension movements in these ends. These studies were also the subject of research by other scholars at work in Italy at the time, such as Johann Peter Frank (1745–1821), who had the opportunity to know of and appreciate the works of Bellingeri. In *De Vertebralis Columnae in Morbis Dignitate*, Frank referred to the pathologies of the spinal cord with the term "rachialgia," as a consequence of venous congestion causing inflammation of the spinal cord (Frank, 1791; Riva, Anghileri, Belingheri et al., 2019). In his studies on cranial nerves, Bellingeri tried to isolate nerve bundles by delineating their origin, course, connections, and terminations. His first works concerned the anatomy and physiology of the fifth and seventh cranial nerves, leading to the dispute over the claim of their discovery with the Scotsman Charles Bell.

With regards to the comparative merits of Bellingeri and Bell, on the functions of the fifth and seventh pairs of cerebral nerves, the observations of the Italian physiologist Gaetano Negri (1797–1849), member of the medico-surgical society of Bologna, are of great interest, analyzing the studies of the two contenders. A review of the contexts of Negri's works were also reported in Volume 42 of *The Edinburgh Medical and Surgical Journal*. The dissertation was published in a series of papers in 1834 on The London Medical Gazette and later in a booklet in the 1835 entitled, *Bellingeri and Sir C. Bell's Writings and Opinions on the Functions of the Fifth and Seventh Pairs of Cerebral Nerves* (Negri, 1834; 1835). See Figure 3.1, right.

He drew inspiration from an article published by the Scotsman Alexander Shaw (1804–1890), in the *Medical Gazette* on July 19th, 1834, titled, *'Sir C. Bell's Discoveries in the Nervous System*, and discussed the physiology of the fifth and seventh cranial nerves and the dispute in question (Shaw, 1834).

Negri reported that Shaw admitted the first description of the anatomical-physiological features of the two nerves was made by Bellingeri. In this regard, Shaw writes:

It is a remarkable fact that five years, at least, before Sir Charles Bell communicated to the Royal Society of London his peculiar doctrines on the uses of the fifth and seventh pairs of nerves, Bellingeri had published a most minute and elaborate view of the anatomical distribution and physiological uses of these nerves, and on many of the most important points of the latter department, had anticipated the British physiologist [. . .]. *We have no doubt that everyone who peruses the dissertation with attention, will be satisfied that the Italian has given a much clearer and connected view of the anatomical and physiological history of these two nerves (the fifth and the portion dura of the seventh) than any one of the writers who have yet attempted the task.* (Shaw, 1834)

Shaw reported, however, that Bell submitted some notes to his colleagues, only as a sketch of his area of research on the brain and printed them privately in 1811. In these notes, Bell pointed out that spinal nerves were double, the anterior and the posterior roots serving different functions, and he performed experiments to ascertain this. He still considered the fifth as a single nerve, separated by other cerebral nerves. Only in March 1821 did Bell examine the functions of the fifth pair and classified it with the spinal nerves (Bell, 1821). From his first paper, read before the Royal Society in July 1821, to the last one, in 1826, Bell considered the fifth pair a mixed nerve of sensory and voluntary motion, generally distributed to the face, both for mastication and sensation; but he never mentioned the smaller portion of the fifth as a peculiar nerve, merely for the voluntary muscular action of the lower jaw (Bell, 1826). This had been described in 1784 by the Piedmontese anatomist Giovanni Battista Paletta (1748–1832), who observed that the anterior portion of the fifth pair, which he termed *nervus crotaphitico et buccinatorius*, was distributed exclusively to the jaw muscles and must therefore be a nerve of motion. Paletta identified it to be the nerve that is affected in trismus (Paletta, 1874).

As already mentioned, Bellingeri published a more detailed and accurate account of the fifth and seventh pairs of nerves in 1818. In his original observations, he inferred that the voluntary motion of the facial muscles, and the animal sense of touch, depended on the influence of the seventh. He also showed that the seventh pair of nerves, or facial nerves, presided over the animal functions of the head, face, and neck, namely, over sensation and motion. He also performed experiments in rabbits resulting in complete palsy of the eyelids and upper and lower lips; moreover, the sensitivity of the face appeared very much impaired and upon plucking out hairs by the roots, the rabbit gave no signs of sensitivity or pain. Bellingeri, besides conferring sensation and numerous other qualities usually assigned to nerves, understood the distinctive physiological properties of the two divisions of the fifth pair, several years before the theory of the influence of these parts was explained by Bell (Bellingeri, 1834a). Although he followed the natural intricacy of the nerves of the face from their origin to their last terminations, he deduced their functions anatomically and physiologically, and somehow even from a pathological viewpoint, experimenting on animals such as dogs, horses, goats, pigs, and sheep (Shaw, 1834; Negri, 1835).

According to Bellingeri, the fact that the temporal and pterygoid muscles in facial paralysis are under voluntary control showed that these are innervated only by the fifth pair: The smaller portion of the trigeminal represented an exclusively motor nerve and not a sensory nerve due to different brain origins, and he proposed that it should be called a masticating nerve. Paletta had rightly observed that the crotaphytid and the buccinator nerves had a distinct innervation from the trigeminal. Bellingeri noted that the smaller portion of the V pair is distinct from the larger portion. With regard to the observation that sometimes the muscles innervated by this minor portion also perform involuntary movements, in addition to voluntary, Bellingeri experimentally proved that this occurs because the smaller portion of the V receives filaments or "surculi" from the lower jaw nerve in the territory where it is distributed, the jaw being a branch of the largest portion of the trigeminus and a nerve exclusively of the senses. This led him to be able to describe neuralgia of the hemiface or, as it was called at the time, "proposalies." The French anatomist, Jean Léon Testut (1849–1925), in his treatise, *Traité d'Anatomie Humaine* [Human Anatomy Traite] of 1889, recognized the eponymous *Bellingeri nerve* to indicate the "chewing nerve" (Testut, 1889).

In his *dissertatio inauguralis* in 1818 (Figure 3.1, left), Bellingeri considered facial nervous prosopalgia to be linked to both the fifth and the seventh pairs of cerebral nerves, and he gave three distinct levels of severity to its form: mild, severe, and irremediable. He also identified neuralgia to be idiopathic, general, sympathetic, symptomatic, or primary and secondary in form (Bellingeri, 1834b). According to Bellingeri, the nerve-related disease appeared more frequently in the spring or autumn. He stressed the difficulties inherent in clinical practice and in the therapy of these forms. In particular, the treatment of inflammatory prosopalgia was somewhat problematic, and only anti-inflammatory drugs had any effect. According to him, the treatment of the irritant was based on methods that had to remove the extraneous and disturbing cause, and for this purpose, topical, revellant, epispastic, and caustic remedies were useful. In some cases, it was necessary to resort to cutting the infected nerves as an *extrema ratio*.

Bellingeri reported more than 40 cases of severe facial neuralgia related to the involvement of the fifth or the seventh pairs of cerebral nerves. He also observed cases with a frequency of three times per day, which he treated with Peruvian bark. In some cases, the disease lasted for years, whereas on other occasions it disappeared on its own after multiple remedies had been vainly applied. Of the 40 cases of neuralgia he treated effectively, 36 of them showed the healing to be definitive. He excised the supraorbital nerve in only four cases. In severing the affected nerve, Bellingeri recommended a double section and the removal of a small piece of nerve to prevent scarring the juxtaposition of the two cut pieces and the recurrence of the disease. The second cut had to be made toward the end of the nerve to avoid severe pain. Bellingeri was against the cauterization of the nerve proposed by Paletta (Arrigoni, 1842; Govoni, Granieri, & Menini, 1996).

Another important study by Bellingeri resulted in his description of a nerve involved in taste; this was approximately 1,600 years after Galen's first description (Finger, 1994; Witt, 2019). Bellingeri reported that the timpani cord of the facial nerve (VII) was the nerve that mediated taste in the anterior portion of the tongue. This finding was later confirmed by experimental observations conducted in the 19th century, which observed that the nerve passed through the mid cavity of the ear to enter the brain (Lussana, 1872; Lorusso et al., 2012). In addition to this, clinical observations indirectly confirmed its involvement in taste perception, because a condition affecting the middle ear causes the loss of taste in the front of the tongue (Snyder & Bartoshuk, 2016).

STUDIES ON NEURO-INFECTIOUS DISEASES

Bellingeri was also interested in the study and research of encephalitis, which was the subject of his work titled, *Storia delle Enepfaliti Epidemiche in Torino* [History of the Encephalitis Epidemic in Turin], published in 1824. He provided one of the first descriptions of lethargic encephalitis, an infection later nosologically defined by the Austrian, Costantin von Economo (1876–1931) in his famous *Encephalitis Lethargica* (von Economo, 1917; Pistacchi, 1998; Foley, 2011).

He categorized encephalitis into four forms, based on the involvement of various parts of the brain: the cephalalgic, the delusional, the lethargic, and the trembling. He also recognized two frequent forms of headache, the frenetic or delusional and the lethargic or soporific. The latter was characterized by a mild (or nonexistent) delusion, stupor, sopor, lethargy, and an almost apoplectic state, widely described previously by Hippocrates (460 BC–377 BC), Gerolamo Fracastoro (1483–1553), John Caius (1510–1573), Thomas Sydenham (1624–1689), François Boissier de Sauvages de Lacroix (1706–1767), Giovanni Battista Borsieri (1725–1785), and Joseph Frank (1772–1842). From an autoptic point of view, Bellingeri mentioned the hyperemia of the parenchyma and the cerebral membranes. He wrote:

> *encephalic mass tends to swell and inturgitate, but being entirely surrounded and locked within the nonyielding bone, it therefore ensues that the effect of tumefaction is exerted on the brain substance and as the inflammation itself progresses, more pressure is produced on the encephalic organ and nerves that arise from it: an immediate effect of that pressure is to produce syndromes of paralysis or deficient nerves.* (Bellingeri, 1825b)

He stressed that encephalitis can be accompanied by mild fever and that in the absence of other inflammatory indexes, including blood, it can have an epidemic character (Bellingeri, 1825b; Levi, 1833). He also described 18 cases of encephalitis with lethargy, which occurred in Piedmont between July and August 1824, demonstrating hyperemia of the parenchyma and brain membranes on autopsy examination. In his words:

> *It should be kept in mind that these comatose fevers had a favorable prognosis because with appropriate care (bloodletting, blisters on the back of the neck, light feeding, enemas), avoiding that the patients were lying down to prevent congestion and the accumulation of fever material in the head, in two weeks healed, without any postencephalitic symptoms.* (Bellingeri, 1825b)

Another area that occupied him was the confirmation of his theory of nervous antagonism and tetanic manifestations, by remarking that this was consequential to the localization of the pathological process in the various areas of the central nervous system (Bellingeri, 1833b). According to him, opisthotonos, the violent extension of the whole body, could result from an illness of the cerebellum, or only the hind cords of the spine; whereas the emprostono, or spasmodic flexion, could be the result of a disease of the brain hemispheres. We now know that this subdivision is not invariable and cannot be physiologically justified.

His monograph titled, *Statistica Nosologica dello Spedale Maggiore dell'ordine Mauriziano per il biennio 1843–44* [Nosological Statistics of the Spedale Maggiore of the Mauritian order for 1843–44] was dedicated to the influence of environmental conditions on the working classes and testified to his commitment to the epidemiology of infectious diseases. Not only did he write that living in damp places and in newly built houses led to more frequent rheumatic or arthritic conditions, but he also observed that insulation or overheating caused an excess of blood with consequent nosebleeds, headaches, and encephalitis. These were more frequent in farmers, masons, cooks, and bakers. Venereal infections were also among the most common diseases, and he had the opportunity to follow a case with exostosis headache, slow thrustitide, frontal neuralgia, and heart disease with angina. According to Bellingeri, carbonic acid vapors, especially when very intense, could generate burdensome headaches. The inhalation of acrid vapors, if breathed for a long time, also could give rise to bronchitis, of which he was able to study several cases among matchmakers (Bellingeri, 1825b, 1842). He also focused on the various forms of involvement of the nervous system and its complications such as encephalitis, meningitis, thornitis, epilepsies, apoplexy, headaches, dizziness, and neuralgia (Bellingeri, 1825b, 1842, 1843, 1844).

Galvanism and Animal Electricity

Bellingeri also investigated the functions of the living organism on the basis of the laws of electrical, galvanic and magnetic polarities, by carrying out multiple experiments on the tissues and organs of animals. He was familiar with the experimental studies of Luigi Galvani (1737–1798), and he complemented these with texts by Johann Peter Frank and Alessandro Volta's (1745–1827) studies on the frog. But he was also influenced by the theories on muscle irritability and nervous sensitivity by the Swiss doctor Albrecht von Haller (1708–1777) (von Haller, 1769).

He attempted to determine the nature and the degree of electricity in different animal tissues by comparing them with various metals. For example, he put the animal viscera and organs in contact with the frog's muscle and nerve. This resulted in the detection of contractions, hence, Bellingeri concluded that the various viscera and organs had no opposing electrical current when prepared in the absence of humidity and, therefore, they must be placed in an aqueous environment. He concluded that the electricity of the various tissues and organs is supplied by the biological fluids of the human body, such as arterial or venous blood and urine, bile, saliva, mucus, and pus. The animal organism could be compared to a galvanic battery in which liquids are motors and the only conductors of electricity. The electricity of biological liquids is similar to that supplied to metals through their mutual contact, and therefore it can be concluded that we can speak of animal electricity. He presented his observations on the electricity of mineral liquids several times to the Academy of Turin.

In a first paper, presented in 1819, Bellingeri showed that urine has an electrical gradient comparable to that of water when the animal is healthy. In 1827, he assessed the electricity of blood, urine, and bile, and concluded that biological liquids represented mostly conductors and interpose, to use his words: "between the circle that takes place, through an iron arch, between the nerves and muscles of a frog" demonstrating that humid materials can promote the electro-physiological contraction (Bellingeri, 1827; Grimelli, 1849; Scoutetten, 1870). Through his research, he sought to demonstrate that the electricity of biological liquids changes in healthy and sick subjects and, in particular, it is reduced in inflammatory diseases and those diseases associated with fatigue (Bellingeri, 1828). He found that arterial blood has a lower electrical charge than venous blood; moreover, the former changed in terms of electrical charges more rapidly and coagulated more properly than venous blood. Bellingeri also attempted to exploit knowledge relating to the electrical properties of tissues and biological liquids for diagnostic use in clinical practice. An attempt in this direction is described by the Piedmontese physician Mauro Ricotti (1766–1831), who reported the case of a patient suffering from a probable form of encephalitis in which Bellingeri set out to examine the patient's urinary electrical properties using electrotherapy as a treatment (Ricotti, 1818).

As quoted by Schiff in *The Lancet*, Bellingeri also aimed to identify: "if the sensory nerve could be considered as a motor nerve which runs in an inverse direction, and of which the action is expressed by a reflex movement." (Schiff, 1876). This aspect also was recognized by Carlo Matteucci (1811–1868), who is considered a pioneer for the development of modern electrophysiology (Matteucci, 1844; Moruzzi, 1996). Bellingeri confirmed that electrical currents directed along the nerves cause the contractions of the respective muscles. He researched circuits composed of neuromuscular tissues on the one side and extrinsic electromotor materials on the other: The muscles separated from the nerves did not contract under the influence of the electric current, while the nerves did (Grimelli, 1849).

CONCLUSIONS

This chapter pays tribute to the memory of a scientist, clinician, and socially involved figure of 19th-century Italy who was unjustly forgotten. Bellingeri was a remarkable pioneer in neurology. He combined experimental research with clinical observation and made a series of original contributions that were based on and prompted further collaborations in Piedmont and throughout the Italian Peninsula.

ACKNOWLEDGMENTS

We would like to thank the descendants of Bellingeri, Carlo Francesco Bellingeri, Leopoldo Bellingeri and Silvia Bellingeri; Dr. Diego Camatti, mayor of Sant'Agata

Fossili; the fellow citizens of Bellingeri's birthplace, and the historian Dr. Eraldo Canegallo.

REFERENCES

Arrigoni R (1842) *Storia Prammatica della Medicina di Curzio Sprengel*. Seconda Edizione, Vol. 5, Prima parte. Firenze: Tipografia La Speranza.

Balestrasse F (1968) *Un grande e dimenticato neurologo dell'Ateneo Torinese: Carlo Francesco Bellingeri*. Pisa: Casa Editrice Giardini.

Banchieri F R (1963) Il neurologo Carlo Francesco Bellingeri. *La Provincia di Alessandria*, 5, 33–34.

Bell C (1821) On the nerves; giving an account of some experiments on their structure and functions, which lead to a new arrangement of the system. Philosophical Transactions of the Royal Society, 111: 398–424.

Bell C (1826) On the nervous circle which connects the voluntary muscles with the brain. *Lond Med Phys* 1: 44–50.

Bellingeri C F (1811) *Bellingeri Caroli Francisci Joseph . . . De novis chinae-chinae succedaneis: In febrium intermittentium curatione dissertatio . . . anno 1811, die 31 decembris, hora 4 pomeridiana* (Doctoral dissertation, in aedibus academia typis Vincentii Bianco).

Bellingeri C F (1818) Caroli Francisci Iosephi Bellingeri dissertatio inauguralis, quam publice defendebat in Regio Athenaeo die 9 maii anno 1818. Augustae Taurinorum. Translation in *Medical Chirurgical Review*, 1834: 413–424.

Bellingeri C F (1823) De medulla spinali, nervisque ex ea proeuntibus. Annotationes anatomico-physiologicae. Taurini.

Bellingeri C F (1824) *Experimenta in nervorum antagonismum. Experimenta physiologica in medullam spinalem*. Torino.

Bellingeri C F (1825a) Experimenta in Nervorum Antagonismus habita; a Carolo Fr. Bellingery, Reg. Acad. Scientiarum et Collegii Med. Taurinii Membr [Experiments performed on the Antonizing Power of the Nerves, by Charles Francis Bellingeri, Member of the Royal Academy of Science, and of the College of Medicine of Turin]. *The Lancet* 7: 147–148.

Bellingeri C F (1825b) *Storia delle encefalitidi che furono epidemiche in Torino nell'anno 1824 con considerazioni sopra di esse e sulla encefalitide in generale*. Torino: Pietro Maletti librajo e negoziante di stampe in via Po.

Bellingeri C F (1826) *Experimenta Physiologica in Medulla Spinalen. Augustae Taurinorum*. Torino: Ex Tipographia Regia.

Bellingeri C F (1827) In electricitatem sanguinis, urinae, et bilis animalium experimenta, Memorie della Reale Accademia delle Scienze di Torino, 36: 295–318.

Bellingeri C F (1828) Experiments on the Electricity of the Blood, the Urine, and the Bile of Animals, In a Healthy and Diseased State. *The Lancet*, 9: 809–810.

Bellingeri C F (1833a) *Ragionamenti esperienze ed osservazioni o patologiche comprovanti l'antagonismo nervoso*. Torino: Il Librajo Gaetano Balduzzi.

Bellingeri C F (1833b) *Karl Franz Bellingeri's Anatomisch-physiologische Untersuchungen über das Rukënmark und seine Nerven*. Gedruckt bei den gebrüdern Mäntler.

Bellingeri C F (1834a) Fisiologia. In *Biblioteca Italiana o sia Giornale di Letteratura Scienze* ed Arti Compilato da Varj Letterati, 74, Milano: Imperiale Regia Stamperia.

Bellingeri C F (1834b) *Storia di nevralgia sopra-orbitario curata con taglio e successica cauterizzazion del nervo con osservazioni fisico-patologiche sopra le medesima. Opuscoli della Società Medico-Chirurgica di Bologna*, IX, 246.

Bellingeri C F (1838) *Sugli emisferi cerebrali dei mammiferi: annotazioni anatomico frenologiche*. Torino: Cassone, Marzorati, Vercellotti.

Bellingeri C F (1839) *Paragone fra la vista e l'udito*. Torino: Alessandro Fontana.

Bellingeri C F (1842/1843) *Memorie originali delle febbri tifoidi che corsero in Torino nell'autunno.*
Bellingeri C F (1843) Utilità dell'estratto di stramonio nell'epilessia. *Scienze Mediche,* 6: 1–9.
Bellingeri C F (1843–1844) *Statistica nosologica del venerando spedale maggiore del Sacro Ordine equestre Mauriziano.* Torino: Stamperia degli Eredi Botta.
Belloni L (Ed.) (1963) Essays on the history of Italian neurology. Proceedings of the International Symposium on the History of Neurology, Varenna,
Bentivoglio M, & Mazzarello P. (2009). History of neurology in Italy. In Handbook of clinical neurology (Vol. 95). Elsevier.
Bostock J (1836) *An elementary system of physiology. Third Edition.* London: Baldwin and Cradock, Paternoster Row.
Brown-Séquard C E (1860) *Course of Lectures on the Physiology and Pathology of the Central Nervous System.* Philadelphia: Collins Printer.
Chiari A (1835) *Del senso del gusto.* Tesi di laurea in Medicina e Chirurgia. I. R. Università di Pavia, Tipografia Bizzoni.
Fine EJ & Darkhabani MZ. (2009). History of the development of the neurological examination. Handbook of Clinical Neurology, 95: 213–233.
Finger S (1994) *Origins of Neuroscience.* Oxford and New York: Oxford University Press.
Foley P B (2011) Encephalitis lethargica-like disorder prior to Von Economo. In J A Vilensky (Ed.), *Encephalitis Lethargica: During and After the Epidemic,* pp. 55–82. Oxford and New York: Oxford University Press.
Frank J P (1791) *Delectus Opuscolorum Medicorum.* Vol. XI. Paviae: Pietro Galeazzi.
Govoni V, Granieri E, & Menini C (1996) The history of the tic douloureux: Autopathograph of an Italian lawyer who suffered from trigeminal neuralgia from 1803 to 1824. *The Journal of History of Neurosciences,* 5: 169–189.
Grimelli G (1849) Memoria sul Galvanismo. Nuovi commentari Academiae Scientiarum. *Instituti Boniensis,* 10: 1–194.
Harris W (1952) Fifth and seventh cranial nerves in relation to the nervous mechanism of taste sensation: A new approach. *British Medical Journal,* 1: 831–836.
Kaulla H (1773) *Karl Franz Bellineri's. Anatomisch-Physiologische Untersuchunger uber das Ruchenmark un seine nerve.* Stuttgart: W. v. Ludvig.
Leidesdorf M (1865) Lehrbuch der psychischen Krankheiten. Enke.
Levi M G (1833) *Dizionario classico di Medicina Interna ed Esterna.* Vol. 10. Venezia: Giuseppe Antonelli Editore.
Lewis D, & Dandy W E (1930) The course of the nerve fibers transmitting sensation of taste. *Archives of Surgery,* 21: 249–288.
Lorusso L, Bravi G O, Buzzetti S, & Porro A (2012) Filippo Lussana (1820–1897): From medical practitioner to neuroscience. *Neurological Sciences,* 33: 703–708.
Lussana F (1872) Sur les nerfs du gout. Observation pathologique. *Archives de physiologie normale et pathologique,* 2: 151–167.
Matteucci C (1844) *Traité des Phénomènes Électro-Physiologiques des Animaux Suivi d'Études Anatomiques sur le Système Nerveux et sur l'Organe Électrique de la Torpille par Paul Savi.* Paris: Fortin, Masson et Cie.
Mazzarello P (2018) Brief Profile of the Neurological Sciences in Italy From the End of the Nineteenth to the First Half of the Twentieth Century. Medicina nei Secoli, 30: 75–104.
Moruzzi G (1996) The electrophysiological work of Carlo Mateucci. Brain Research Bulletin, 40: 69–91.
Negri G (1834) On the comparative merits Dr. Bellingeri's and Sir C. Bell's writing and opinion on the functions of the fifth and seventh pairs of cerebral nerves. The London Medical Gazette, 14: 749–751; 784–787; 845–848; 881–885; 913–915.
Negri G (1835) *On the comparative merits Dr. Bellingeri's and Sir C. Bell's writing and opinion on the functions of the fifth and seventh pairs of cerebral nerves.* London: John Churchill, Princes Street, Soho.

Ng A L C, Rosenfeld J V, & Di Ieva A (2019) Cranial nerve nomenclature: Historical vignette. *World Neurosurgery*, 128: 299–307.
Paletta J B (1874) *Nervus Crotaphiticus et Buccinatorius*. Mediolani, Ludwing, Tome 3.
Pistacchi E (1998) L'encefalite letargica di Costantin Von Economo. *Le Infezioni in Medicina*, 3, 164–167.
Ricotti M (1818) *La storia d'una rara malattia nervosa con varie annotazioni*. Pavia: Presso Fusi e Comp. Success. Galeazzi.
Riva M, Anghilieri F, Belingheri M, & Zatti G (2019) Johann Peter Frank (1745–1821) and the Pathogenesis of Back Pain. *Spine*, 4: E1159–E1160.
Shaw A (1834) Question of the originality of Sir C. Bell's discoveries in the Nervous System The London Medical Gazette, 14: 559–565.
Schiff M (1876) Carlo Matteucci: His merits in physiological and medical physics. *The Lancet*, 108: 150–151.
Scoutetten H (1870) *Évolution Médicale de l'électricité du sang chez les animaux vivants de l'anesthésie et de l'unité des forces physiques et vitales*. Metz: Imprimerie F. Blanc.
Silvano M (1987) Ricordando il bicentenario della nascita di Carlo F. Bellingeri. Discorso commemorativo in occasione tenuto a Sant'Agata Fossili l'11 ottobre 1987.
Snyder D J, & Bartoshuk, L M (2016) Oral sensory nerve damage: Causes and consequences. *Reviews in Endocrine and Metabolic Disorders*, 17: 149–158.
Testut J L (1889) *Traité d'Anatomie Humaine*. Paris, Octave Doin Èditeur.
The Edinburgh Medical and Surgical Journal (1834). Part II. Critical Analysisi. Caroli Francisci Bellingeri . . . Vol. 42, n. 120, pp. 111–138.
Tomey M I, Komotar R J, & Mocco J (2007) Herophilus, Erasistratus, Aretaeus, and Galen: Ancient roots of the Bell–Magendie law. *Neurosurgical Focus*, 23: 1–3.
von Economo C (1917) Encephalitis lethargica. *Wiener Klinische Wochenschrift*, 30: 581–585.
von Haller A (1769/1959) Elementa physiologiae corporis humani. Lausanne: Sumptibus Franciscis Grasset et Sociorum [The discovery of animal electricity and its repercussions on them]. In Stefanutti Ugo's *Facts and Figures of the History of Medicine*. Venice: Alfieri.
Walker A (1834) The nervous system, anatomical and physiological. London: Smith, Elder and Co., Cornhill.
Witt M (2019) Anatomy and development of the human taste system. In R I Doty (Ed.), *Handbook of Clinical Neurology. Smell and Taste*, pp. 147–171. Amsterdam, The Netherlands: Elsevier.
Zanchin G, & Premuda L. (Eds.) (1990) Lo sviluppo storico della neurologia italiana: lo studio delle fonti. Padova: Garangola.

CHAPTER 4

Exploring the Museum of Human Anatomy

GIACOMO GIACOBINI, CRISTINA CILLI, AND
GIANCARLA MALERBA

THE ORIGIN OF THE MUSEUM OF HUMAN ANATOMY

The Museum of Human Anatomy, and its associated historical archives and library, preserve the memory of the Turin anatomical school, in particular with regards to the 19th century.

The museum dates back to 1739, when Professor of Anatomy Gian Battista Bianchi sketched the project of the *Museo Accademico* (Academic Museum). Turin was the capital of the Kingdom of Sardinia, and King Carlo Emanuele III welcomed the project. The museum was housed in the University building, which is currently the home of the Rectorate, and hosted diverse scientific collections, including the anatomical ones (Di Macco, 2003). But the collections were soon separated, and the Anatomical Museum underwent various displacements during the second half of the 18th century. Between 1830 and 1837, the museum was placed in the *Palazzo dei Regi Musei* (Palace of the Royal Museums), together with the Natural History Museum, the Egyptian Museum, the Museum of Antiquities, and the Academy of Sciences, and opened to the public. Between 1837 and 1897, it was housed in the Ospedale di San Giovanni (Saint John's Hospital).

The year 1898 was a crucial year: the museum was re-established in the Building of the Anatomical Institutes, which had been inaugurated in the same year; its monumental halls were designed to echo the importance of science in the positivist Turin of the late 19th century. In the same year, however, Carlo Giacomini, the former director of the Anatomical Institute and Museum, who had greatly enriched the collections, died. His successor, Romeo Fusari, oriented his research toward histology and embryology. As a consequence, the collections had no significant enrichment, and the museum was closed. During the 20th century, it did not undergo any noteworthy changes, rather, it remained "crystallized" until the beginning of the 2000s, when a restoration project took place. The museum finally opened to the public in 2007 (Abbott, 2008) and now belongs to the *Sistema Museale di Ateneo* (University Museum System).

More than 200 anatomical wax models enrich collections of the museum. Many of these were produced in Turin, Florence, and Naples during the second half of the 18th and the first half of the 19th centuries (Giacobini, 1997). The second hall of the museum is dedicated to neuroanatomy, which had been the main research interest in the Turin anatomical school. The preparations and models on display retrace the history of the discovery of the organization of the nervous system. Few objects date back to the 18th century, but most of them are from the 19th century. Each object tells a story, which is linked to the lives of the people who had realized them or used them for teaching or research purposes (Giacobini et al., 2003, 2015).

When discussing people who made pioneering contributions to neuroanatomy in Turin, Luigi Rolando and Carlo Giacomini need to be mentioned. But while Luigi Rolando has been the subject of numerous historical scientific publications, Carlo Giacomini is less known, especially outside Italy, and he will be given more space here.

LUIGI ROLANDO, THE MAN BEHIND THE SCISSURE

Luigi Rolando (1773–1831) integrated data of gross and microscopic anatomy and embryology with functional and experimental observations. In doing so, he modernized the methods used to study the nervous system.

During the Napoleonic period, when he was a Professor of Anatomy at the University of Sassari, in Sardinia, he published the *Saggio sopra la vera struttura del cervello* [Essay on the True Structure of the Brain] (Rolando, 1809). With the Restoration, Rolando returned to the University of Turin, and in 1828 published a second revised edition of his *Saggio* (Rolando, 1828). Rolando's name is mentioned in several eponyms, such as the central sulcus of the brain (fissure of Rolando, Rolando's sulcus, rolandic fissure; see Pearce, 1999; Figure 4.1, top) and Rolando's *substantia gelatinosa* of the spinal cord. Yet, there is more than that: less used, but still relevant, are the eponyms of the Rolandic and pre-Rolandic arteries (central and precentral sulcal arteries) and the Rolandic operculum (postcentral operculum). However, even though Rolando contributed significantly to the development of the Anatomy Museum of Turin, which is also named after him, the objects related to his scientific activity are relatively few.

Much more prominent are the objects testifying to his commitment to teaching and his willingness to further develop the museum, according to his plan of enriching it with new collections and suitable halls for their display. Michele Lessona, in his book *Naturalisti Italiani* (Italian Naturalists), tells of an anecdote about Rolando's search for a proper exhibition space. A large hall located in the Palace of the Royal Museums had been assigned by the King to the zoologist Franco Andrea Bonelli to house zoological collections. In 1830, "when the hall was ready, one of Bonelli's colleagues and close friends, a distinguished Anatomist, without the knowledge of Bonelli, got the hall for the exhibit of anatomical preparations. The day he knew

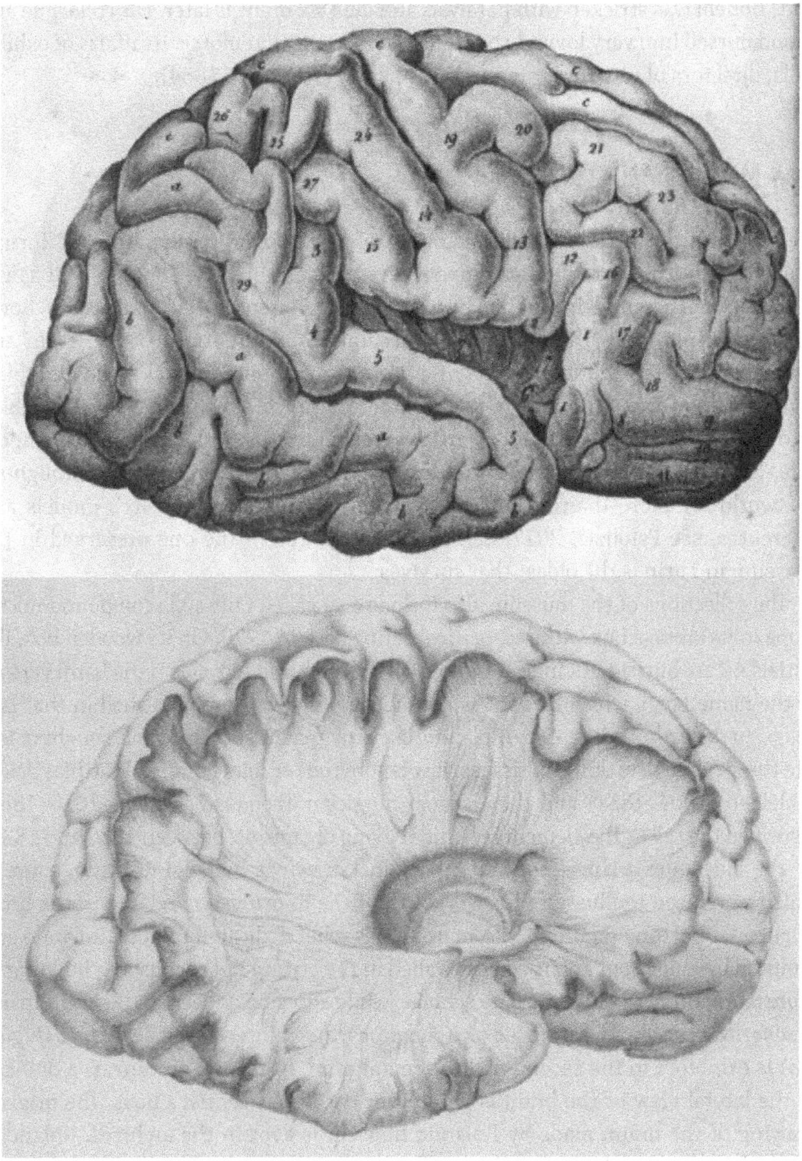

Figure 4.1. Top: lateral view of the right cerebral hemisphere by Luigi Rolando, from his *Della struttura degli emisferi cerebrali* (On the Structure of Cerebral Hemispheres, Figure 1, 1830. Museum of Human Anatomy, University of Turin (Library).
Bottom: dissected right hemisphere of the brain by Luigi Rolando, c. 1825, black and red crayon drawing on paper. It was published as Fig VI in his *Della struttura degli emisferi cerebrali* (On the Structure of Cerebral Hemispheres), 1830. Museum of Human Anatomy, University of Turin (Historical archives).

that, Bonelli was stricken with paralysis and died six months later. His colleague and friend nursed him very lovingly but, I dare not say, with remorse. In affairs of exhibit halls, directors of museums are merciless people" (Lessona, 1884).

WAX MODELS AND DRAWINGS

We also owe to Rolando the development of the ceroplasty laboratory of Torino, which continued to produce wax models even after he died in 1831, as well as the purchase of other models that had been realized in Florence (Giacobini, 1997). Some of those displayed in the museum are accurate representations of the brain and spinal cord. In 1830, Rolando bought a life-size anatomical model made of papier-mâché and produced in Paris by Louis Jérome Auzoux, which can be disassembled into 129 pieces, illustrating 1,115 anatomical details. Even the brain is decomposable. The models produced by Auzoux, and by the firm he created, spread throughout the world for more than a century (for information about Auzoux's models and references, see Palouzié, 2017; de Merode et al., 2017): the one preserved in the Museum in Turin is the oldest that survives.

The collections of the museum also include a so-called Cuff-style compound microscope in its storage box with accessories, dating back to 1770. On its wooden box, the initials AR are burned. AR indicates Aloysius Rolando, and Aloysius is the Latin version of the name Luigi, which he used when scholarly papers were published in that language. In the early 19th century, Rolando, like other scientists of his time, sought to isolate the structures making up tissues, just before the German botanist Matthias Jakob Schleiden (1804–1881) and the German physician Theodor Schwann (1810–1882) identified the cell as the elementary unit of living organisms, between 1838 and 1839.

The museum's archives contain 19 original drawings by Luigi Rolando, some of which were used to illustrate his works; 16 of the drawings are related to the brain (Figure 4.1 bottom; Figure 4.2). A marble bass relief dedicated to Luigi Rolando and sculpted by Luigi Bogliani in 1847 is walled in the atrium of the museum building. It represents Minerva crowning the scholar, while showing a disciple the brain inside a calvarium cut skull. A portrait of Rolando by the painter Pasquale Baroni (Figure 4.3) is exhibited in the second hall of the museum. In this oil on canvas, a drawing of the lateral view of the brain is painted next to the scientist's bust. The original drawing of the brain, made by Rolando himself, is kept in the archives. Rolando's life and works have been the object of many publications, starting from the very first detailed biographies published by Lorenzo Martini (1831), Carlo Francesco Bellingeri (1834), and Carlo Demaria (1846) (for recent contributions, see Manni, 1973; Pogliano, 1988; Caputi et al., 1995; Dini, 2001; Sammet, 2007).

GIACOMINI'S ANATOMY

Carlo Giacomini (1840–1898) (Figure 4.4) developed his scientific activity at the University of Turin during the last decades of the 19th century (Loreti, 1963;

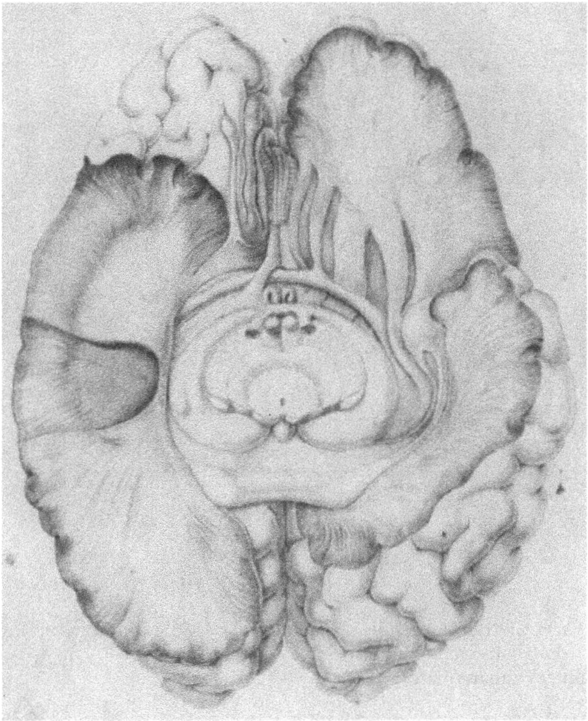

Figure 4.2. Dissected brain (inferior view) by Luigi Rolando, c. 1825, black and red crayon drawing on paper. It was published as Fig IX in his *Della struttura degli emisferi cerebrali* (On the Structure of Cerebral Hemispheres), 1830.
Credits: Museum of Human Anatomy, University of Turin (Historical archives)

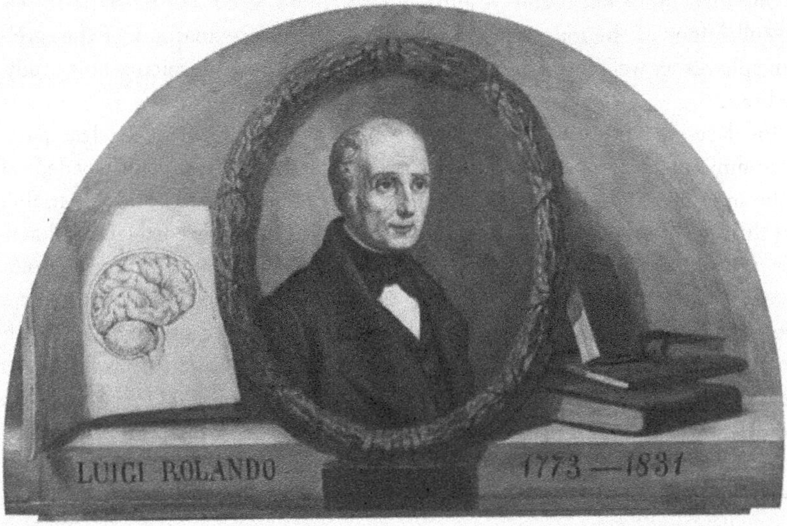

Figure 4.3. Portrait of Luigi Rolando by Pasquale Baroni, c. 1898. Oil on canvas. Museum of Human Anatomy, University of Turin.
Credits: Roberto Goffi.

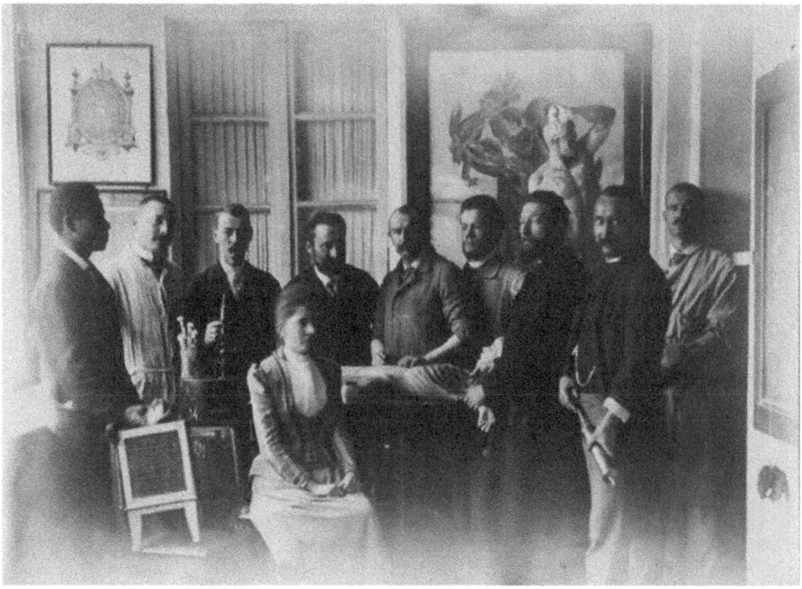

Figure 4.4. Carlo Giacomini and his collaborators, c. 1885. Museum of Human Anatomy, University of Turin (Historical Archives).
Credits: Museum of Human Anatomy.

Giacobini et al., 2003; Perrini et al., 2013). His activity spanned various fields of anatomy, but the investigation of the nervous system had been his preeminent interest. Within neuroanatomy, various research lines caught his attention, including brain pulsations and microcephalic brains (Loreti, 1963). The areas where he obtained more noticeable results, however, and left more relevant traces in the collections of the museum, are related to the surface anatomy of the cerebral hemispheres as well as to the sections he produced for the microscopic study of the brain.

The last part of the 19th century, which overlapped with the last part of Giacomini's life, was a period of intense research activity. It was primarily dedicated to the accurate description of the morphology of the brain surface and its variability, and this was often accompanied by theories on the putatively correlated behaviors. This research benefitted from the development of new preparation techniques to overcome several challenges. Among them, the preservation in liquid, expensive glass jars occupying a lot of space, the need to remove specimens from their containers for research or educational purposes, and the periodic controls that were necessary to ensure that the preservation liquid did not evaporate. Several scholars had developed technical procedures for dry preservation of the brain. Importantly, the preparations made with those techniques not only gave the anatomical specimen greater consistency but also eliminated deformations, thus making the observations more reliable.

A NEW TECHNICAL PROCEDURE

Carlo Giacomini developed a new technical procedure, one that could apply to various anatomical parts and not just to the brain, which was presented at the Royal Academy of Medicine of Turin and distributed as an offprint (Giacomini, 1878a; see also Giacobini et al., 2016). In the text, Giacomini refers to the procedures that others had developed "to give the brain consistency and make it easy to handle, without any of its most essential characteristics being lost." However, he considered those results unsatisfactory. This was mostly due to the formation of cracks and to a marked reduction in the volume, up to a quarter of the original. He then described his new method as follows: "It can be divided into two stages: the first concerns the hardening of the nervous substance; the second, the immersion of the suitably hardened brain in glycerol." Giacomini proposed alternative procedures, which involved the use of different substances for the hardening phase (such as solutions of zinc chloride or potassium dichromate). Hardening was followed by immersion in alcohol, where the preparation would float avoiding deformations. The hardened brain then would have been transferred to glycerol, which would have gradually replaced the alcohol. At this point, it was possible to extract the brain from the liquid and let it dry (for further details see Giacomini, 1878a; Giacobini et al., 2016). The reduction in volume appeared minimal, unlike the one caused by the techniques devised by others. Giacomini concluded his presentation by stressing the importance of creating collections of brains prepared with his method for research on individual variability, for comparative anatomy studies, and to document those cases with pathological lesions, supported by the patient's medical history.

Giacomini prepared a thousand brains using this method. Approximately 800 of them are conserved in four vitrines in the Museum of Human Anatomy in Turin. A series of brains of other vertebrates, preserved with the same technique, is also displayed in a fifth vitrine. Some of these preparations were presented at the Italian General Exposition in Turin in 1884 and at the exhibition that took place in Turin in 1906 during the 6th International Congress of Criminal Anthropology. Others were donated to the Museum of Comparative Anatomy in Turin. Moreover, in the Lombroso Museum, "around 50 brains prepared with the Giacomini method, which had belonged to criminals and mostly came from the prisons in Turin" were displayed in a vitrine, and some are still conserved in the storerooms (Montaldo, 2015). Other collections are housed in the Museum of Anatomy in Modena (made by Giuseppe Sperino, who was a pupil of Giacomini) and in the Museum of Biomedicine in Parma (made by Lorenzo Tenchini).

CONVOLUTIONS AND CIRCUMVOLUTIONS

Based on these types of preparations, in 1877–1878, Giacomini compiled a *Guida allo studio delle circonvoluzioni cerebrali dell'uomo* [Guide to the Study of the Cerebral

Convolutions of Man], which was published in a monograph "with figures inserted in the text," where the furrows and convolutions of the various lobes were accurately described (Giacomini, 1878b). The aforementioned drying technique for preparing the brain was instrumental in making those observations. In fact, "in certain seasons of the year the brain is so soft when it is extracted from its cavity 24 hours after death, that it would be almost impossible to remove its membranes to make the convolutions more visible, if it was not suitably prepared beforehand [. . .]. In such a way, the brain, which is an extremely delicate organ that must be prepared and handled with great care, becomes resistant and is accessible to everyone."

In his conclusions, Giacomini reveals that, as previously stated by Rolando (1828), "The cerebral convolutions [. . .] always prove to be constant in number and direction, in their mutual relationships and their development [. . .] and the variations never radically alter the general type of conformation, except in cases where the brain has seriously deteriorated."

This monograph was followed by a richly illustrated volume titled *Varietà delle circonvoluzioni cerebrali dell'uomo* [Varieties of the Cerebral Convolutions of Man] (Giacomini, 1882a). This research also was published in French, albeit in a shorter version, and this contributed to the international circulation of the results (Giacomini, 1882b). In the preface, the author anticipates some considerations, which he elaborates on in the closing chapter: "It would give me great pleasure if I could demonstrate through this that many peculiarities found in the convolutions of the brain—to which great importance has been attributed by virtually considering them deviations from the usual type of structure or characteristics of particular mental dispositions, thus threatening to raise extremely serious issues in the anatomical and psychic field—are nothing but frequently observed individual variations, and not linked to particular attitudes of the individuals in which they appear." Giacomini's study was based on the observation of "168 brains belonging to individuals of different sex and age which had lived in various social conditions [. . .]. They include 22 brains of individuals considered to be a threat to society, who died in prison, and some of which were obtained through Lombroso's friendship." Some brains on display at the museum are still accompanied by the legend "Cervelli di criminali" [Criminals' brains]. In his conclusions, Giacomini wrote: "What do these many variations tell us? Can we relate them to specific conditions of the individual? Can we consider them as characteristics of particular psychic manifestations?" The answer is straightforward: "The present state of our knowledge does not permit us to say whether these variations are linked to particular dispositions of the mind or to specific development of the faculties of intelligence [. . .]. We cannot arrive at an [. . .] even approximate, diagnosis of the way in which psychic functions were performed through an examination of the cerebral surface, without distorting the facts." He then goes on to say: "we do not find that the brains of social misfits have a specific type of conformation [. . .] and we can in no way relate these variations to their malevolent actions."

CRIMINALS AND CARNIVORES

Giacomini criticizes claims of "similarities between the brain of a criminal and that of a carnivore" made by other authors, especially Moritz Benedikt (1879): "While most of the findings resulting from our observations are completely in contrast with respect to what has been reported by other observers, this should in no way discourage scholars. Indeed, it should make them wary of the a priori method, which can be extremely useful in studying the physiology and pathology of the central nervous system when applied with great caution and moderation, but can easily lead to false impressions and often disappointments, and even cause us to deviate from the rightful path of study, thus impeding the slow and gradual acquisition of precise and positive knowledge." This comment exhibits a rather modern methodological approach.

Benedikt replied to these criticisms in an open letter that was published "with a note by Prof. Giacomini" (Benedikt, 1883). At the beginning of the text, Benedikt stresses the potential controversy of the subject: "When I published my studies on criminal brains three years ago, I decided to discuss the issue as little as possible [. . .] otherwise, I would have always had to live like an Indian ready to fight." He concluded: "Among the anatomists concerned with the brain there are still many theologians and fearful individuals who do not wish to recognize the definitive facts of cerebral anatomy because they are afraid of going against dogmas and their social power."

Lorenzo Tenchini, the director of the Institute of Human Anatomy in Parma, also explored the subject. He published a series of four memoirs on *Cervelli di criminali* [Brains of Criminals] (Tenchini, 1885–1895), which he preserved using Giacomini's method. In the preface to the first, he states: "Benedikt's fundamental idea that the criminal brain corresponds to a characteristic anatomical type [. . .] finds no support. In this, my researches concur with those recently conducted by Flesch, Giacomini, Rüdinger and others, who are presently concerned with the subject. However, I found that anomalies were frequently and variously manifest in criminal brains, in greater proportion than in those of law-abiding men, which were examined for comparison."

Giacomini's findings also were destined to come into conflict with Cesare Lombroso's beliefs, who was then working on the third edition of his *L'uomo delinquente* [Criminal Man]. Published in 1884, in that work Lombroso emphasized the importance of cerebral anomalies he believed were linked to criminal behaviors. Importantly, references to the brain are almost nonexistent in the two previous editions, published in 1876 and 1878. Lombroso commented on Giacomini's work as follows: "But Giacomini [. . .] gave far less importance to these anomalies because he had found similar ones in noncriminal individuals [. . .]. The one objection that can be raised is that the normal ones were gathered in a hospital where the majority of patients were from the dubious and imbecile classes" (Lombroso, 1884).

In the fifth edition of the book, an entire chapter, titled *Anomalie del cervello dei delinquenti* [Anomalies of the Criminal Brain] (Lombroso, 1896), was devoted to this.

Lombroso made personal observations and cited those of various authors, also providing an extensive bibliography including works by Giacomini and by Tenchini. The concluding paragraph, however, sounds extremely cautious: "These observations enable us to state that there is no special type of criminal brain, just as there is no special type of normal brain. However, we have seen that in the former the anastomoses between one fissure and another are generally less frequent than in normal brains [. . .]. We may legitimately say that degenerative and abnormal characteristics are present more frequently in the criminal brain and cranium than in normal ones."

Giacomini died in 1898. In his will he had written: "Being neither an advocate of cremation nor cemeteries, I would like my bones to be laid to rest in the Anatomical Institute where I spent the best years of my youth and to which I have devoted all my energies [. . .]. I would also like my brain to be preserved with my method and placed in the museum together with the others." His skeleton, with the brain positioned at its feet, is displayed in a vitrine in the second room of the museum (see Figure 4.8).

ROLANDO'S DOUBLE SCISSURE IN GIACOMINI'S BRAIN

A year after Giacomini's death, his pupil Giuseppe Sperino presented a study on Giacomini's brain at the Royal Academy of Medicine of Turin. Giacomini's brain had been prepared using Giacomini's method, as penned in his will. His brain had a double fissure of Rolando in the right cerebral hemisphere. As written in the report that came out after the presentation (Sperino, 1900), this was a very rare variation, one that Giacomini had come across only once (Giacomini, 1882a). The session at the Royal Academy of Medicine was attended by Cesare Lombroso, who did not miss the chance to remark that "the observation concerning the criminal type is not contradicted, but on the contrary confirmed, by this anomaly found in Giacomini, because he was a genius" (Giacobini et al., 2003, 2016).

Lombroso referred to Giacomini's brain in the second volume of his *Nuovi studi sul genio* [New Studies on Genius] of 1902, where he enclosed a photograph of it. He added: "It should be noted that he, who was the first to illustrate this anomaly, was one of the most forthright opponents of the pathological theory of genius and of the criminal. Oh, is it not one of those symbolic instances designed to show us that truth will out and to consolidate it, that one of the most unusual cerebral anomalies [. . .] was found in that great man who most strongly contested the degenerative theory and the existence of cerebral atypias in criminal man and the genius ones?" (Lombroso, 1902).

While working on the gross anatomy of the brain, Giacomini began to scrutinize its microscopic organization. He considered the histology of the nervous system to be a logical evolution of the research he had carried out until then. Around 1880, knowledge of the microscopic structure of the nervous system was still very inaccurate (Galloni, 1994). Since a few years before, techniques for the inclusion of tissues and for the creation of thin sections had been developed, and the possibility of using some dyes, such as carmine, hematoxylin, and eosin also had been discovered. In 1873, Camillo Golgi had perfected his "black reaction" technique to highlight nerve cells. In those years, growing attention was paid both to the gross anatomy of the nervous system and to the study of nerve cells. Observations at an intermediate level, however, were lacking, and they could have allowed the evaluation of the distribution of gray (cortex and nuclei) and of white matter as well as the distribution of nerve cells and fibers (Galloni, 1994).

"It is quite easy"—stated Giacomini in 1882—"to demonstrate at the microscope the component elements, for example, of the red nucleus, of the roof nucleus and of other gray matter clusters [. . .] but sometimes it is difficult to establish their precise position, the relationships and the connections between them and with the surrounding parts, the changes in form, volume, direction taken by them [. . .]. Histological sections of large parts of the brain are thus essential, and from them not only must we begin before entering into the most intimate study of the different parts, but their careful examination can provide us with knowledge that we cannot otherwise obtain, and often without the aid of instruments. This is perhaps a little too neglected by the great majority of observers. In fact, in the study of the central nervous system, too often observers resort to the most powerful enlargements, to the most complicated stainings, while sometimes they neglect data which can be obtained by directly examining a conveniently prepared part" (Giacomini, 1882c).

Nevertheless, this project was challenged by technical problems, given that it was necessary to find a way to make large sections of the brain. In 1882, however, Giacomini succeeded in obtaining thin sections of the human brain in toto. These sections, which were between 100 and 200 μm thick, were mounted between two glass plates, thus allowing both naked-eye and microscopic observations. Fixation was made in Muller's fluid followed by alcohol, and sections were obtained with a Gudden's microtome modified by Forel and stained with carmine (Giacomini, 1882c; see also Galloni, 1994), as Giacomini highlighted in the paper presenting this preparation technique.

The observation of those large sections of the brain required a microscope with a large stage. Such an instrument (Figure 4.5), of which two specimens are preserved (one is on display in the museum), was constructed in 1883 by Francesco Koristka in Milan, based on Giacomini's project. It has a large stage and a modified arm with forward displacement of the optic tube. The description of the microscope was published by Giacomini (1883), and the original manuscript is held in the museum's archives. Among the results of the research made by Giacomini with this microscope, the most important one is represented by a detailed description of the ventral hippocampus (Figure 4.6) in humans and other mammals. Giacomini was the first who described the uncus band of the hippocampus (Giacomini, 1882d), which was later named "band of Giacomini" or "limbus of Giacomini" by Gustav Retzius (1896).

TALKING BRAINS

The Museum of Human Anatomy of Turin preserves almost 200 of these brain sections, stored in a specially built cabinet. It is a valuable piece of furniture in eclectic neoclassical style, made of pear wood in 1882, equipped with over 300 drawers.

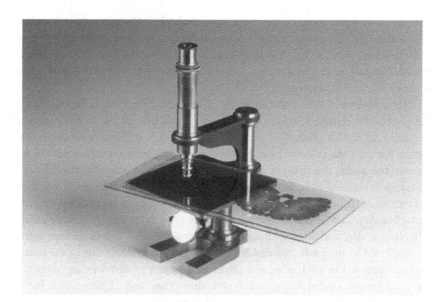

Figure 4.5. Francesco Koristka (Milan), microscope for the observation of large sections of the brain based on Carlo Giacomini's project, 1883. Museum of Human Anatomy, University of Turin. Credits: Roberto Goffi.

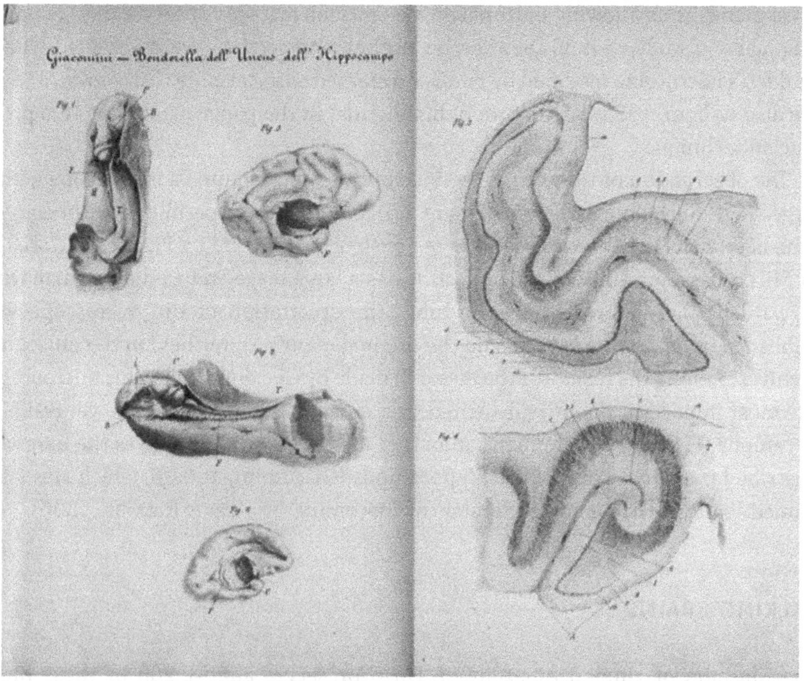

Figure 4.6. Dissection and microscopic sections of the ventral hippocampus. Figures published by Giacomini (1882). Museum of Human Anatomy, University of Turin (Library). Credits: Museum of Human Anatomy.

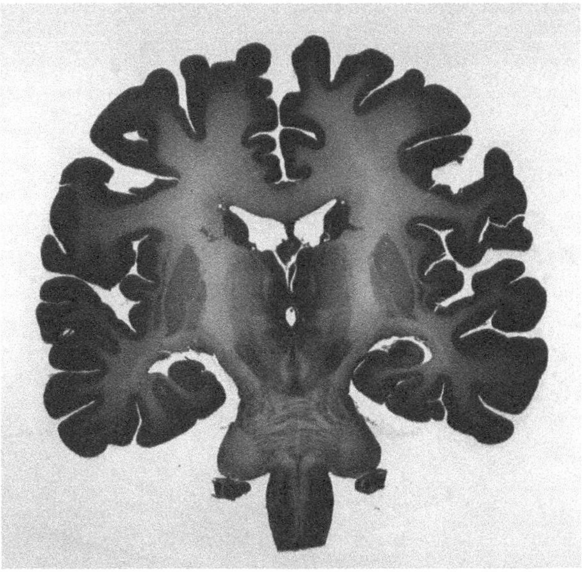

Figure 4.7. Coronal section of the brain stained with carmine and prepared by Carlo Giacomini for low magnification microscopic observations, c. 1880. Museum of Human Anatomy, University of Turin.
Credits: Museum of Human Anatomy.

A Latin sentence engraved on the top of the cabinet, quoted from an 18th-century publication by the Turinese anatomist Giovanni Fantoni, refers to the brain: *Exigua est capitis moles, sed immensa recondit misteria. Omnis molecula divinum exhibet artificium* [Small is the size of the head, yet it conceals immense mysteries. Each molecule is an expression of divine power]. Almost a century and a half after their preparation, these sections are still in excellent condition (Figure 4.7). They maintained their color: the gray substance is in dark red and the white substance in a pink color. They were perfectly suited to the type of observation for which they had been made: a microscopic study at a small magnification and an examination with the naked eye to precisely define the limits between gray and white matter. At higher magnification, cells are also identifiable. Their conservation status is still relatively good, considering that the brains were extracted from cadavers destined for the dissection room, and then fixed several hours after the death of the individual.

In the museum, a large glass pane set in front of a window and made up of 24 glass panels with painted brain sections fixed on a metal frame is supported by a walnut base. In the lower part of the wooden structure, real backlit brain sections are exposed, visible by means of a mirror. This showcase was crafted in 1897 by the leading Turinese cabinetmaker G. Negri in anticipation of the renovated museum in the new premises under construction at that time. It celebrates Giacomini's research, which at that time had notable resonance.

The museum still has several documents of that period, including purchase invoices of the microscopes, furniture, and stained-glass window; microscope description published by Giacomini (and related manuscript); Giacomini's publications

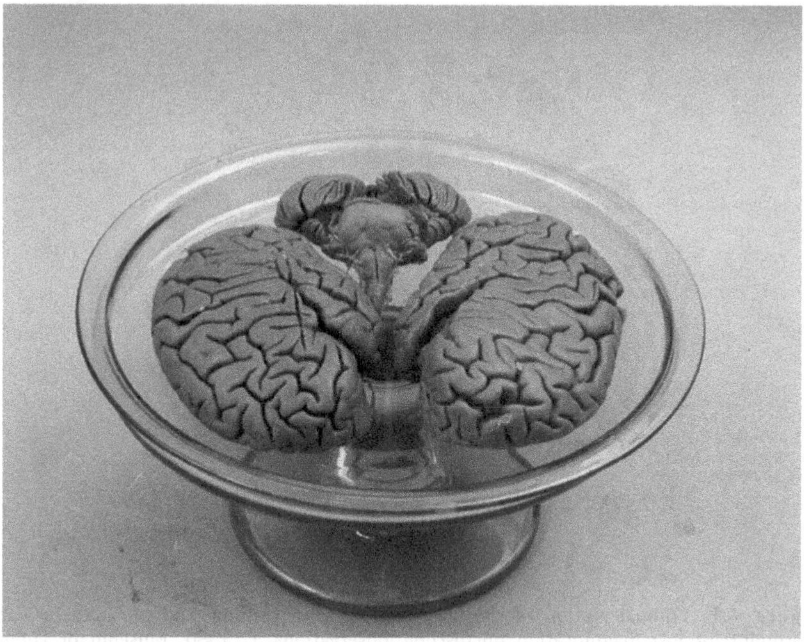

Figure 4.8. Carlo Giacomini's brain preserved with his method. Museum of Human Anatomy, University of Turin.
Credits: Roberto Goffi.

of observations made with the microscope (including description of the hippocampus), and the original *camera lucida* drawings.

From a museological point of view, the objects related to Carlo Giacomini's activity play a crucial storyteller function. Among them, they make visible the interactions among various categories of cultural heritage. Think about the collections of dry brain specimens, his microscope, other related instruments, the microscopic preparations for whose observation the microscope had been designed, the scientific furniture, manuscripts, photographs, drawings, and administrative documents (Giacobini et al., 2011). These interrelated objects and documents are enriched by an unusual component: the skeleton of the author of the research on brain anatomy, Professor Giacomini himself, in accordance with his last will and testament.

ACKNOWLEDGMENTS

The authors are indebted to Giulia Alice Fornaro for kind revision of the English text and to Alessandro Riva for help in compiling the bibliography on Luigi Rolando.

REFERENCES

Abbott A (2008) Turin's Anatomy Museum. *Nature*, 445: 736.

Bellingeri C F (1834) Elogio storico del professore Luigi Rolando. *Memorie della Regia Accademia delle Scienze di Torino*, 37: 153–193.

Benedikt M (1879) *Anatomische Studien an Verbrecher-gehirnen für Anthropologen, Mediciner, Juristen und Psychologen bearbeitet*. Wien: Braumüller.

Benedikt M (1883) Sulla questione dei cervelli dei delinquenti. Lettera aperta al prof. Carlo Giacomini, in Torino (con note del prof. Giacomini). *L'Osservatore, Gazzetta delle Cliniche*, 19: 141–143; 156–159; 174–176.

Caputi F, Spaziante R, Divitiis E, & Nashold B S (1995) Luigi Rolando and his pioneering efforts to relate structure to function in the nervous system. *Journal of Neurosurgery*, 83 (5): 933–937.

Demaria DC (1846) Elogio storico di Luigi Rolando. *Giornale della Regia Accademia di Medicina di Torino*, 1: 277–325.

De Merode L, Gonriveau M, & Hanse A-S (2017) *Les modèles d'anatomie clastique du docteur Auzoux (1787–1880). Etude, restauration et mise en valeur*. Bruxelles: Presses Universitaires.

Di Macco M (2003) Il "Museo Accademico" delle Scienze nel Palazzo dell'Università di Torino. Progetti e istituzioni nell'Età dei Lumi. In G Giacobini (Ed.), La memoria della Scienza. Musei e collezioni dell'Università di Torino, pp. 29–52. Torino: Editris.

Dini A (2001) Introduzione. In L. Rolando (Ed.), *Saggio sopra la vera struttura del cervello dell'uomo e degli animali e sopra le funzioni del sistema nervoso*. Firenze: Giunti.

Galloni M (1994) Carlo Giacomini e l'istologia dell'encefalo. *Journal of Biological Research*, 70 (7): 15–24.

Giacobini G (1997) Wax model collection at the Museum of Human Anatomy of the University of Turin. *Italian Journal of Anatomy and Embryology*, 102: 121–132.

Giacobini G, Cilli C, & Malerba G (2003) Il Museo di Anatomia umana. In G Giacobini (Ed.), *La memoria della Scienza. Musei e collezioni dell'Università di Torino*, pp. 143–154. Torino: Editris.

Giacobini G, Cilli C, & Malerba G (2011) Le fonti archivistiche per la museologia scientifica. Il caso del Museo di Anatomia umana dell'Università di Torino. In S Montaldo, P Novaria (Eds.), *Gli archivi della scienza. L'Università di Torino e altri casi italiani*, pp. 24–31. Milano: Franco Angeli.

Giacobini G, Cilli C, & Malerba G (2015) *"Luigi Rolando" Museum of Human Anatomy, University of Turin*. Torino: Edizioni Libreria Cortina.

Giacobini G, Cilli C, & Malerba G (2016) Carlo Giacomini, his "new process for preserving the brain" and the dispute with Lombroso over "criminal brains." In R Toni, E Bassi, S Montaldo, A Porro (Eds.), *Lorenzo Tenchini and His Masks. An Anatomical Clinical Collection of the late 19th Century at the Universities of Parma and Turin*, pp. 33–37. Milano: Skira33.

Giacomini C (1878a) *Nuovo processo per la conservazione del cervello*. Torino: Tip. Vercellino e Comp.

Giacomini C (1878b) *Guida allo studio delle circonvoluzioni cerebrali dell'uomo*. Torino: Tip. Camilla e Bertolero.

Giacomini C (1882a) *Varietà delle circonvoluzioni cerebrali dell'uomo*. Torino: Ermanno Loescher.

Giacomini C (1882b) Varietés des circonvolutions cérebrales chez l'homme. *Archivi Italiani di Biologia.*, 1 (2–3): 1–64.

Giacomini C (1882c) Sezioni microscopiche dell'intero encefalo umano adulto. *Giornale della Regia Accademia di Medicina di Torino*, 30: 1–18.

Giacomini C (1882d) Benderella dell'uncus dell'ippocampo nel cervello umano e di alcuni animali. *Giornale della Regia Accademia di Medicina di Torino*, 30: 3–28.

Giacomini C (1883) Nuovo microscopio per l'esame delle sezioni dell'intero encefalo umano adulto. *Giornale della Regia Accademia di Medicina di Torino*, 31: 1–8.
Golgi C (1873) Sulla struttura della sostanza grigia del cervello. *Gazzetta Medica Italiana*, 33: 244–246.
Lessona M (1884) *Naturalisti italiani*. Roma: Sommaruga.
Lombroso C (1876) *L'uomo delinquente, studiato in rapporto all'antropologia, alla medicina legale ed alle discipline carcerarie* (1st Ed.). Milano: Hoepli.
Lombroso C (1878) *L'uomo delinquente, in rapporto all'antropologia alla giurisprudenza ed alle discipline carcerarie* (2nd Ed.). Torino: Fratelli Bocca.
Lombroso C (1884) *L'uomo delinquente, in rapporto all'antropologia, giurisprudenza ed alle discipline carcerarie, Delinquente-nato e pazzo morale* (3rd Ed.). Torino: Fratelli Bocca.
Lombroso C (1896) *L'uomo delinquente, in rapporto all'antropologia, alla giurisprudenza ed alle discipline carcerarie* (5th Ed.). Torino: Fratelli Bocca.
Lombroso C (1902) *Nuovi studii sul genio. Da Colombo a Manzoni*. Milano-Palermo-Napoli: Remo Sandron Editore.
Loreti F (1963) Contributo alla storia dello studio anatomico dell'Università di Torino. Carlo Giacomini (1840–1898). *Memorie dell'Accademia delle Scienze di Torino*, 4 (2): 1–69.
Manni E (1973) Luigi Rolando, 1773–1831. *Experimental Neurology*, 38: 1–5.
Martini L (1831) *Necrologia del chiarissimo Professore Luigi Rolando*. Torino: Regia Tipografia.
Montaldo S (2015) *Il Museo di Antropologia criminale 'Cesare Lombroso' dell'Università di Torino*. Milano: Silvana Editoriale.
Palouzié H (2017) *Prodiges de la nature. Les créations du docteur Auzoux (1797-1880). Collections de l'Université de Montpellier*. Montpellier: Direction Régionale des Affaires Culturelles.
Pearce J M S (1999) The fissure of Rolando, Historical note. *Journal of Neurosurgery and Psychiatry*, 67: 528.
Perrini P, Montemurro N, & Iannelli A (2013) The contribution of Carlo Giacomini (1840-1898): The Limbus Giacomini and beyond. *Neurosurgery*, 3: 475–482.
Pogliano C (1988) Il "nobilissimo viscere." Luigi Rolando anatomista e fisiologo dell'encefalo. *Piemonte Vivo*, 4: 42–49.
Retzius G (1896) *Das Menschenhirn. Studien in der Makroskopischen Morphologie*. Stockholm: Norstedt & Söhne.
Rolando L (1809) *Saggio sopra la vera struttura del cervello dell'uomo e degli animali e sopra le funzioni del sistema nervoso*. Sassari: Stamperia di S. S. R. M. Privilegiata.
Rolando L (1828) *Saggio sopra la vera struttura del cervello e sopra le funzioni del sistema nervoso* (Seconda Edizione). Torino: Pietro Marietti.
Rolando L (1830) Della struttura degli emisferi cerebrali. *Memorie della Regia Accademia delle Scienze di Torino*, 35: 3–79.
Rolando L (1974) *Saggio sopra la vera struttura del cervello dell'uomo e degli animali e sopra le funzioni del sistema nervoso*. Bologna: Arnaldo Forni.
Rolando L (2001) *Saggio sopra la vera struttura del cervello dell'uomo e degli animali e sopra le funzioni del sistema nervoso*. Firenze: Giunti.
Sammet K (2007) Luigi Rolando (1773–1831). *Journal of Neurology*, 254 (3): 404–405.
Sperino G (1900) L'encefalo dell'anatomico Carlo Giacomini. *Giornale della Regia Accademia di Medicina di Torino*, 63: 737–805.
Tenchini L (1885–1895) *Cervelli di delinquenti. Superficie metopica (Memoria Prima, 1885); Superficie parieto-temporo-occipitale (Memoria Seconda, 1887); Superficie interna (Memoria Terza, 1891); Superficie inferiore (Memoria Quarta, 1895)*. Parma: Luigi Battei.

CHAPTER 5

Cesare Lombroso

An Unconventional Biography

PAUL KNEPPER

In the decades preceding World War I, Cesare Lombroso (1835–1909; Figure 5.1) became an international celebrity. A medical doctor with an interest in psychiatry, Lombroso insisted that physical characteristics could explain all mental activities. He claimed to have identified biological markers for a range of behaviors and conditions, including criminality, terrorism, prostitution, insanity, and genius (Figure 5.2). His new approach, criminal anthropology, spread across the emerging social and behavioral sciences. Lombroso's studies inspired international conferences, appeared in newspaper columns and literary magazines, and found their way into artwork, operas, and novels (Becker & Wetzell, 2006; Knepper & Ystehede, 2013).

Assessing Lombroso's legacy in neuroscience is not a simple task. For some, he promoted a pseudoscience comparable to phrenology or astrology and merited nothing more than a footnote in the history of science (Gould 1981; Jarkko et al., 2015). "The term 'lombrosian' is often referred to as the idea of identifying a criminal from his face," Musumeci (2013, p. 132) observes: "the adjective itself, 'lombrosian,' is used as an 'insult' or a 'joke'." For others, Lombroso is no laughing matter. He instigated a sinister science that framed the structure of criminal biology as implemented in National Socialist Germany (Rafter, 2008). Horn (2003, p. 2) concludes that "criminal anthropology has been limited to a supporting role in a cautionary tale about a deviant or spurious science." Yet, others would nominate Lombroso as the founder of modern neurocriminology. "The racial side of Lombroso's theory fell into justifiable disrepute after the horrors of World War II," Raine (2013a) says, "but his emphasis on physiology and brain traits has proved to be prescient. Modern-day scientists have now developed a far more compelling argument for the genetic and neurological components of criminal behavior" (see further Raine, 2013b; Sirgiovanni, 2017; Savopoulos & Lindell, 2018).

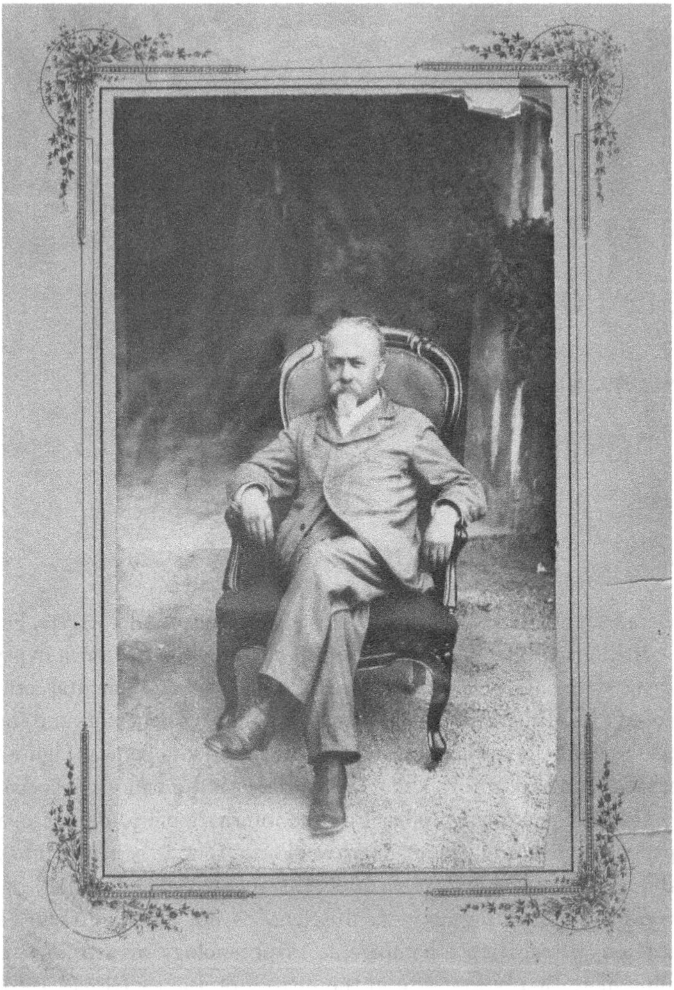

Figure 5.1. Cesare Lombroso seated in a chair, looking into the camera lens (property of the Museo di Antropologia criminale "Cesare Lombroso" dell'Università di Torino). Courtesy of Silvano Montaldo.

Lombroso wanted to be remembered as a scientist who explored the deep origins of behavior. Still, criminal anthropology moves beyond the history of science to broader social, political, and cultural accounts. To understand Lombroso, it is essential to examine his motivation, the range of his interests, and changes in his outlook during his life. This chapter will not develop a conventional biography written in chronological order. Instead, four aspects of *La Scuola Lombrosiana* will be investigated: the criminal type, methodology, crime prevention, and scientific racism. Assessing a scientific career that involves tattoos, a crime museum, haunted houses, Nazis and Count Dracula is not a straightforward summary of theory, research, and discovery.

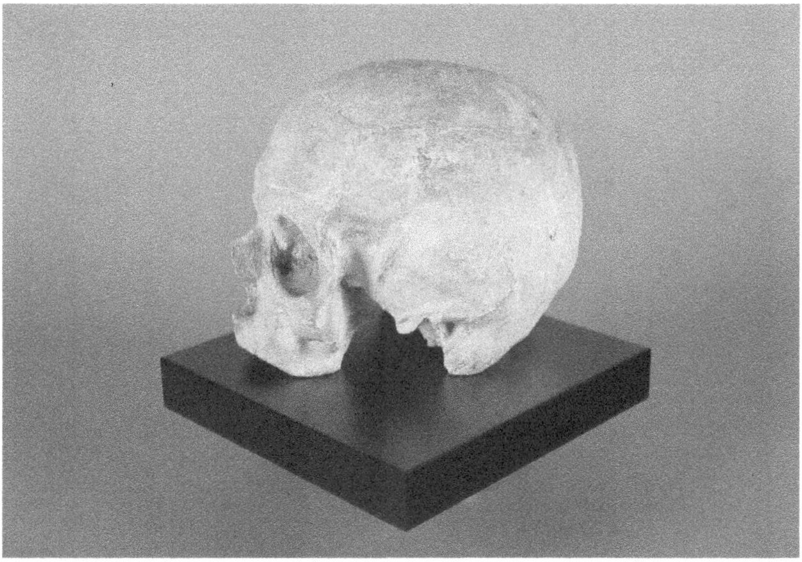

Figure 5.2. Plaster cast of Alessandro Volta's skull as evidence of Lombroso's studies on genius (photo by R. Goffi, property of the Museo di Antropologia criminale "Cesare Lombroso" dell'Università di Torino). Courtesy of Silvano Montaldo and Cristina Cilli.

THE CRIMINAL TYPE

The Lombroso Museum reopened in 2009 (Figure 5.3), and, like its founder, it has been the recipient of some controversy. In 2012, a judge ordered the museum to hand over one of its treasured possessions, the skull of Giuseppe Villella, to the mayor of Motta Santa Calabria, for burial at the site where he was said to have been born. The University of Turin appealed the court order. The director of the museum, Silvano Montaldo, argued that the skull is protected under Italian Cultural Heritage law as an important object for the history of science. "It is difficult to consider Villella's skull scientifically irrelevant and thus unworthy of display in a museum," Montaldo has explained, "That is, unless one believes that science must destroy the traces of its past" (Ystehede, 2016).

For Lombroso, this skull held a position in the history of science equivalent to Newton's apple. Villella's skull revealed the criminal type, one of the significant scientific findings in an age of scientific discovery. Lombroso continued to insist it was real, that he had been first to identify it, and that no one could take that away from him. He preserved the concept of the criminal type, or "born criminal," even while he expanded his ideas about crime in society (Gibson, 2006). Lombroso theorized that the causes of criminal behavior were found in the distant past. He advanced the concept of atavism, "the reversion of criminals to a lower state of physical and psychological evolution" (Gibson, 2006, p. 139). Criminals were an anachronism, a residual element from a previous epoch in the natural history of the earth. Lombroso also claimed that vestiges of this prehistoric past could be detected through physical

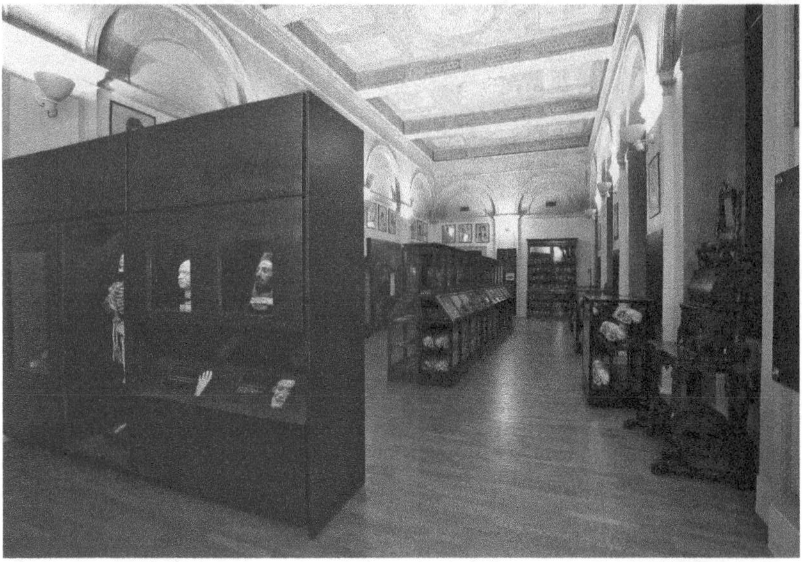

Figure 5.3. Hall of the Museo di Antropologia criminale "Cesare Lombroso" dell'Università di Torino (photo by R. Goffi, property of the Museo di Antropologia crimianle "Cesare Lombroso" dell'Università di Torino). Courtesy of Silvano Montaldo and Cristina Cilli.

peculiarities, including the size of the skull. *L'uomo delinquente* opens with an introduction to craniometry, in which he explains how the shape of some human skulls resembles that of monkeys, rodents, and lemurs (Lombroso, 2006, p. 49).

Lombroso was interested in brain anomalies, particularly in relation to psychiatric pathologies, but he did not pursue a microscopic analysis of internal structures. Rather, he emphasized other external features of the body: the shape of ears, distance between toes; location of eyes, gait, and body hair. His inquiry included tattoos and jargon among prisoners, as well as prisoner writing, graffiti, and handcrafts. He explored epilepsy, mental illness, and genius concerning inherited criminality. With the assistance of colleagues, students, and prisoners, including future Nobel Laureate Camillo Golgi, he conducted experiments in "electric algometry," the attempt to measure sensitivity to pain across normal and pathological individuals (Mazarello 2010, pp. 40–41).

Lombroso studied medicine at the University of Pavia, the University of Padova, and the University of Vienna before completing a medical degree at the University of Pavia in 1858 and a degree in surgery from the University of Genoa in 1859. He volunteered for the medical service in the Piedmontese army and served at various posts, including Calabria. While quartered in peacetime Pavia, he developed his interest in clinical psychiatry. He received permission to study the people with mental health conditions at the hospital of St. Euphemia, and in 1862 he presented a series of lectures in psychiatry and anthropology. For the next 10 years, Lombroso was in charge of the insane at hospitals in Pavia, Pesaro, and Reggio Emilia. In 1876, he won the chair of legal medicine and public hygiene at the University of Turin, where he would remain for the rest of his career. Later, he became professor of criminal anthropology and director of the Institute of Legal Medicine and Criminal Anthropology (Wolfgang, 1961).

Lombroso told the story of his scientific breakthrough in different ways; it takes place at different times and contains various elements (Gibson, 2006). Near the end of his life, he recalled that his "fundamental idea" had not come from a single moment but a series of intuitions. The first inkling occurred to him in 1864, working on his studies of Italian soldiers, in trying to distinguish the honest soldier from his dishonest colleagues. He developed the idea further in 1866 as he began his study of insanity at asylums. By the time he made his autopsy of Villella in 1870—or was it 1871?—he had more than an "idea." It was a "revelation." On that cold, gray November morning, cutting open the base of the neck to expose the skull where it attaches to the spine, "I seemed to see all of the sudden, lighted up as a vast plain under a flaming sky, the problem of the nature of the criminal—the atavistic being who reproduces in his person the ferocious instincts of primitive humanity and the inferior animals" (Lombroso, 1910).

The idea of the criminal type of brain as a throwback to an earlier stage in human evolution did not originate with Lombroso. He may have borrowed it from Darwin's comment about "black sheep" in *The Origin of Species* (1859). Mazzarello (2011) notes that Lombroso could have acquired a French translation of the book in Pavia as early as 1862. But, as Pancaldi (1991) points out, the concepts of evolutionary development in Lombroso's work, as well as the citations in his texts, suggest the influence of pre-Darwinian evolutionary theory. In the early 19th century, science as a profession for specialists in particular areas was not yet established. Nor did science require the equipment of a scientific laboratory and the resources of a university. Amateurs contributed to public discussions, often incorporating scientific findings within ethical or religious understandings of the world.

In 1844, for example, a Scottish publisher, Robert Chambers, produced *Vestiges of the Natural History of Creation*, which situated the creation of the earth within the natural history of the universe. Chambers assembled material from astronomy, geology, chemistry, physics, phrenology, and anthropology to show how isolated findings in these areas added up to a grand history of evolutionary development. In a chapter on the "mental constitution of animals," he explored the idea of how individuals could be born into the world, come of age in a civilized nation, and become malefactors. "Does God, it may be asked, make criminals? Does he fashion certain beings with predestination to evil? He does not do so; and yet the criminal type of brain, as it is called, comes into existence following laws which the Deity has established" (Chambers, 1844, pp. 355–356).

The significance of Villella's skull had less to do with producing the insight concerning evolutionary theory than with what Garland (2002) characterizes as the "Lombrosian project." Unlike others who speculated about atavism as a source of behavior, Lombroso promoted criminal anthropology as a specialist science of the criminal (Garland, 2002, p. 25). Chambers published his ideas anonymously to shield himself from criticism (which he received from scientists as well as clergy). Lombroso championed his cause, as his son-in-law Guglielmo Ferraro (1908) observed, in the style of a Jewish prophet. He produced five editions of *L'uomo delinquente* between 1876 and 1896; the final edition swelled to four volumes. He founded a journal, *Archivo di Psichiatria e Antropologia criminale* [Archive of Psychiatry and Criminal Anthropology], along with Enrico Ferri and Raffalae Garafalo. Lombroso put his name to 30 books and a thousand articles, not only in Italian, but French, Spanish, English, and German. He attracted individuals in different countries who diffused and amplified his ideas, including John Wigmore in the United States, Pauline Tarnovsky in Russia, Havelock Ellis in Great Britain, and Hans Kurella in Germany (Rafter, 2006; Knepper, 2018). Not to mention Leo Tolstoy, Josef Conrad, Arthur Conan Doyle, and Bram Stoker who wrote him into their novels. In *Dracula*, Mina Harker informs van Helsing that Lombroso would classify the evil count as a criminal type.

Lombroso initiated the international congresses of criminal anthropology. Every four years or so before World War I, lawyers, doctors, judges, and prison administrators met to discuss the application of science to criminality and criminal law. The first congress took place in Rome at the *Palazzo delle Belle Arti* in 1885. Other congresses took place in Paris (1889), Brussels (1892), Geneva (1896), Amsterdam (1901), Turin (1906), and Cologne (1911). The participants gave reports, joined discussions, and viewed exhibitions. The congresses attracted participants from across Europe, as well as South America and Asia. Reports of Lombroso's exchanges with Alexandre Lacassagne at the Rome congress and Leonce Manouvrier in Paris echoed in the academic literature long after the meeting had closed. Reports of fierce battles between the Italian School of the criminal body and the French School of social milieu became the stuff of academic legend central to the formation of a new science of the criminal (Kaluszynski, 2006).

METHODS OF INQUIRY

Lombroso did not invent the account of Villella's skull, but he embellished it to establish a scientific provenance for his theory. He insisted on providing empirical evidence for each aspect of his work, although his narrative ranges across anecdotes and proverbs. Early on, critics attacked him for his failure to follow the experimental method and for his casual approach to statistics. Lombroso's missteps are easy to spot, not only because he produced his material quickly, but also because his methods do not work and his conclusions do not adhere to a coherent argument. His writings display contradictions, inconsistencies, and mistakes (Gatti & Verde, 2012).

Whenever a patient or a prisoner died at an institution where Lombroso was employed, the corpse would find its way into his hands. Lombroso conducted thousands of postmortem examinations. Early in his medical career, he began the practice of carefully documenting the physical peculiarities of patients: physical aspects such as bones, teeth, nails, ears, and hair. He became known as *l'alienista della stadera*, "the scales-and-weights surgeon" (Kenney, 1910, p. 221). His books and articles report numerical data, comparative analyses, and historical statistics, "but it is essentially the minute and detailed examination of the individual that characterizes his most basic tool of investigation and gathering data" (Wolfgang, 1961, p. 258).

Lombroso's persistent carelessness and growing celebrity made him an irresistible target. Britain's Home Office commissioned an inquiry led by Charles Goring, a medical officer attached to various English prisons. With the assistance of other prison medical officers, and statistical advice from Karl Pearson at University College London, Goring analyzed anthropometric and psychological measurements for some 3,000 prisoners. His report, completed in 1913, and reissued after the war, denounced Lombroso's studies as more "superstition" than "science" (Goring, 1919, pp. 20–25). He found none of the "extraordinary number of anomalies" Lombroso claimed to have witnessed. The Italian professor routinely confused "technical criminals," that is, those who happened to be in prison, with "anthropological" or "real" criminals who existed solely in his imagination (Goring, 1919, pp. 84–85). The legend of Goring having delivered the definitive refutation of criminal anthropology began early. *The New York Times* (1913) offered a lengthy description of Goring's report under the headline, "'There is no criminal type,' says prison expert."

Later critics reprised the theme of Lombroso as an incompetent researcher who failed to follow the scientific method. Gould (1981, p. 125) ridiculed the opening section of the third edition of *L'uomo delinquente* as "what must be the most ludicrous excursion into anthropomorphism ever published." Lombroso "twisted all these stories into his system" of thought and constructed his statements in such a way as to preclude their falsification by empirical testing. Gould recalculated Lombroso's data concerning the size of brains to demonstrate the fatal flaw in his empirical method. Lombroso argued that criminals have smaller brains than most people, although some criminals have very large brains. "Yet Lombroso's data show no such thing" (Gould, 1981, p. 130). The implication is that Lombroso's research amounts to little more than popular prejudices wrapped in a veneer of scientific jargon, which is why even the proponents of recent studies of the criminal body, whether evolutionary psychology or biosocial criminology, insist that modern science has nothing to do with Lombroso (DeLisi, 2013). Although Italy became the first nation in Europe where technologies concerning brain activation patterns, such as functional magnetic resonance imaging (fMRI), have been used in insanity defenses in courtrooms, Italian neuroscientists have kept their distance from Lombroso (Sirgiovanni, 2017, p. 168).

Challenging the data in Lombroso's texts is useful, but misses something important about his method. To understand what Lombroso was trying to do, it is necessary to explore why he established his museum. The *Museo di antropologia criminale "Cesare Lombroso"* was the first of its kind in Italy, and became the model for similar institutions in European cities. It began with a collection of skulls he acquired while working as a medical doctor in prisons and asylums (Lombroso, 1906a). Lombroso revealed his collection to the public for the first time in 1884 as part of the anthropology exhibition at Turin's *Esposizione Generale Italiana*. When the international congress of criminal anthropology convened in Rome a year later, he set up an extensive display: skulls arranged on tables, body parts floating in alcohol-filled jars, and faces revealed in photographs and death masks. The exhibition contained some 70 skulls of criminals, the entire skeleton of a thief, and swatches of tattooed skin extracted from prisoners. He presented aspects of the criminal's body in 300 photographs, life-size sketches, and handwriting samples (Montaldo, 2013).

In 1892, Lombroso learned that the director-general of prisons, Count Bertrani-Scalia, had a collection of skeletons stored at Regina Coeli and was thinking of starting a museum. It was just the thing Lombroso had in mind (Lombroso, 1910). The Museum of Psychiatry and Criminal Anthropology at the University of Turin opened in 1889, and it included a corridor of skeletons, allegedly those of notorious brigands from Southern Italy. The largest room contained a scale model of Eastern State Penitentiary in Philadelphia, surrounded by portraits on the walls of criminals and epileptics. Lombroso displayed criminal types obtained from government authorities in Spain, Mexico, Portugal, Chile, and Australia. He filled glass display cases with daggers used by Camorra; crucifixes of prisoners seeking redemption; and pottery pieces containing inscriptions of robbers and murderers. He displayed items made by prisoners, including a court scene molded from clay and sketches of shootouts with Carabinieri (Lombroso, 1907).

The museum seems nothing more than a jumble of trivial, odd, and sinister items (Regener, 2003). But for Lombroso, it provided a medium for inquiring into the origins of criminality. As Mario Carrara, who succeeded Lombroso as the director of the Institute, explained, the museum combined criminal anthropology and medico-legal training. Adjacent to the room devoted to criminal anthropology, the Institute housed a space dedicated to forensic materials, including body parts in jars on wooden shelves revealing the effects of a gunshot, stabbing, or other wounds. Students needed to recognize "through the traces" of lesions the cause of death, the nature of the instrument used, and whether it was a case of suicide, homicide, accident, or other cause (Carrara, 1928, p. 11). Forensic science was not a discrete form of inquiry, but part of Lombroso's thinking.

Lombroso established criminal anthropology as a historical science. As Cleland (2001) explains, researchers working in the "historical sciences" of geology, astronomy, paleontology, and evolutionary biology pursue a different method than those working in the "experimental sciences" of physics, chemistry, and biology. Because the problems they study result from causes in the remote past, investigators in the historical sciences cannot create experimental conditions in a laboratory. Instead, they try to reconstruct past events from physical traces that have survived into the present. The historical sciences pursue a three-step method. First, assemble a collection of traces; second, propose a common cause; and, third, provide a unifying explanation. Cleland refers to the third step as a search for a "smoking gun," the discovery of a trace that clinches the case for a particular causal story (Cleland, 2002, 2011). Forensic science can be categorized as a historical science. The events in question have already occurred. Forensic scientists do not create data through experiments in laboratory settings, but can only study proxy data; that is, the remains of those events left behind (Houck, 2009).

For Lombroso, the causes of criminality have already taken place; they occurred in a previous epoch of natural history that cannot be reconstructed in conventional time. The objects in his museum represented traces of deep time, remnants of the prehistoric past that survived into the present. Lombroso pursued each of Cleland's steps. He assembled a puzzling collection of traces: the shape of ears, distance between toes, the thickness of hair, and other characteristics of the body. He identified a common cause in atavism, and in his autopsy of Giuseppe Villella he found his smoking gun.

So, what went wrong? According to the logic of historical science, there should be multiple traces of natural causes from the past, but "the trick is finding them" (Cleland, 2002, p. 492). There needs to be something puzzling about the traces to suggest a common cause or source; simple correlations can result from separate causes (Cleland, 2011, p. 574–575). The speed at which Lombroso worked, the ambiguity of his concepts, and his casual approach to statistics meant that he accepted even superficial connections as justification for presuming a common cause. He quickly absorbed various material into his narrative, which left mistakes, contradictions, and nonsense. There is no definitive proof of a smoking gun (Cleland, 2002). It is always possible that further discoveries will dislodge the leading theory from the top shelf. Further, many of the factors that contribute to finding a smoking gun are "sociological or psychological, as well as theoretical and empirical" (Cleland, 2002, p. 482). In other words, there is room for prejudice, politics, and other subjective factors in the designation of a leading explanation.

Lombroso began his search for the natural origins of crime within a racist view of human development, and this led to many false assertions. For Lombroso, degrees on the evolutionary scale of human development corresponded with racial divisions. In *L'uomo bianco e l'uomo di colore* (*The White Man and the Man of Colour*, 1871), he explained that, originally, all people had dark skin. As evolution took place, lighter skin emerged, eventually leading to the emergence of the "white man." At the present state, the "coloured man" remained closer to the primate than other races. This "science" confirmed the political affairs in which European powers operated colonial empires; as the most highly evolved, the European races displayed the most highly advanced civilizations. He revealed a contemptible dismissal of non-white races, native peoples of the Americas, Asia, and especially Africa as inferior beings. Lombroso's racist outlook applied to Europe as well, specifically, to the southern tip of the Italian peninsula. He judged the inhabitants of Calabria and Sicily to be racially inferior owing to the mixture of African and Arab blood (Lombroso & Ferrero, 2004, p. 289). So, Villella's skull provides the smoking gun owing to the racist psychological and sociological lens through which Lombroso sees it.

CRIME PREVENTION

The introduction of brain imaging techniques in recent years has raised concerns about a return to "Lombroso's vision" of crime prevention. Munthe and Radovic (2015) explain that recent advances in genetics and neuroscience have revived ethical worries about screening individuals at risk for future criminal behavior. Lombroso encouraged early intervention. Using the techniques of his science, teachers could "identify in children the incurable signs of inborn criminality" (Lombroso, 2006, p. 335). Because punishment had no effect, preventive isolation was needed. "Born criminals . . . " Lombroso (1902, p. 2138) advised, "should be sequestered from their earliest years to avoid greater misfortunes."

To accompany his new science, Lombroso championed a new legal philosophy. He wanted to replace moral and religious foundations of criminal law with the scientific study of criminals, which he referred to as *la difesa sociale*, or "social defense." The criminal law should no longer focus on moral responsibility, requiring punishment for wrongdoing, but implement measures of security to contain the dangerousness of the criminal threat. In other words, the severity of response would not be judged according to intent as revealed by a particular action, but according to the degree of harm the individual presented to society. Enrico Ferri, who spent a year at Turin with Lombroso, championed social defense in Italy. At the first congress of criminal anthropology in 1885, Ferri insisted that the scientific study of the criminal provided the foundation for social defense. The task was to write the theory of criminal anthropology into a penal code. At the fifth congress in Amsterdam, the participants voted for permitting the judge to include at trial the "bio-physical facts" of the defendant's personality (Cantor, 1936, pp. 21–22).

The philosophy of social defense has already had a career as curious as its originator. Legal measures during the Stalin era of the Soviet Union went the farthest toward replacing legal responsibility with social dangerousness, although Hitler's Germany and Mussolini's Italy took some steps in this direction (Cantor, 1936). During the interwar period, the International Penal and Penitentiary Commission (ICPC) promoted *La Scuola Lombrosiana*, and during the 1930s, urged governments to develop criminal biology using anthropometrical and biological information. Following the Second World War, the United Nations dissolved the ICPC for its Nazi affiliation. Nevertheless, in 1948, the UN's Economic and Social Council adopted social defense as its guiding philosophy for the prevention of crime and the treatment of offenders. The current social defense movement seeks to take advantage of the human sciences to study the individual, this time without neglecting individual human rights; it also credits the Italian positivist school with taking the first step away from punishing the individual to protecting society (Rozès, 1995, p. 313).

Lombroso's vision of crime prevention was broader than the identification of atavistic criminals. His colleagues in *La Scuola positiva*, Enrico Ferri and Raffaele Garafalo, prompted him to acknowledge that the search for the etiology of crime extended beyond the body. Ferri formulated a classification of criminal types that included not only the atavistic or "born criminal" but also the "occasional criminal" (Sellin, 1961). In the fourth edition of *L'uomo delinquente*, Lombroso affirmed his confidence in science as the route to biological explanation, but he accepted Garafalo's proposal that some thieves were motivated exclusively by opportunity. He also expressed his anxiety about the speed and direction of modern civilization, which would pull him further toward opportunity as an explanation (Lombroso, 2006, p. 288).

Lombroso lived and worked during a period of scientific and technological achievement. Between 1870 and 1909, the invention of the telegraph, the telephone, airplane, and motor car made the world a smaller place and accelerated the speed of daily life. Lombroso took a keen interest in technology, whether burglars' tools or burglar alarms, and he realized that technology brought new forms of crime and new possibilities for crime prevention. In an article written before 1909, Lombroso predicted that, although the volume of crime would decrease owing to preventive measures, the complexity of crimes would increase. The "crimes of the coming century" would involve extensive stock swindles, frauds using fake newspaper advertisement, and murder by less traceable poisons. This new type of criminal would "make use of all progress along technical, scientific, and economic lines"; crimes would be committed with the assistance of bicycles, automobiles, and trains, as well as the telephone, telegraph, and newspaper advertising. Social defense likewise would require all these methods, "the most powerful agents for their discovery, apprehension, and repression" (Lombroso, 1912).

So important was the bicycle to criminal activity, Lombroso mused, it was necessary to replace the old adage *cherchez la femme*—a woman was the source of any conflict between men—with the phrase *cherchez la bicyclette*. The bicycle was a cause of crime, Lombroso said, as young men would stoop to any level of immorality to get their hands on one. Theft often led to violence among otherwise reasonable men. It was also an instrument of crime; the bicycle provided a new means of highway robbery. The bicycle also brought about "minor or pseudo crimes." The Italian government, for example, had decided to levy a bicycle tax. Each machine would need to bear a stamp indicating it had been registered and the tax paid, and this led to petty crimes related to forged registration cards, fraudulent dealings with bicyclists visiting from foreign countries, and trading registration cards from one machine to another. At the same time, the bicycle brought changes in society likely to bring about a reduction in crime. Bicycling offered an alternative to alcohol, and public houses, especially in rural areas, adapted to the changing business environment. Many sold mineral waters, syrups, and coffee. Bicycling contributed to physical fitness and reduced stress and various forms of emotional depression (Lombroso, 1900).

No longer does the atavistic criminal type represent the main objective of social defense. The objects of scientific crime prevention are not a residual population of cave-dwellers with a mental capacity limited to stone tools, but the masses of modern minds capable of gaining an unfair advantage from every scientific and technological marvel. The emerging generation of criminals made of "normal" or "ordinary" people without physiological or psychological deficiencies. Social defense cannot rely on legal reforms, whether scientific policing or preventive isolation. Rather, it will require innovative defenses against the new weapons afforded criminals by modern life. Lombroso offered examples. In England, where politicians talked about preserving personal liberties, a recent authority advocated suppression of criminal safe houses. The Americans had invented a more practical solution: security companies. An American firm had devised an alarm that could signal the presence of an intruder from a switch fixed near the bedstead. The turn of a key activated a telegraph link to the telegraph office, which notified the police. Trains and telegraphs represented advances in the fight against crime as well as offering tools to commit crime (Lombroso, 2006, pp. 135–136).

Lombroso anticipates research in evolutionary psychology and biosocial criminology in proposing evolutionary development as the source of rationality. Recent work about evolutionary psychology does not attempt to find pathological conditions in a particular population, but aims to account for the formation of "rationality" in the masses of human beings. Lombroso becomes the founder of research into the evolutionary foundations of moral or pro-social behavior, from Wilson's sociobiology (1975) to Pinker's "better angels" (2011).

SCIENTIFIC RACISM

Much has been made of Lombroso's military service, anthropometric research, and subsequent theory of crime. Pick (1989) explains how Lombroso "volunteered for the new national army" and conducted his anthropometric research into the "ethnic diversity of the Italian people." The "problem of criminality was part of the problematic of 'making Italy'" (Pick, 1989, pp. 110–119). This implies that given Lombroso's view as an intellectual from the "advanced" industrialized north of Italy, he was interested in how to incorporate the "backward" agrarian South, and so he was eager to put his racialized science to work in the service of the emerging Italian nation-state. Criminal anthropology appears as scientific racism in the service of state-building (D'Agostino, 2002; Salvatore, 2006).

But this critique presents Lombroso as an Italian scientist and Lombroso was an Italian-Jewish scientist. He was born into a Jewish family in Verona in 1835, a city ruled by the Habsburg Kingdom of Venice. The Catholic authorities allowed Jews to attend the gymnasium and, for a time, Lombroso studied at the public school controlled by the Jesuits. He supported the emerging Italian state for the same reason many Jews did: The *Risorgimento* held the promise of emancipation from centuries-old restrictions on Jewish life. Emancipation had come to Jews first in Piedmont and extended to other areas as Piedmont became the basis for the emerging Italian state (Knepper, 2011, p. 357).

It is chilling to read statements from *L'uomo delinquente* knowing about the horrors of Auschwitz and Dachau. Lombroso insisted that the death sentence for the criminal type was consistent with the laws of nature: "progress in the animal world, and therefore in the human world, is based on a struggle for existence that involves hideous massacres." In the fifth edition, Lombroso says that society need spare no sentiment for atavistic criminals, who are "programmed to do harm" and reproduce in their being "not only savage men but also the most ferocious carnivores and rodents" (Lombroso, 2006, p. 348). Rafter (2008, p. 179) identifies Lombroso as the "strongest influence on German criminology" during the interwar period. "Lombroso's key writings, translated into German by the end of the 19th century, shaped the contours of the emerging science of criminal biology." She (2008, pp. 193–194) also says that Lombroso's criminal anthropology "deeply stamped" developments in Mussolini's Italy, such as eugenicist measures in the penal code of 1927.

Some of those within Lombroso's circle sided with fascist regimes. Salvatore Ottolenghi completed his medical degree at Turin and studied with Lombroso for 10 years. He became professor of legal medicine at the University of Rome and director of scientific policing at Regina Coeli prison, where he turned Lombroso's ideas into a teachable and practical technology for the national police (Dunnage, 2017). He became a "Jewish fascist." He praised Mussolini for grasping Lombroso's teaching that "one cannot understand crime if one does not study the criminal" (Gibson, 2002, p. 141). Others did not. Mario Carrara, Lombroso's son in law, became one of only 13 academics who refused to swear allegiance to Mussolini in 1929 and was dismissed for his opposition. In 1936, Mussolini abolished all chairs in criminal anthropology at all universities in Italy in reprisal for visible opposition to his government. Lombroso's daughter Gina, and her husband Gugliemlo Ferrero, who also opposed the regime, established a safe house in Geneva for Italians fleeing the fascists (Monaco & Mula, 2011, p. 686; Montaldo, 2013, p. 105).

What Lombroso himself would have done is another question. Lombroso did not live to experience the rise of fascism in the interwar period. He did witness the wave of prejudice against Jews that swept across Europe in the late 19th century. In Germany and Austria, anti-Semitic political parties contested elections; in France, the Dreyfus affair exposed a reservoir of anti-Jewish prejudice. Its proponents referred to themselves as "anti-Semites" to emphasize that they did not object to Judaism as a religion, but to Jews as a matter of racial characteristics. A flurry of anti-Jewish pamphlets, books, and articles drew on emerging race science, and it was in one of these libraries, the National Socialist Institute in Munich, that Hitler found material for his rants (Ryback, 2009, p. 50).

One group of Jewish intellectuals responded with a Jewish-oriented social science. Arthur Ruppin, Joseph Jacobs, and Maurice Fishberg led a countermovement that came to be known as "Jewish social science" or "Jewish statistics." They did not avoid racial language, but rather, used "facts" from anthropometry and craniometry to challenge anti-Semitic statements. In one version, favored by Zionists such as Max Nordau, Jewish social scientists presented statistics to demonstrate the poor physical condition of Jews, the accumulated effects of confinement in ghettos, and the need for a Jewish homeland away from urban squalor. Lombroso contributed to Jewish social science.

Along with Ruppin, Jacobs, and Fishberg, he produced material about Jewish characteristics. He wrote articles challenging anti-Semitic claims and exposing prejudice in the accusations against Dreyfus. He wrote a short book, *L'antisemitismo e le Scienze Moderne* [Anti-Semitism and the Modern Sciences] (1894), as well as several articles in which he consistently defended Jews from racist attacks (Knepper, 2013). Consistent with the strategy of Jewish social science, he countered race science with his own science. He invoked atavism to characterize the "anti-Semitic wind" gusting across Europe. "Anti-Semitism is an atavistic phenomenon," Lombroso wrote in 1897, "which has its basis in the lowest passions of mankind" (Lombroso, 1897).

From the opening pages of the first edition of *L'uomo delinquente*, Lombroso displayed his contempt for "primitive peoples." The characteristics of the criminal skull are similar to the "black American and Mongol races, and above all, prehistoric man much more than the white races" (Lombroso, 2006, p. 49). He retained this through all five editions. Near the end of his life, however, he reversed his view. In his studies of spiritualism, Lombroso declared new respect for so-called backward societies.

He began his studies of spiritualism in the late 1880s with visits to several "haunted houses." Given his reputation as a secular intellectual pursuing a scientific explanation, his reports attracted wide attention (Ferraculti, 1996, p. 134). As Lombroso recounted, the Pavarino family in Turin heard the sound of a water basin being overturned, yet no one else was in the room. The following morning, the bell attached to the entrance began to ring on its own. Members of the family heard continual groans. The youngest daughter awoke to the feeling of blows, but saw no one; by morning, the sunlight revealed bruises on her body. The most curious aspect of Lombroso's account is not his thoughts about poltergeists, but about the people who make these statements. They were, Lombroso said, "a family of working people" and—the curious part is that—he believed them. Lombroso said that he had the occasion to report facts about hauntings, now so frequently reported and well-attested. Centuries had passed without anyone taking notice of them, except among the lower classes, which are not in communication with the educated classes. "It is not that they did not occur; but that the educated classes no longer believed in them" (Lombroso, 1906b).

Lombroso managed to write a book, shortly before his death, on spiritualism. In the preface to *After Death—What?*, he compared scientific knowledge to mapping the islands across a wide sea; science could grasp what could be observed, but there was much more to be known. He had been wrong about science; scientific facts were neither as permanent nor as objective as they appeared. He also suggested that he had been wrong about people; specifically, the people who came to him with ghost stories. He had dismissed their accounts as superstition or mental illness; now he thought there was more to them than this. "Perhaps the proof that appeals to me with most insistent force is the universality of the belief among all peoples (at least in humble classes who are nearer to the foundation of truth than they seem) in the existence not only of mediums and magicians . . . but of spirits, and especially the souls of the dead" (Lombroso, 1909, p. 204). He devoted an extensive chapter to the spiritual beliefs of people across Africa, India, and the Americas. Although he refers to them as "primitive peoples" he insists that they possess deeper and more important knowledge than the advanced peoples of Europe. In making such an observation, he retreated from the racist hierarchy he established in his early work.

CONCLUSIONS

Cesare Lombroso was a crucial figure in making Turin the site for emerging neuroscience. He filled his books and articles with superficial correlations, sloppy comparisons, and extraneous information. Nevertheless, he made his inquiries within the framework of historical science. From this perspective, the human body presented a museum, a collection of artifacts revealing what had taken place in an earlier epoch.

Lombroso's energy and imagination in pursuing a scientific understanding of criminal behavior made many others aware of the possibilities. He promoted dangerous proposals based on overconfidence in the certainty of science. He encouraged early intervention and preventive confinement without an understanding of how these policies would be used by authorities. Scientific racism infused his outlook throughout his career, warping his theories, data collection, and interpretation of findings. Yet Lombroso acknowledged his Jewish identity and turned his science against anti-Semitism. Near the end of his life, he acknowledged his mistaken beliefs about so-called primitive peoples. On reflection, he decided their understanding of the world offered another route to discovering realms beyond the grasp of science.

REFERENCES

Becker P & Wetzell R (2006) *Criminals and Their Scientists: The History of Criminology in International Perspective*. Cambridge: Cambridge University Press.

Carrara M (1928) *Institute of Legal Medicine and Criminal Anthropology Royal University of Turin. Methods and Problems of Legal Education: Institutes of Legal Medicine* (Ninth Series). New York: Rockefeller Foundation.

Chambers R (1844) *Vestiges of the Natural History of Creation*. London: John Churchill.

Cleland C (2011) Prediction and explanation in historical natural science. *British Journal of the Philosophy of Science*, 62: 551–582.

Cleland C (2002) Methodological and epistemic differences between historical science and experimental science. *Philosophy of Science*, 69: 474–496.

Cleland C (2001) Historical science, experimental science, and the scientific method. *Geology*, 29: 987–990.

Cole S & Campbell M (2013) From subhumans to superhumans: Criminals in the evolutionary hierarchy, or what became of Lombroso's atavistic criminals? In P Knepper & P Ysehede (Eds.), *The Cesare Lombroso Handbook*, pp. 147–170. New York: Routledge.

D'Agostino P (2002) Craniums, criminals, and the 'cursed race': Italian anthropology in American racial thought, 1861–1924. *Comparative Studies in Society and History*, 44: 319–343.

Del Lago E (2011) Italian national unification and the *Mezzogiorno*: Colonialism in one country? In D Healy & E De Lago (Eds.), *The Shadow of Colonialism on Europe's Modern Past*, pp. 57–72. London: Palgrave Macmillan.

DeLisi M (2013) Revisiting Lombroso. In F T Cullen & P Wilcox (Eds.), *The Oxford Handbook of Criminological Theory*, pp. 5–21. New York: Oxford University Press.

Dunnage J (2017) The legacy of Cesare Lombroso and criminal anthropology in the post-war Italian police: A study of the culture, narrative and memory of a post-fascist institution. *Journal of Modern Italian Studies*, 22: 365–384.

Ferrero G (1908) Lombroso, prophet and criminologist. *Century Illustrated Monthly Magazine*, 76: 925–929.

Foucault M (1978) About the concept of the 'dangerous individual' in 19th-century legal psychiatry. *International Journal of Law and Psychiatry*, 1: 1–18.

Garland D (2002) Of crimes and criminals: The development of criminology in Britain. In M Maguire, R Morgan, & R Reiner (Eds.), *The Oxford Handbook of Criminology*, pp. 7–50. London: Oxford University Press.

Gatti U & Verde A (2012) Cesare Lombroso: Methodological ambiguities and brilliant intuitions *International Journal of Law and Psychiatry*, 35: 19–26.

Gibson M (2002) *Born to Crime: Cesare Lombroso and the Origins of Biological Criminology*. Westport, CT: Praeger.

Gibson M (2006) Cesare Lombroso and Italian criminology: Theory and politics. In P Becker & R Wetzell (Eds.), *Criminals and their Scientists: The History of Criminology in International Perspective*, pp. 137–158. Cambridge: Cambridge University Press.
Gibson M (2013) Cesare Lombroso, prison science and penal policy. In P Knepper & M Ystehede (Eds.), *The Cesare Lombroso Handbook*, pp. 30–46. London: Routledge.
Gibson M & Rafter N (2007) Introduction. In M Gibson & N Rafter (Eds.), *Criminal Man*, pp. 1–41. Durham, NC: Duke University Press.
Goring C (1919) *The English Convict*. London: HMSO.
Gould S (1981) *The Mismeasure of Man*. New York: W.W. Norton.
Horn D (2003) *The Criminal Body: Lombroso and the Anatomy of Deviance*. New York: Routledge.
Jarkko J, Griffiths S, & Maraun M (2015) *The Myth of the Born Criminal: Psychopathy, Neurobiology and the Creation of the Modern Degenerate*. Buffalo, NY: University of Toronto Press.
Kenney C (1910) The death of Lombroso. *Journal of the Society of Comparative Legislation*, 10(2): 220–228.
Knepper P (2018) *Second science? The future historical science in criminology*. In G Farrell and A Sidebottom (Eds), *Realist Evaluation for Crime Science: Essays in Honour of Nick Tilley*, pp. 119–137. London: Routledge Taylor & Francis.
Knepper P (2011) Lombroso's Jewish identity and its implications for criminology. *Australian and New Zealand Journal of Criminology*, 44: 355–369.
Knepper P (2013) Lombroso and Jewish social science. In P Knepper & P J Ystehede (Eds.), *The Cesare Lombroso Handbook*, pp. 171–186. London: Routledge.
Knepper P (2018) Laughing at Lombroso: Positivism and Criminal Anthropology in historical perspective. In R Triplett (Ed.), *Wiley Handbook of the History and Philosophy of Criminology*, pp. 51–66. Hoboken, NJ: John Wiley.
Knepper P & Ystehede PJ (2013) *The Cesare Lombroso Handbook*. London: Routledge.
Lombroso C (1902) Precocity in crime. *The Independent*, 54: 2136–2138.
Lombroso C (1907) My museum of criminal anthropology. *New York Times*, February 17, 1907.
Lombroso C (1910) The criminal. *Putnam's Magazine*, 7: 793–796.
Lombroso C (1911) *Criminal Man, summarized by G Lombroso Ferrero*. New York: G.P. Putnam's Sons.
Lombroso C (1912) Crime and insanity in the twenty-first century. *Journal of Criminal, Criminology and Police Science*, 3: 57–61.
Lombroso C (2006) *Criminal Man*. (M Gibson & N Rafter, Trans.). Durham, NC: Duke University Press.
Looney J W (2010) Neuroscience's new techniques for evaluating future dangerousness: Are we returning to Lombroso's biological criminality. *University of Arkansas at Little Rock Law Review*, 32: 301–314.
Mazzarello P (2010) *Golgi: A Biography of the Founder of Modern Neuroscience*. New York: Oxford University Press.
Mazarello P (2011) Cesare Lombroso: An anthropologist between evolution and degeneration. *Functional Neurology*, 26: 97–101.
Montaldo S (2013) The Lombroso Museum from its origins to the present day. In P Knepper & P J Ystehede (Eds.), *The Cesare Lombroso Handbook*, pp. 98–112. London: Routledge.
Munthe C & Radovic S (2015) The return of Lombroso? Ethical aspects of (visions of) preventive forensic screening. *Public Health Ethics*, 8: 270–283.
Musumeci E (2013) New natural born killers? The legacy of Lombroso in neuroscience and law. In P Knepper & P J Ystehede (Eds.), *The Cesare Lombroso Handbook*, pp. 131–146. London: Routledge.
New York Times (1913) "There is no criminal type," says prison expert. November 2, 1913.
Pancaldi G (1991) *Darwin in Italy: Science Across Cultural Frontiers*. Bloomington: Indiana University Press.

Pick D (1989) *Faces of Degeneration: A European Disorder*, c. 1848–1918. Cambridge: Cambridge University Press.
Rafter N (2008) *The Criminal Brain: Understanding Biological Theories of Crime*. New York: New York University Press.
Raine A (2013a) The criminal mind. *Wall Street Journal*, December 13, 2018.
Raine A (2013b) *The Anatomy of Violence: The Biological Roots of Crime*. New York: Pantheon.
Regener S (2003) Criminological Museums and the Visualization of Evil. *Crime, History and Societies*, 7: 2–13
Rozès S (1995) ISSD: International Society of Social Defence. In M C Bassiouni (Ed.), *The Contributions of Specialized Institutes and Non-Governmental Organizations to the United Nations Criminal Justice Program*, pp. 313–226. The Hague: Martinus Nijhoff.
Savopoulos P & Lindell A (2018) Born criminal? Differences in structural, functional and behavioural lateralization between criminals and noncriminals. *Laterality: Asymmetries of Body, Brain and Cognition*, 23: 738–760.
Sellin T (1958) Enrico Ferri (1856–1929). *Journal of Criminal Law, Criminology and Police Science* 48: 481–492.
Sirgiovanni E (2017) Criminal heredity: The influence of Cesare Lombroso's concept of the "born criminal" on contemporary neurogenetics and its forensic applications. *Journal of the History of Medicine*, 29: 165–188.
Wetzell R (2000) *Inventing the Criminal: A History of German Criminology, 1880–1945*. Chapel Hill: University of North Carolina Press.
Wolfgang M (1961) Pioneers in criminology: Cesare Lombroso (1835–1909). *Journal of Criminal Law, Criminology and Police Science*, 52: 361–391.
Ystehede P (2013) Demonizing being: Lombroso and the ghosts of criminology. In P Knepper & P J Ystehede (Eds.), *The Cesare Lombroso Handbook*, pp. 72–97. London: Routledge.
Ystehede P (2008) *In the Twilight of Good and Evil: Cesare Lombroso and the Criminological Imagination*. Saabrücken: VDM Verlag.
Ystehede P (2016) Contested spaces—on crime museums, monuments and memorials. In P Knepper & A Johansen (Eds.), *The Oxford Handbook of the History of Crime and Criminal Justice*, pp. 338–352. New York: Oxford University Press.

CHAPTER 6

Seeing the History of Neuroscience in Turin through the Lenses of Its Instruments/Part 1

MARCO R. GALLONI

If Turin is one of the cradles of modern neuroscience, its excellence is due to the people, to the instruments, and how the former interacted with the latter. The city of Turin still preserves many of the instruments used to achieve the breakthrough discoveries mentioned in the chapters that precede and follow. Such instruments have been either upgraded to widely used procedures or to new inventions. Seeing the history of neuroscience in Turin through the lenses of some among its key instruments might add a new dimension to the stories narrated so far, and explain the geographical influence that Turin experienced over the centuries.

Let's start with Michele Vincenzo Malacarne (1774–1816), one of the main characters in Chapter 2. Born in Saluzzo, he was a genuinely eclectic scholar: He was appointed as a professor of surgery in the Universities of Pavia and Padua, but wrote about art, literature, and the history of medicine (Malacarne, 1786). He studied the anatomy of the brain not only by compiling a three-volume book on dissection in man (Malacarne, 1780), but also by exploring comparative anatomy (Figure 6.1). Among others, he assessed the encephalon of the seal (Malacarne, 1805) and birds, particularly of goose and duck (Malacarne, 1782). He followed the methods previously proposed by authors such as Galen and Andreas Vesalius, Costanzo Varolio, Franciscus de le Boë Sylvius, Nathaniel Highmore, and Guichard Joseph Duverney. His macroscopic observations were accurate, and Malacarne wrote a handbook describing all the steps of his work to allow other anatomists to follow his lead.

Contrary to what one might expect from a handbook, no particular mention was made of the saws, scalpels, scissors, trephines, and tweezers he used. They might likely have been those typical of the pre-aseptic era. Yet, as proof of his personal experience, he recommended knives with large and thin blades such as those that gradually became the standard tools for brain sectioning. To make the dura mater

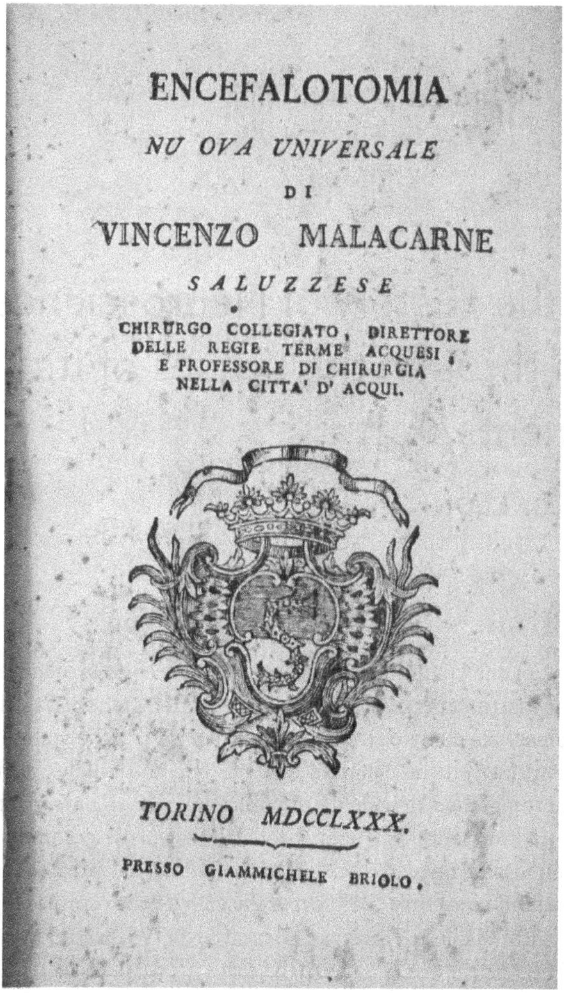

ENCEFALOTOMIA

NUOVA UNIVERSALE

DI

VINCENZO MALACARNE

SALUZZESE

CHIRURGO COLLEGIATO, DIRETTORE DELLE REGIE TERME ACQUESI, E PROFESSORE DI CHIRURGIA NELLA CITTA' D' ACQUI.

TORINO MDCCLXXX.

PRESSO GIAMMICHELE BRIOLO.

Figure 6.1. Frontispiece of Vincenzo Malacarne's book on the dissection of the brain, 1780. Courtesy of Marco Galloni.

blood vessels more visible, Malacarne injected them with vegetal-mineral water, wine, wine spirit, vinegar, melted wax and tallow stained with vermillion and mercury. The latter materials had to be injected warm and could even damage the preservation of the native anatomy. In the same years and for the same purpose, Paolo Mascagni (1755–1815) in Siena developed the perfusion of vessels—mostly the lymphatic ones—with mercury. This method took advantage of the peculiar weight of the liquid metal, which could make its way more easily in the circulatory system, even in the presence of coagulation (Mascagni, 1787). Another technical detail in Malacarne's work is the explicit reference to the *pied de Roi* (the foot) and its minor divisions (inches) as far as linear measures are concerned. The introduction of the metric system was decreed in France in 1795, upon the recommendation of a specific committee chaired by the Turin-born mathematician Luigi Lagrange (1736–1813). Despite this, the standardization process within the Reign of Sardinia began more than 50 years later, in 1850, and proceeded even more slowly.

In the fourth chapter, we met the anatomist Luigi Rolando (1773–1831), who advanced the knowledge of the central nervous system and whose name is still attached to many of the specific brain structures he pioneeringly described. From a merely technical perspective, Rolando did something novel yet straightforward when he cut brain slices along vertical planes and not, as more commonly done, via horizontal incisions (Stefanutti, 1974). In a book published in 1828, he summarized his research on morphology and physiology, with the latter being the most interesting source of information about the actual work he performed (Rolando, 1828). For example, Rolando understood the functions of the various parts of the encephalon after damaging or entirely destroying specific anatomical regions. But at a later time, he developed methods for local electric stimulation that were even more efficient. He used wires linked to the poles of Volta's pile and, observing the extent and the nature of the movements caused by the electrical stimulation of cerebellum, he thought of a correspondence between the superimposition of metallic discs in the pile and the lamellar architecture in that part of the brain. Both these complex and similar structures produce "fluids"—galvanic and nervous—that transmit energy and produce effects such as muscular movement; indeed, Volta's pile was often called "Volta's engine." The cerebellum lamellae already had been the object of consideration by Malacarne, who observed that idiots had a smaller number of these structures (De Renzi, 1848). Moreover, Rolando compared the *cerebellum lamellae* to Giuseppe Zamboni's (1776–1846) pile. Introduced in 1812, that pile was a dry battery that generated a low-intensity electrical current for a very long time so that it was applied to electrical clocks and considered a source of perpetual motion.

It makes quite an impression to read the long list of animals, belonging to many different species, which were sacrificed in that research as well as the operating procedures described in a disquieting way. We have to consider that, unfortunately, at that time, the sensitivity for the pain suffered by animals was very different from our days and almost nonexistent. This partially explains, but certainly does not justify, the often-naïve approach to the descriptions we can read today. The neurological signs recorded during observations and experiments were often of deep suffering, ending in a fast and merciful death. The physiological procedures usually needed a local demolition of the skull with a trephine. Still, for the cerebellum and the pons, a trocar was directly inserted through the mouth to perforate the palate and the base of the skull. Many old trephines, showing the typical rounded crown-shaped cutting blades, are preserved in medical collections as they were needed in case of skull wounds caused by accidents or war injuries. They could indeed help the removal of bone fragments and make the edges of the breach more regular, thus facilitating the healing. Another, more problematic, application of the trephine was the cure of severe headache, of epilepsy, and even of melancholy. In an attempt to relieve the head from noxious fluids, this hazardous procedure was practiced in several areas from the Renaissance to the beginning of the 19th century (Gross, 1999). But let's come back to Rolando for a little while.

When the French army invaded Piedmont in 1804, Rolando decided to follow the king Carlo Emanuele IV when exiled to Sardinia. On the way to Sardinia, he spent two years in Florence, where he acquired competence in iconographic techniques, such as anatomical drawing and wax modeling. He could have experienced a similar exposure under the guidance of Paolo Mascagni (1755–1815) and Felice Fontana (1730–1805), who had a master of molding in their workshop: Clemente Susini (1754–1814). When Rolando came back to Turin in 1814, he started the collection of more than two hundred wax models, among which the nervous system is widely represented. A great help in sketching anatomical specimens came from the invention of the "camera lucida," devised in 1806 by William Hyde Wollaston (1766–1828). Although the camera lucida significantly improved the likeliness of the drawings (Figure 6.2), we have no information on the use of a similar optical instrument by Rolando. Therefore, it is likely that the high quality of his images of the brain relies completely on his artistic talent, which was undoubtedly remarkable.

In Turin, there is also an unsigned microscope of John Cuff's (1708–1772) design that bears the initials of Luigi Rolando on the wooden case. Although this is a typical model of the 18th century, in the Anatomy Institute there are also two magnificent microscopes made by Giovanni Battista Amici (1786–1863). Amici started making

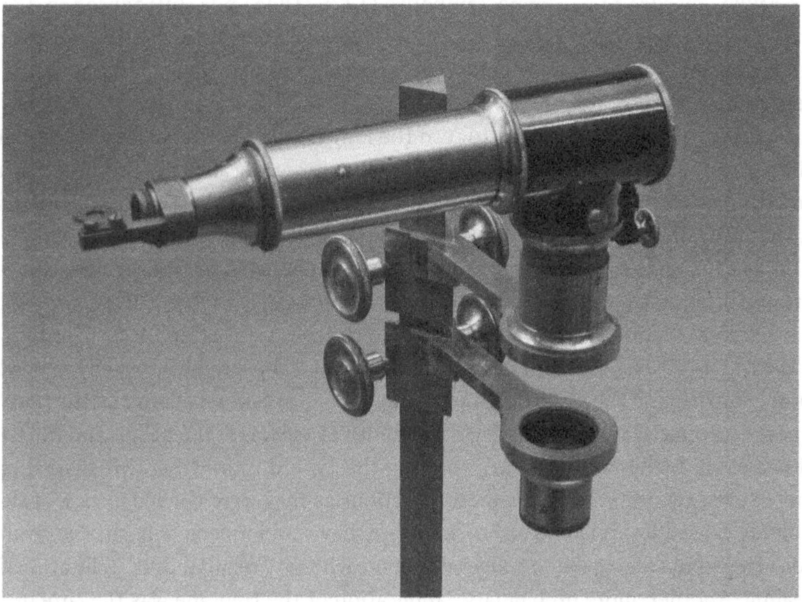

Figure 6.2. Wilhelm His's embryograph is a low-magnification microscope introduced in 1880 for drawing embryos, with a camera lucida invented by Chevallier & Oberhauser with a range of magnification from 4 to 40. It was used in many fields of anatomy, in particular in neurology. Courtesy of Marco Galloni.

optical instruments in Modena, which is almost 300 kilometers away from Turin, in 1825. The first and bigger one was sold in 1828 (Meschiari, 2003) for 750 francs. It had six eyepieces and four achromatic lenses, which were carefully calculated with regard to the thickness of the cover glass in the histological specimens, and it was provided with a simple camera lucida. Such a microscope was undoubtedly an outstanding tool to have and demonstrated Rolando's interest in the study of the fine structure of living matter. This is a rather new approach if compared to the opinion of François Xavier Bichat (1771–1802), who is remembered as the founder of histology. But Bichat never relied on the microscope because the observed images were too obscure and misleading, given that they were deeply affected by the aberrations of the lenses. The techniques of preparation of anatomic specimens for the microscope were then quite simple. Many of them consisted of the maceration in the water of the organs, and this procedure allowed the separation of the various tissue components. The other typical approach was the injection of fixing agents and stains through veins and arteries. A small wax model of a group of cells, possibly adipose tissue, is present in the collection of the Anatomy Museum and seems to be a witness to Rolando's microscopic studies and his awareness that macroscopic models were not sufficient anymore for teaching purposes.

While Rolando was in Sardinia, a relatively new experimental "model" was offered for the studies of physiology in Turin: the bodies of beheaded victims of the guillotine. Among its declared human rights, the French Revolution had introduced the exclusion of pain in the execution of capital punishments; the invention introduced in 1789 by Joseph-Ignace Guillotin (1738–1814) was the embodiment of this. Nevertheless, adverse opinions and some rather emotional witnesses induced many scientists to study the persistence of consciousness in the severed heads via sensorial and electric stimuli (Chamayou, 2008). Similar tests were carried out in Turin in 1802 by Antonio Maria Vassalli Eandi (1761–1825), professor of physics, who helped with galvanic instruments, the physicians Carlo Stefano Giulio (1757–1815) and Francesco Rossi (1769–1841), who made their observations on the heads and trunks of three beheaded bodies (Vassalli et al., 1802). Such an exceptional and transient situation was apparently favorable for neurological studies, but no exhaustive results were obtained.

When Rolando came back to Torino, he put great effort into teaching activities, organizing the Museum of Anatomy, and writing some of the volumes in which he summarized his discoveries. Also, with the collaboration of the physiologist Lorenzo Martini (1785–1841), he started to compile a dictionary of biomedical knowledge (Rolando et al., 1822–1828). Martini was a scholar with a broad scientific culture, but he was not an experimental scientist. His old-fashioned attitude was testified to by the fact that he always gave lessons in Latin. Yet a capacity to synthesize complex concepts probably allowed him to foresee topics that would have later become popular, including the chemical nature of the signal transmission in the nervous system.

Four years after being appointed as a professor of Anatomy in Turin, Carlo Giacomini (1840–1898) proposed a systematic classification of the brain's "convoluted" appearance (Giacomini, 1878). As a keen representative of scientific positivism, Giacomini correctly used his knowledge against the ideas of one of the most influential scientists of that time: Cesare Lombroso (1835–1909), the founder of criminal anthropology, who believed that the shape of the brain could explain behavioral deviance. He introduced microscopy in the neurological field and contributed to innovating the available methods and instruments, including the definition of histological structures of the brain (Giacomini, 1882). He made large cerebral slides and developed a specific microscope to observe them. In those years, fixative agents for biological tissues were mostly alcohol and chromic acid solutions. Still, both of them were causing the hardening of the specimens, and formaldehyde as a preservation medium was only proposed in 1892 by the French chemist Jean-Auguste Trillat (1861–1944), who was born in Pont-de-Beauvoisin (Isère), 240 kilometers away from Turin. The following step was the thin sectioning with the use of the microtome, but the specimens, which consisted of thick slices of whole brains, needed an uncommonly large instrument such as the one that had been proposed in 1875 by Johann Bernhard Aloys von Gudden (1824–1886) and realized in the workshop of Hermann Katsch (1837–1891) in München.

Von Gudden was a psychiatrist and a neuroanatomist who championed the combined use of macroscopic observations with microscopic studies. The available techniques could only process small specimens, however, and he had to envisage an original, wider microtome (von Gudden, 1875). But he could benefit from the discovery of the "black reaction," made by Camillo Golgi (1843–1926) in 1873, which allowed him to recognize different pathways of optical fibers and the consequences on thalamic nuclei of damages in specific cortical areas. We know that Giacomini took advantage of von Gudden's work and followed a similar scientific approach. But we also know that he introduced original improvements: When he ordered a new microtome in 1878, Giacomini asked Hermann Katsch to modify the surfaces for the sliding of the knife, as the glass allowed a smoother cut. Although the first microtome had been built in 1770 by George Adams, Jr. (1750–1795), the use of this instrument became a standard procedure in laboratories only a hundred years later, namely after 1875, as stated in a handbook of histology published in 1885 (Friedlander et al., 1885). The inclusion in hard materials to facilitate the cut was often obtained with boiled egg-white or soap, with the drawback they could not be removed from the sections. Paraffin was proposed by Edwin Klebs (1834–1913) in 1864 and had the advantage was of melting with benzene, but it did not become a standard protocol until the end of the century. Giacomini did not use any embedding medium and cut human brains deeply fixed in Müller solution and hardened in alcohol, as the staining was with ammoniac carmine.

But the exceptionally large slides could not be seen with a traditional microscope because of the insufficient dimensions of the stage (Figure 6.3). Therefore, Giacomini asked Francesco Koristka (1851–1933), who, in 1880, had launched a new factory for the production of scientific instruments in Milan, for a modified version of a microscope with a wider stage (Giacomini, 1883). The need for special microscopes to observe large slides was also recognized by the German firm Zeiss, which produced specific adaptations of the 1c and 1d stands in the first decade of the 20th century.

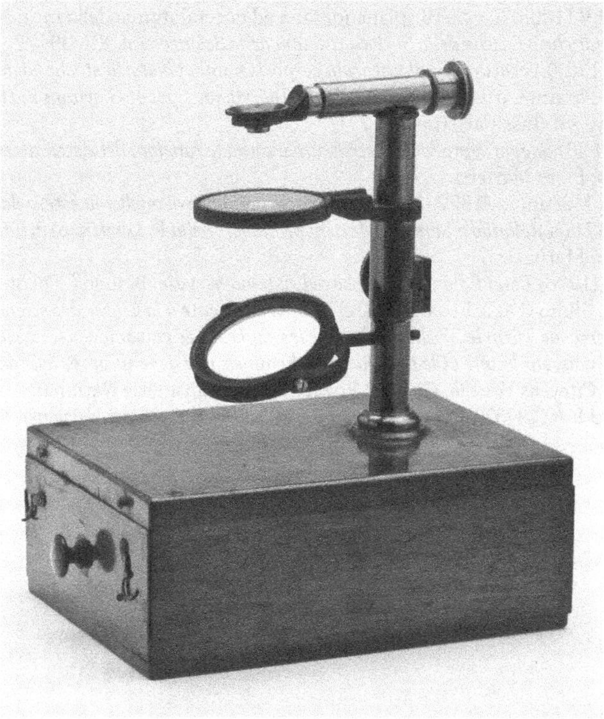

Figure 6.3. A simple microscope with different low magnification lenses, which can be mounted on the wooden box containing all its parts, was used for fine anatomical dissections. Courtesy of Marco Galloni.

REFERENCES

Chamayou G (2008) The debate over severed heads: Doctors, the guillotine and the anatomy of consciousness in the wake of the Terror. *Revue d'histoire des sciences*, 61: 333–365.

De Renzi S (1848) *Storia della medicina in Italia*. Napoli: Tip. Filiatre-Sebezio.

Friedlander C, & Martinotti G (1885) *La tecnica microscopica applicata alla clinica ed all'anatomia patologica*. Torino: UTET.

Giacomini C (1878) *Guida allo studio delle circonvoluzioni cerebrali dell'uomo*. Torino: Camilla e Bertolero.

Giacomini C (1882) Sezioni microscopiche dell'intero encefalo umano adulto. *Giornale R. Accademia Medicina di Torino*, anno XLV: 3–18.

Giacomini C (1883) Nuovo microscopio per l'esame delle sezioni dell'intero encefalo umano adulto. *Giornale R. Accademia Medicina Torino*, anno XLVI: 412–420.

Gross C G (1999) A hole in the head. *History of Neurosciences*, 5(4): 263–269.

Malacarne M V (1780) *L'encefalotomia nuova universale* (3 voll). Torino: Giammichele Briolo.

Malacarne M V (1782) Esposizione anatomica delle parti relative all'encefalo degli uccelli. *Memorie Matematiche e Fisiche della Società Italiana delle Scienze*, vol. I: 747–767.

Malacarne M V (1786, 1789) *Delle opere de' medici, e de' cerusici che nacquero, o fiorirono prima del secolo XVI negli Stati della Real Casa di Savoja* (2 voll). Torino: Stamperia Reale.

Malacarne M V (1805) Saggio di splancnografia ed encefalotomia della foca. *Memorie Matematiche e Fisiche della Società Italiana delle Scienze*, vol. XII: 39–72.
Mascagni P (1787) *Vasorum lymphaticorum corporis humani historia et ichonographia.* Siena: Pazzini Carli.Meschiari A (2003) *The Microscopes of Giovanni Battista Amici.* Firenze, Ed. Tassinari, (pp. 26–27).
Rolando L (1828) *Saggio sopra la vera struttura e sopra le funzioni del sistema nervoso.* Torino: Piero Marietti.
Rolando L, & Martini L. (1822–1828) *Dizionario periodico di medicina esteso dai signori dottori Luigi Rolando e Lorenzo Martini professori nella R. Università di Torino* (14 voll). Torino: Marietti.
Stefanutti U (1974) *Luigi Rolando studioso del sistema nervoso.* Bologna: Forni.
Vassalli A M, Giulio C S, & Rossi F (1802) *Rapport prèsentè à la Classe des sciences exactes de l'Academie de Turin le 27 thermidor, sur les expèriences galvaniques faites les 22 et 26 du mème mois, sur la tète et le tronc de trois hommes, peu de tems après leur décapitation, par les Citoyens Vassalli, Giulio et Rossi.* Torino: Imprimerie Nationale.
von Gudden J B A (1875) Über ein neues microtom. *Arch Psychiatr Nervenkr,* 5: 229–234.

CHAPTER 7

Enrico Morselli in Turin

Expectations, Challenges, and Disappointment

ALESSANDRO BARGONI

In the context of the life of the psychiatrist and anthropologist Enrico Morselli (1852–1929; Figure 7.1), joining Turin represented something more than just a chance to achieve, finally, national visibility. It meant, for him, the opportunity to focus on research topics that would have later defined his career and become his signature. The period spent in Turin started with high expectations, proved to be challenging, and ended in complete disappointment. His arrival in Piedmont was motivated by practical reasons connected with the management of the Asylum and the need to connect the clinic administration and University teaching even more strongly. But, to fully understand this and contextualize his years in Turin, we need to take one step back.

The Turin Asylum had two main sections, so close yet so far: one in via Giulio in Turin and another one housed in the Chartreuse of Collegno, just kilometers away from the Turin city center. At the end of the 1870s, Giovanni Stefano Bonacossa (1804–1878), the director for the previous 25 years, who was also a professor of Mental Illnesses Clinical Medicine, died. His death destroyed the already tricky balance between the various groups sitting on the Asylum Administrative Board, representing a clash between the clinical and the academic worlds. Giovanni Stefano Bonacossa embodied both souls, being a clinician and an academic. His dual role emphasized the attention given by the State to the complex intertwining of knowledge about alienation and the treatment and custody of the insane, slightly after the creation of the first professorship of this kind in Florence (CISO, 2007).

But this is just part of the story. Although the chair, granted by the Administration, was housed in the via Giulio, the professorship was funded by the Ministry. Thanks to a new regulation that came into place in 1832, the professorship was given to the consultant doctor, Stefano Bonacossa, who was a well-known psychiatrist. This established an interdependence between the academic and clinical functions.

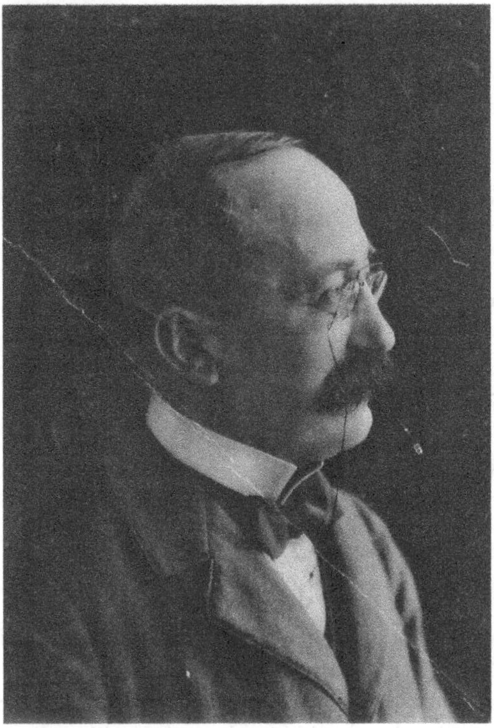

Figure 7.1. Portrait of Enrico Morselli.
Credits: Archivio dell'ex ospedale psichiatrico San Lazzaro di Reggio Emilia—Ausl RE. Da Fotografia E. Rossi Genova. Thanks to Nicoletta Natalini.

Nevertheless, when Bonacossa's retirement from the Asylum administration came, the mediocrity of his successor induced the Faculty to call Bonacossa back to continue delivering his teaching activities. When he died in 1878, the quest for a new director started. And the whole situation exploded.

The chair was initially given to the new director of the Asylum, Michelangelo Porporati. But the Faculty Board, after a heated (and somewhat divisive) discussion, did not confirm his professorship, and even denied his request to continue his teaching. The teaching load for 1879–1880 was then given to the criminologist Cesare Lombroso (1835–1909). Porporati, who felt hurt in his professional credibility, resigned from the Asylum administration, but kept his position as Advisor on the Asylum Administration Board. In 1879, the positions of Director of the Asylum and the Chair of Mental Illnesses Clinical Medicine were both vacant. In this context, a suitable candidate for both the positions was needed. Thanks to an agreement between the Asylum and the University, the latter was granted the Faculty to propose a candidate for the professorship of Mental Illnesses Clinical Medicine, who would also be consultant (Bargoni, 2008).

Traditionally, the Asylum management was not very open toward new therapies: the custody of the "insane people" was actively pursued, thus subordinating the medical and clinical aspects to this issue. The European "hospital Grand

Tours" visitors, since the very beginning of the 19th century (e.g., Luis, Esquirol) unanimously reported that Piedmont had some of the strictest asylum management practices in Italy, barely masked by a superficial diplomatic condescendence. In addition to this, another critical factor was the (real or supposed) limited means of the Asylum, which very often reduced an inmate's food to bare subsistence. This also happened shortly before Morselli's arrival (Moraglio, 2002).

The Asylum atmosphere in the last months of 1879 was particularly tense because of the friction with the University and the non-attribution of the professorship to Porporati, a physician who had spent his career in the Hospital and was not connected with academia. This tension was further ignited by his resignation from the role of a Consultant, which was ill-received by both the Asylum Administration Board and Porporati himself. Therefore, there was resentment toward the University; although initially it was hidden and somehow limited, it then became apparent.

Enrico Morselli represented the University in the Asylum. His call in Turin was supported by his acquaintance with Lombroso, given that they were both pupils of the neurologist and anthropologist Paolo Mantegazza (1831–1910). Moreover, he was esteemed and supported by many psychiatrists, including Augusto Tamburini (1848–1919), a supporter of the anthropologic trend in psychiatry.

Morselli arrived in Turin in 1880: he was 28 years old, director of the Asylum and adjunct professor of Psychiatric Clinic. Despite his young age, his credentials were impressive: from a clinical perspective, he had successfully directed the Macerata Asylum; academically, he had been Professor of Psychiatry in Pavia. In 1874, he was the editor and the cofounder, with Livi and Tamburini, of the *Rivista Sperimentale di Freniatria e di Medicina Legale in relazione con l'Antropologia e le Scienze Giuridiche e Sociali*. He was also an anthropologist, having attended Paolo Mantegazza's school in Florence. His experience in Macerata anticipated what he would have found in Turin but with a substantial difference. The Administrative and Management Councils were not against him in Macerata.

Moreover, some politicians supported him openly and encouraged his work toward modernization of the asylum. The lessons learned from his teacher Livi, who reformed two asylums, came in handy and proved to be instrumental when he directed the Macerata asylum. Enrico Morselli became a Consultant in a challenging atmosphere. In essence, the Administration was against him, the means were limited, the asylum often resorted to segregation, contention and guards ordinarily prevaricated the inmate (Cassata & Moraglio, 2005).

Morselli tried to change this situation with the same enthusiasm he had in Macerata. Still, the intense hostility and the preconceptions toward him exhibited by the Administration Board frustrated his efforts. While directing the Asylum, the Administration often denied him the possibility of selecting patients for practical clinical teachings. The administration prevaricated him and expected to choose the patients on his behalf, because, according to regulations, they had the duty to supervise the inmate's treatments. This was a significant limitation, and not only a formal one, given that the "professor" had a double role.

Moreover, Morselli desired a laboratory with modern medical instruments for his research, but the Hospital, given its limited means, could not provide him with one.

Such a working environment prevented him from carrying on the scientific research he desired. In addition to this, the Administration was not missing a single chance to make the life of the new Director almost impossible. On the Governing Board, two physicians were particularly hostile to Morselli. One was the resentful Porporati, who had been humiliated by the Faculty, and the other one was Angelo Perotti, a former jail physician. His provenance made clear the Institution's intentions: he was an obscure character. He joined the Administrative Board of the Asylum thanks to the support of the state administration he was mainly tied to because he observed all the regulations and all the orders blindly.

Morselli's enthusiasm in his clinical activity was coupled with a parallel interest in teaching, with the publication of *Introduzione alle lezioni di psicologia patologica e clinica psichiatrica* [Introduction to the Lessons of Pathological Psychology and Psychiatric Clinics] for his Turin course, in 1881 (Morselli, 1884). Turin's social environment was very different from the one Morselli was used to while in Macerata: Turin was an industrial city, with all the incongruences and social problems to which this could lead. Marginalization, poverty, beggary, deviance, alienation, and exploitation were factors in social pathologies, and the Asylum acted as a safeguard of public security. It is thus understandable that the confiscation of padlocks and straitjackets, as well as the use of new noncoercive methods, raised concerns about the loss of control over internal order by the Governing Board of the Hospital. This created an atmosphere of mistrust regarding the actions of the Clinician and Consultant, and originated a more profound break, which became irremediable.

On the 18th of April 1885, Morselli wrote a letter to the Rector. He explained his difficulties and decided to create a new relationship with the Asylum through a new agreement, to avoid the end of "the existence and the future itself of the Mental Illnesses University clinic." In this letter, Morselli expressed his strong wish to leave the Asylum administration. Some days later, on the Register of the Deliberation of the Asylum Direction, his resignation was acknowledged for "personal reasons." Morselli was *de facto* forced to resign from his role as an Asylum Consultant because of the misunderstanding and the boycott by a conservative and bigoted establishment, which was utterly impervious to the new trends of Italian phrenology.

Yet Morselli did not leave Turin, and he continued to teach Psychiatry, still hoping for a reconciliation with the Asylum administration. However, the attacks against the University by the Asylum administrators and by Porporati continued. The latter presented the Rector a memorandum, shifting the debate to a personal level, accusing Morselli of arrogance, due to the bold tones he had used against the Asylum administration. This was coupled with another accusation, of superciliousness, because Morselli tried a more "technical" and "scientific" psychiatry, which, according to Porporati, was against the main concern and responsibility of the Direction, which should, instead, operate for the sake of a patient's well-being. Porporati's tone gives the idea of the mystification of reality and his intentions. This summarizes the inadequacy of the institution, wherein an incompetent character such as Porporati, supported by the political and administrative establishment, tried to put a cultural giant like Morselli into a corner. Porporati, in his memorandum, accused Morselli of bullying his patients with experimental psychology or hypnosis, saying that: "when physicians are not overseen, when they are absolute masters without effective control, without someone who protects the patient against some perversions, how can we know if an excessive passion for science could push over some of his followers? The famous motto is: *faciamus experimentum in corpore vili*. Now, who will protect the poor inmate against those experiments?" (Montaldo & Novaria, 2011). Porporati continued to discredit Morselli's work, stating that the administration had to prevent him from discharging some of the inmates, whom the Director-Consultant considered perfectly dischargeable, but that the administration, which only aimed at the patients' well-being, considered wrong. All the administrators came from the upper bourgeoisie or were notables who strongly wanted to protect the public order. Porporati concluded by adding that the administration had interrupted the visits from the families, ended the outgoing mobility of the inmates, and eliminated work in the Asylum, all inopportune measures taken by Morselli.

But despite all the attacks instituted by his detractors, Morselli's scholarly fame was consolidated thanks to the many initiatives he undertook in Turin. He wrote articles for the *Rivista sperimentale di freniatria* and the *Archivio per l'antropologia e l'etnologia*. He actively took part in the works for the Lombrosian *Archivio di scienze penali e antropologia criminale*, and twists and turns marred even his personal and professional relationship with Cesare Lombroso. He was also interested in some aspects of hygiene, following the scientific project of Luigi Pagliani and his *Giornale della Società Italiana di Igiene* [Journal of the Italian Society of Hygiene]. Morselli was also a member of the Management Board, and he contributed multidisciplinary studies with a plethora of scientific figures, such as engineers, architects, clinicians, biologists, and naturalists, thereby facilitating their dialogue (Guarnieri, 1986).

His activities connected him to esteemed faculty colleagues, including Giulio Bizzozzero (1846–1901) and Angelo Mosso (1846–1910). With the latter, he shared some studies on experimental psychology, often made in the physiology laboratory. He also met Pagliani, mentioned earlier, who would become, shortly after, the technical writer of the first sanitary law of the Italian Kingdom, presented by Francesco Crispi in 1888. Thanks to his dialectic abilities, he became a brilliant speaker who gave popular lectures, as did other Turin scientists, including Jacob Moleschott (1822–1893), Giulio Bizzozero, Angelo Mosso, and Pio Foà (1848–1923). They were all great science communicators, who believed in the social value of explaining science through popular conferences. Morselli kept alive the cultural enterprise of the *Rivista di Filosofia Scientifica* [Journal of Scientific Philosophy], which promoted reflection on the theoretical elaboration of positive science topics and their experimental nature across the whole country. He was helped by two valid collaborators: Gabriele Buccola (1854–1885) and Eugenio Tanzi (1856–1934). Another motivation induced him to stay at the same university: he was waiting for the Ministry selection to become a full professor (Roux, 1910).

Psychiatry was at the core of Morselli's investigation, but other interests included anthropology, biology, psychology, neurology, experimental psychology, sociology, criminology, sexology, hypnotism, parapsychology, evolutionism, statistics, and pharmacology (Figure 7.2). After his experiences in Reggio and Macerata, Morselli was oriented toward a psychiatric taxonomy based not only on the symptom, but

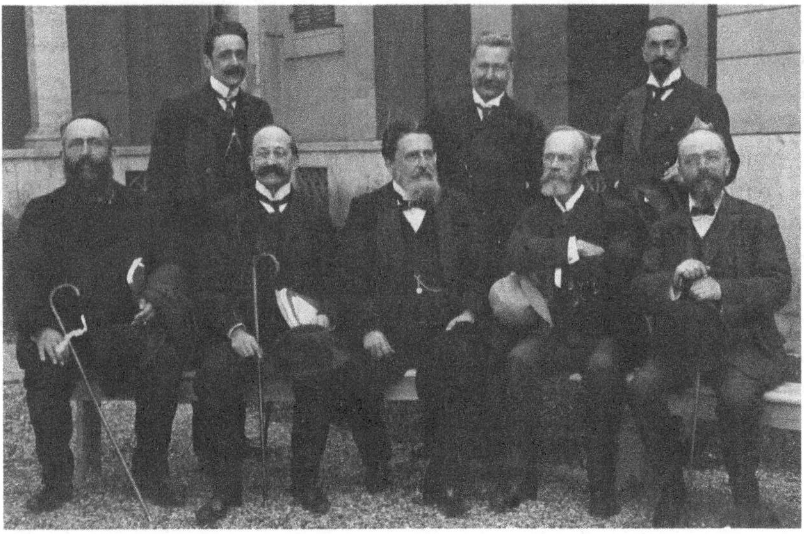

Figure 7.2. Group picture with Enrico Morselli. Standing, on the right side: Giulio Cesare Ferrari; standing on the left, probably Luigi Patrizi. Seated, from the second one on the left: Enrico Morselli, Luigi Luciani, William James, and Giulio Fano.
Credits: Aspi—Archivio storico della psicologia italiana, Università di Milano-Bicocca, Archivio Giulio Cesare Ferrari, b. 57, fasc. 10. Thanks to Paola Zocchi.

also on etiology. Seen from this perspective, the psychic issue was an answer to the practical and theoretical instances of the new specialist approach of clinical medicine at the end of the 19th century, assuming its experimental aspects. When Morelli arrived in Turin in 1880, he began a great new enterprise: the *Rivista di filosofia scientifica* [Journal of Scientific Philosophy] (Ciocca, 1984). His enterprise was an important event for Italian culture, a sort of showcase for Italian Positivism. Morselli's tenacious attitude allowed the preparation of two volumes per year. Hundreds of authors and collaborators, among the most important representatives of Italian Positivism, were involved. Foreign authors, including Herbert Spencer (1820–1903), Ernst Haeckel (1834–1919), Emil Kraepelin (1856–1926), and Gustav von Bunge (1844–1920), were among the contributors, too.

Morselli had a vision: "the constitution in Italy of a group of scientists and philosophers, independent from every dogma, tradition and authority, free from every idea of school or system, but who all use the positive and experimental method" (Tagliavini, 1986).

The *Review* was an innovative tool to understand the relationship between positive philosophy and science, where, as M.T. Monti observes: "there is a common method in both, as well as contents are concerned, since the scientific problems have an inner dignity as a philosophical problem. From this point of view, there is maybe a naïve optimism in imagining a sort of agreement between scientists and philosophers, but in concrete terms, he suggests scientists to discuss the methodology of scientific research avoiding coarse empiricism, using factual empirical reality, through logic correlations" (Monti, 1983).

Morselli promoted positive science in a confident monistic perspective, and he did so by contributing, as he penned in the presentation for the first number, "with his modest but active part to the diffusion of positivism." His contribution was two-faced: on the one side, his scientific research; on the other side, his effort to re-establish what was needed by empirical and positive science. In other words, the *Review* was the concrete implementation of Morselli's cultural and methodological project, at least for some time (Morselli, 1885). After he left the problematic seat of Turin, the *Review* survived only for a year in Genoa, probably because of the death of the Milanese editor Dumollard, who was instrumental to the organization and the funding of the *Review*. But this was also likely due to Morselli's fatigue, openly admitted in his farewell to the readers, expressed in a "biological" fashion, where growth is followed by flourishing, decline, and death (Morselli, 1891).

Due to the vacancy of the chair of Mental Illnesses at University of Genoa, after the passing of Dario Maragliano who was of the same age and with whom he had shared the experience of the asylum in Reggio Emilia under the direction of Carlo Livi, Enrico Morselli asked to be reassigned to Maragliano's chair in 1889. In November, Morselli began his courses in Genoa where Eugenio Tanzi followed him.

Morselli's stay in Turin was filled by works, monographs, and publishing initiatives. Among them were some articles he wrote after his lectures at the *Reale Accademia di Medicina* of Turin [Royal Medicine Academy] (Garbiglietti, 1872). In what looks like a rather unusual event, Morselli was accepted among the members of the prestigious Turin Academy, first as a corresponding member. This was possible thanks to the introduction of President Garbiglietti, a famous anthropologist. Morselli had sent a memorandum the previous year, *On a rare anomaly of the malar bone*, studying the skulls collected by Gaddi, who was his anatomy professor in Modena (Morselli, 1872), followed by *Some observations on the Sicilian skulls of the Modena museum and on Sicily ethnography* (Morselli, 1873). When he joined Turin, and became a professor of Mental Illnesses Clinical Medicine, his status upgraded to full membership. As a member, he published valuable articles in the *Giornale dell'Accademia di Medicina* [Journal of the Academy of Medicine]. Some are noteworthy, including *Experimental Psychology researches on brain circulation changes due to different simple perceptions*, with the physiologist G. Bordoni Uffreduzzi; *Contribution to the doctrine of systemic primitive madness*, with G. Buccola; and *Circulation and breath modifications during hypnosis* with Tanzi. These are three experimental psychology reports, written when Angelo Mosso and Cesare Lombroso studied these phenomena and published the results in the *Giornale* and *Memorie dell'Accademia delle Scienze di Torino*. These works testify to the climate of intense cooperation among various groups of scientists pursuing common research interests.

REFERENCES

Bargoni A (2008) Il lungo viaggio di Stefano Bonacossa tra i mentecatti d'Europa. In *Atti del Congresso SISM*. Firenze: Tassinari.

Cassata F, & Moraglio M (2005) *Manicomio, società e politica. Storia, memoria e cultura della devianza mentale dal Piemonte all'Italia*. Pisa: Edizioni BFS.

Centro italiano di storia sanitaria e ospedaliera, CISO (2007) *Il Regio Manicomio di Torino. Scienza, prassi e immaginario nell'Ottocento italiano*. Torino: EGA Editore.
Ciocca A (1984) Scienza e filosofia in italia fra '800 e '900 attraverso l'esperienza di Enrico Morselli. *Il Veltro*, 28 (5/6): 669–676.
Garbiglietti A (1872) *Note ed osservazioni anatomico-fisiologiche intorno alla memoria del dott. Enrico Morselli sopra una rara anomalia dell'osso malare: relazione del socio dottore collegiato Antonio Garbiglietti alla R. Accademia di medicina di Torino e letta nelle adunanze delli 19 e 26 luglio 1872*. Torino: V. Vercellino.
Guarnieri P (1986) *Individualità difformi: la psichiatria antropologica di Enrico Morselli*. Milano: Angeli.
Montaldo S, & Novaria P (2011) *Gli archivi della scienza. L'Università di Torino e altri casi italiani*. Milano: Franco Angeli.
Monti M T (1983) Ricerche sul positivismo italiano: filosofia e scienza nella "Rivista di filosofia scientifica." *Rivista Critica di Storia della Filosofia*, 38(4): 409–440.
Moraglio M (2002) *Costruire il manicomio: storia dell'Ospedale psichiatrico di Grugliasco*. Milano: UNICOPLI.
Morselli E (1872) Sopra una rara anomalia dell'osso malare. *Annuario della Società dei naturalisti*, 7(1): 25–32.
Morselli E (1873) *Alcune osservazioni sui crani siciliani del Museo modenese e sull'etnografia della Sicilia*. Firenze: Pellas.
Morselli E (1884) *Introduzione alle lezioni di psicologia patologica e di clinica psichiatrica: letta nella R. Università di Torino addì 17 marzo 1881*. Torino: Loescher.
Morselli E A (1885) La filosofia monistica in Italia. Agli amici e collaboratori della "Rivista di Filosofia scientifica." Pag.1–36 *Rivista di filosofia scientifica* (VI): 9–12.
Morselli E A (1891). Agli abbonati e ai lettori della "Rivista di Filosofia scientifica." *Rivista di filosofia scientifica* (X): 781–784.
Roux O (1910) *Illustri italiani contemporanei* (volume III). Firenze: Bemporad.
Tagliavini A (1986) *L'età del positivismo, a cura di Paolo Rossi*. Bologna: Il Mulino.

CHAPTER 8

Neuroimaging before Neuroimaging

Angelo Mosso's Pioneering Experiments

STEFANO SANDRONE

IMAGING THE BRAIN

The development of neuroimaging techniques, such as computed axial tomography (CAT scanning), functional magnetic resonance imaging (fMRI), and positron emission tomography (PET), has been one of the most important biomedical achievements of the past hundred years. These techniques allowed the *in vivo* visualization of the brain and gave new impetus to medicine, neurology, psychiatry, psychology, philosophy, economics, and related fields by providing two unprecedented types of insight. On the one hand, by yielding structural images of brain anatomy, neuroimaging enabled the detection of pathological abnormalities, and hence constituted a breakthrough in medical diagnosis (Sandrone, 2015; Filippi, 2015; Jhaveri et al., 2021; Bandettini, 2012). On the other hand, besides providing functional insights, neuroimaging can shed light on philosophical questions that are intimately linked to "who we are" and are as old as humankind (Dolan, 2008; Papanicolaou, 2017; Gazzaniga, 2009). Nations worldwide made unprecedented investments in neuroimaging-related research: key projects include the European Human Brain Project (started in 2013, funded with $1.2 billion), the US BRAIN Initiative (2013, $1 billion), and the Japanese Brain/MINDS (2014, $310 million; Costandi, 2016).

Due to its recent prominence in the scientific literature, it would be tempting to infer that science based upon neuroimaging techniques has transpired only over the past decades. Still, the development of brain imaging devices has a history spanning more than a century (Catani & Sandrone, 2015). Nobel Laureate Charles Scott Sherrington is often credited with being the first scientist who investigated the physiological relationship between brain function and blood flow changes in 1890 (Roy & Sherrington, 1890; Kullmann, 2014). This concept is at the heart of the subsequent development of neuroimaging techniques. In their seminal work on the cerebral circulation in animals, Roy and Sherrington (1890) mentioned the "Mosso method" as one of the main techniques for investigating brain blood flow in humans.

In the same year, however, William James, while introducing the concept of brain blood flow variations during mental activities (James, 1890), briefly reported some studies of the Italian physiologist Angelo Mosso, who was defined by the journal *Nature* as "the foremost Italian physiologist of his time and generation" (Anonymous, 1946, p. 689; Sandrone et al., 2012). Remarkably, Mosso's studies were realized before 1890.

FROM THE SCHOOL TO THE *FALEGNAMERIA* (AND BACK)

Angelo Mosso (Figure 8.1) was born on the 31st of May 1846, to Margherita Contessa, a seamstress, and Felice, a carpenter. Mosso was born in Turin, but his modest family was from Chieri, a town approximately 15 kilometers away. Days after his birth, Mosso and his family returned to Chieri, where he spent his childhood and his youth (Foà, 1957).

It is in the city of Chieri that Mosso's father had his *falegnameria* (carpentry shop) and the young Mosso started his educational journey. He did so, however, *in modo non proprio lineare* [in a non-linear fashion], as written in the *Treccani Enciclopedia*: in other words, the young Mosso was *not* a model pupil. Reportedly, his mother had to intercede with the headmaster to have her son readmitted to the school. While not in school, his father put him to work in his own falegnameria (Foà, 1957; Sandrone et al., 2012). Within the carpentry shop, Mosso had the chance to learn how to build a machine piece by piece (Foà, 1957). Although it might sound like something of an exaggeration to contemporary readers, this was the place where Mosso could start acquiring and refining his technical skills. Along with a solid academic education, over time these technical skills became "exceptional," as highlighted by the *Nature* piece published a hundred years after Mosso's birth (Anonymous, 1946, p. 690).

Mosso could attend high schools in Asti and Cuneo, two larger cities in Piedmont, thanks to a few scholarships. But then he failed in securing a scholarship from the "Collegio delle Province," which would have been ideal to continue his studies at the University of Turin without being a burden for the family. Nevertheless, his family's savings and Mosso's earnings as an assistant-teacher of natural sciences at a high school in Chieri allowed him to pay the academic fees and join the university. He graduated *magna cum laude* in medicine in 1870 with a thesis entitled *Saggio di alcune ricerche fatte intorno all'accrescimento delle ossa* [An essay on some research on bone growth] (Mosso, 1870), which was published in Naples in the same year. In the meantime, Mosso also managed to become an intern at the Mauriziano Hospital in Turin.

Perhaps Mosso's original plan was to work as an assistant to Jacob Moleschott, who was the Chair of Physiology in Turin. Mosso's exposure to Moleschott's ideas was perhaps also due to Luigi Pagliani, his former flatmate, who was working at Mauriziano Hospital (Nani, 2012; Losano & Pinotti, 2000). Leverage obligations, however, forced Mosso to become a medical officer and work as a military officer

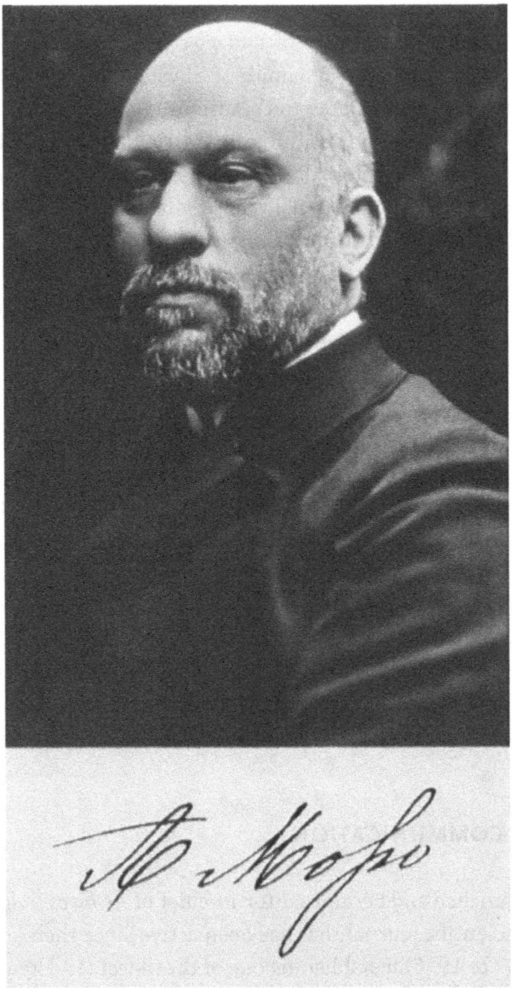

Figure 8.1. Portrait and signature of Angelo Mosso. Courtesy of Marco Galloni.

(*medico di battaglione*), and he was sent to Calabria, Campania, and Sicily. Pagliani, who was one year younger than Mosso, was appointed as an assistant at the Physiology Laboratory directed by Moleschott in 1871.

LEARNING FROM THE MASTERS

In the same year, following Moleschott's advice (and with his recommendation), Mosso moved to Florence and entered the physiology laboratory directed by Moritz Schiff. In Florence, Mosso studied the mechanics of esophageal contraction for two years. Within Schiff's laboratory, Mosso met Giulio Ceradini, a physician who had performed research with Hermann von Helmholtz in Heidelberg and Carl Ludwig in Leipzig (Foà, 1957). Perhaps inspired by Ceradini's experience, in 1874 Mosso decided to go to Leipzig and be part of Ludwig's laboratory. There, he learned the "graphical method" to study the dynamics of physiological phenomena, especially the physiology of visual mechanisms and emotions (Nani, 2012). While in Germany, Mosso was offered two academic positions, one in Heidelberg and one in Kiel, but he preferred to return to Turin. Before doing so, Mosso visited the laboratory of Claude Bernard and Étienne-Jules Marey in Paris, where he met Jean-Martin Charcot, Charles-Édouard Brown-Séquard, and Louis-Antoine Ranvier.

It is difficult to grasp the breadth and depth of the works that Mosso realized during (and after) his European tour. But there is a striking common denominator: the focus on graphical methods to analyze physiological dynamics. Once back in Turin, Mosso continued applying the graphical method to the circulation in the human brain (Sandrone et al., 2012). In the course of time, in chronological order, Mosso started to teach pharmacology (or, as it was called at that time, *materia medica*) in 1875, and he was appointed as a *Professore Straordinario* in 1876. He then became the Chair of Physiology and the Director of the Institute in 1879. He succeeded Moleschott, who was nominated Senator three years before and obtained the academic position of Professor of Physiology at the University of Rome. Finally, Mosso was also awarded the Royal Prize by the *Accademia dei Lincei* for his studies on human brain circulation. The prize motivation was written by Hermann von Helmholz and delivered to Mosso by Quintino Sella, former Minister of Finances, alpinist, and President of the Accademia itself, which Mosso joined as a member (*socio nazionale*) in 1882.

SCIENCE PLUS COMMUNICATION

In 1882 Mosso launched and became editor-in-chief of *Archives Italiennes de Biologie*, a peer-reviewed scientific journal that has been active since then (and was only suspended from 1937 to 1956). Establishing one of the oldest (and longest lasting) neuroscience journals worldwide was a rather modern move. But Mosso's modernity was not limited to this: he decided to write popular science books. In fact, in the 1880s Mosso began a collaboration with the publishing house of *Fratelli Treves*, with whom he published the monograph titled *La Paura* [Fear] (Mosso, 1883). He quickly became a prolific writer and continued writing science books for a general audience. Among them were *Una ascensione d'inverno al Monte Rosa* (1885), wherein he described a climb with the son of Quintino Sella, and the monograph titled *La Fatica* [Fatigue] in 1891. Beyond books, Mosso linked his name to the Treves family by marrying Maria Treves, who gave birth to Emilio (1886), Laura (1889), and Emilia/Mimì (1890). Only Mimì escaped from death at a young age. Two years after Mimì's birth, Mosso delivered the *Croonian lecture* (Oliver, 1896), printed with the title of *Les phénomènes psychiques et la température du cerveau*, on the same theme as his book *La temperatura del cervello* (1894; Nani, 2012).

Mosso's research activity was characterized by eclectic interests ranging from anatomy and physiology to experimental psychology, psychiatry, neuroscience, social and occupational medicine, and archeology. Beyond his contributions to neuroscience, which will be discussed in the next paragraphs, his name also is attached to the many instruments he invented and/or refined. Among others, these included the plethysmograph and the pneumograph, but also the ergograph, which was used to quantify the optimum strength of muscle contraction before the appearance of muscular fatigue, and a sphygmomanometer to measure pulse volume (Sandrone et al., 2012). He also improved "moving carpets (. . .), dummy rowing machines (. . .); rubber tents and iron rooms for reproducing the air rarefactions of the highest mountains, machines to imitate the winds of the Alps" (Foà, 1957, p. 557).

NEW ENVIRONMENTS

Mosso created new research environments, literally and figuratively. He founded the Institute of Physiology close to the Parco del Valentino, a public park along the banks of the Po River. He established the first (and, *bona fide*, even the second) physiology laboratory in altitude by funding the "Regina Margherita Hut," 4,554 meters above sea level, which was opened in the presence of the Queen Margherita of Savoy, as well as the Institute at the Col d'Olen, 2,901 meters above sea level, known as "Istituto Angelo Mosso." In these places Mosso pursued his broad research interests, sometimes with his former flatmate Pagliani. Among the topics explored were the study of breathing (Mosso, 1878; Mosso, 1884a), the physical laws of human muscular fatigue (Mosso, 1891, but see also Giulio et al., 2006; and Di Giulio & West, 2013), the analysis of behavioral reactions, the modifications of sleep architecture in monkeys at high altitude, and some remedies for mountain sickness (Mosso, 1898, 1909). These endeavors made him a forerunner of aeronautical and space medicine (Various Authors, 1912). Mosso studied the diastolic activity of the heart, blood, arterial pressure, temperature of the brain, and the function of the bladder (Foà, 1957). He conducted experiments with silkworms, pigeons, and dogs and studied asphyxiation among railway workers (Nani, 2012; Mosso, 1900).

SPORTS AND ARCHEOLOGY

Mosso was keen on sustaining the health of workers and on promoting physical activity, even on counteracting "negative effects" of urbanization and industrial work (Nani, 2012). Interestingly, his old flatmate Pagliani also played a key role in Italian public health: he held the first Chair of Hygiene established in Italy (1878) and played a leading role at the newly founded "Directorate General of Health" (1886). Both Mosso and Pagliani championed the importance of physical education within the Italian school system, which is a commitment that Mosso also continued as a Senator.

But Mosso's impact went well beyond the bricks and mortar of the elementary school. He promoted the importance of sports activity within and outside school also through congresses, committees, and popular books. In 1896, Mosso became

President of the *Reale Società Ginnastica di Torino*, which was also represented by a football team. Notably, this football team is one of the oldest Italian football teams ever, and one of the four teams that played in the first Italian Serie A Football League. This competition took place within a national congress of physical education organized by Mosso himself in Turin in 1898 (Sandrone et al., 2012). The following year, Mosso visited the United States for a series of academic lectures (Dearborn, 1900) and recollected this experience in the book titled *La democrazia nella religione e nella scienza: studi sull'America* [Democracy in religion and science. Studies on America] (Mosso, 1908). He was also nominated rector of the University of Turin, albeit just for a brief period.

Mosso's health was deteriorating due to the consequences of syphilis. In an attempt to improve his health, Mosso left the Chair in Turin and moved to Rome, where he was nominated as a Senator in 1904 (Nani, 2012) and could benefit from a milder climate. In Rome, he met Giacomo Boni (Foà, 1957), a Venetian-born archeologist who directed the excavation in both *Foro Romano* (Roman Forum) and *Palatino* (Palatine Hill). Thanks to Boni, Mosso met Duncan Mackenzie, Scottish archeologist and assistant to Sir Arthur Evans during the discovery of Crete's palace of Knossos (Foà, 1957). As Mosso's health was further deteriorating, the physicians advised him to spend more time outdoors. Mosso joined the Italian archeological expedition in Crete and then in Apulia and Sicily. At these sites, he could apply his systematic attitude to archeology, a field of investigation he considered insufficiently scientific (Sandrone et al., 2012). He even published peer-reviewed papers on archeology and wrote articles on archeology for a general audience (Nani, 2012). Mosso died in 1910, aged 64. His grave is not too far from those of Luigi Rolando and Cesare Lombroso in the Monumental Cemetery in Turin. According to *Nature*'s obituary, Mosso's school can be considered a "physiological Mecca" (Anonymous, 1946, p. 690) as he trained some of the most influential Italian researchers, including Vittorio Aducco, Aldo Fano, Amedeo Herlitzka, and Mariano Luigi Patrizi (Anonymous, 1946).

NEUROSCIENCE STUDIES BEFORE THE BALANCE

It would be extremely difficult, and perhaps useless, to list and categorize every scientific contribution, given the wide range of his research interest and the numerous instruments Mosso invented and refined. But we can identify three neuroscience subdomains, which are not independent, yet logically concatenated.

Cerebral Temperature

Mosso's interest in the brain probably started with the study of brain temperature, although one of the key works was not published until 1894 (Mosso, 1894). Although the nexus between studying the functional capacity of the brain and measuring its temperature may be elusive at first, this research interest was in line with the scientific climate of the 19th century. At that time, the dominant view was that all forms of movement and activity produce a certain amount of heat. By applying this cause-effect principle to the neuroscientific domain, the underlying hypothesis was that blood supply following mental activity might also reflect an increment in temperature within the brain (Zago et al., 2009). It was, therefore, not unusual for scientists to place thermometers on the scalp, or even in direct contact with the cerebral cortex, to quantify regional changes in temperature; they were often doing so after the administration of pharmacological substances or during mental tasks (Zago et al., 2009; Broca, 1879; Lombard, 1879; Mosso, 1894; Berger, 1901).

The "Mosso Method"

In parallel, to explore the link between blood flow and brain activity, Mosso applied the graphical method he had learned and developed between Florence and the European tour. By doing so, he defined the "Mosso method." The experiments conducted with the "Mosso method" started more than a decade before 1890, which is the year that saw the publication of the widely cited report authored by Roy and Sherrington.

Mosso measured changes in cerebral blood flow in patients by recording brain pulsations, a phenomenon typically observed in the fontanelles of newborns, with the use of a special plethysmograph (Mosso, 1880; Sandrone et al., 2012). A plethysmograph is a tool used to quantify the sphygmic graph amplitude, which is the blood volume pulse following contraction of the heart. By positioning a portion of the plethysmograph in the skin graft, the pulsations of the cerebral blood flow could be observed. Mosso applied his method to patients with skull openings to investigate cerebral blood flow changes during cognitive and emotional tasks (Zago et al., 2009).

Among the first experimental subjects were Caterina X, a 37-year-old peasant who was dying from an infection due to syphilis (Giacomini & Mosso, 1876), and Giovanni Thron, an 11-year-old boy. While Caterina X had lesions of the frontal bone and in the parietal lobes (Giacomini & Mosso, 1876; Albertotti & Mosso, 1878; Zago et al., 2009), Giovanni had temporoparietal damage (Albertotti & Mosso, 1878). Mosso and his collaborator Giacomini applied the plethysmograph to various body parts including arms, feet, and brain (Mosso, 1875; 1876; 1880) to detect the cerebral pulse (namely, cerebral pulsations). Brain pulsations increased when Caterina woke up and when Giovanni was called by his name, even if asleep (Albertotti & Mosso, 1878; Zago et al., 2009).

But it was the third patient, the 37-year-old farmer Michele Bertino, who allowed Mosso to investigate deeply the relationship between brain circulation and brain activity (Mosso, 1880). Bertino had a skull breach of two centimeters in the right frontal region, which proved to be an ideal type of cranial lesion for Mosso's studies (Zago et al., 2009). Brain pulsations were recorded when Bertino was requested to multiply 8 × 12; when the clock of the local church bell struck 12 and the chiming could be heard; and when, subsequently, Mosso asked Bertino if the midday prayers (including the Ave Maria) should have been said. An increase in brain pulsation was recorded in all three tasks; a task-related change in brain blood volume, independent from respiratory changes, occurred. Mosso even documented the "resting state"; as a reference, forearm pulsation was recorded. The emotional state was investigated in a fourth patient called Luigi Cane, a 45-year-old construction worker whose head was hit by a brick that damaged the right parietal-occipital region (Mosso, 1894). First, Mosso replicated with Luigi a mathematical task already done with Bertino (still a multiplication, but in this case 21 × 13). Then, he asked Luigi to think about the emotion he felt the first time he saw his future wife: in both cases, the plethysmograph recorded an increased brain pulsation.

This method allowed Mosso to record local increase in blood flow during tasks of various nature in patients with skull defects. William James stated that these works constituted "the best proof of the immediate afflux of blood to the brain during mental activity" (James, 1890). However, the "Mosso method" had some limitations: it was invasive and could only be applied to subjects with skull defects.

THE "HUMAN CIRCULATION BALANCE"

Mosso trained in Paris with Claude Bernard, the "primer of the second biomedical revolution" (Conti, 2001, p. 703). Bernard planned to explore the physiology of mind and brain, but did not have the proper technology to do so, and he died before Mosso's physiological tools reached fruition. Sherrington was familiar with Mosso's work; he, however, refers only to *some* of Mosso's works in his paper (the reasons behind the oversight of much of his work are still unknown). In his *Principles of Psychology* (1890), James mentioned some of Mosso's recordings of brain pulsations performed in patients with skull breaches (see also Raichle & Shepherd, 2014). In the process, James only briefly referred to another invention of Mosso, the "human circulation balance," whose precise workings and experiments remained largely unknown until I published a paper in 2014 (Sandrone et al., 2014), where a detailed description of the balance can be found.

In the words of William James, this was a "delicately balanced table which could tip downward either at the head or the foot if the weight of either end were increased" (James, 1890). This device could measure the redistribution of blood during emotional and intellectual activity in healthy participants. Breathing, via a pneumatic pneumography, and changes in the volume of feet and hands, via a hydraulic plethysmograph, were co-recorded (Sandrone et al., 2014; Figure 8.2). Mosso studied the circulation of the blood in the human brain with (and without) this balance in several works (Mosso, 1880; 1881; 1882; 1884b). Moreover, there are also indirect accounts from his daughter Mimì (Mosso, 1935). The balance overcame the limitations mentioned above, as it could be used noninvasively on healthy subjects (Mosso, 1884b; Sandrone et al., 2014).

By positioning subjects in equilibrium, with small regular waves due to respiration, Mosso demonstrated that the increase in cerebral blood flow was proportional to the complexity of the task. For example, a simple auditory stimulus prompted the balance to tilt toward the head-side of the participant (Sandrone et al., 2014). But when stimuli of increasing cognitive complexity were used, such as a page from a newspaper or one written in an abstruse language, "the balance tilted faster towards

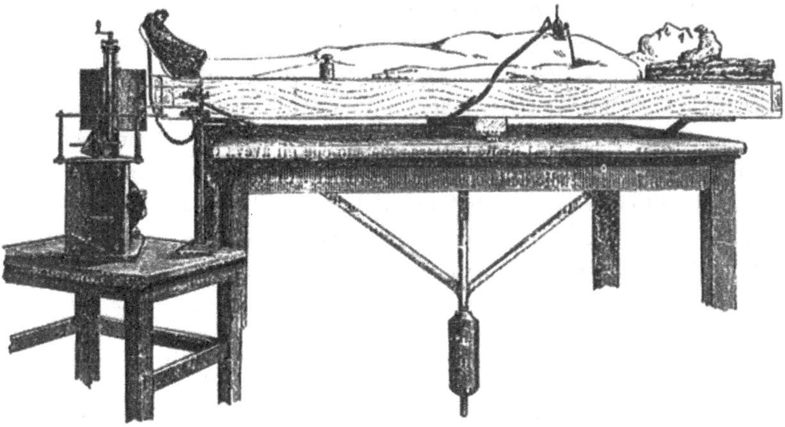

Figure 8.2. Human circulation balance used to measure cerebral activity during resting and cognitive states. Angelo Mosso's original drawing. Credits and source: adapted from Mosso, 1884, Atti della Reale Accademia dei Lincei—Memorie della Classe di Scienze Fisiche, Matematiche e Naturali XIX:534. Thanks to the Accademia dei Lincei for the opportunity to reproduce the figure in this book.

the head side when the subject was reading a page written in an abstruse language or belonging to a manual than it did when the subject was reading a newspaper or a novel" (Sandrone et al., 2014, p. 626, after Mosso, 1935). The same happened with "emotional" stimuli: when Mosso's brother read a letter written by his spouse and when the student read a letter from an upset creditor, "the balance fell all at once" (Sandrone et al., 2014, p. 626, after Mosso, 1935).

Mosso's approach was innovative with regard to the tool used and the number of variables taken into account, which are still extremely relevant in contemporary neuroimaging (Sandrone et al., 2014). In the design of neuroimaging experiments, Mosso's procedures were not too different from the ones of many neuroscientists across the world today. For example, students (and colleagues) were often the subjects of his experiments; this might have introduced a sampling bias, which still affects psychology and neuroscience nowadays (Nielsen et al., 2017; Henrich et al., 2010; Seixas & Basto, 2009; Chiao & Cheon, 2010). Personal comfort for the participants was important for Mosso and it is essential nowadays, with the double aim of avoiding artifacts and creating an ecological set-up that was as close to normal as possible (Mosso, 1884b). The importance of a resting state before recording was not unknown to him either: participants sometimes spent more than one hour on the balance before the experiment took place. While analyzing results, Mosso took into account demographic aspects, including age and education, in a way that resembles today's covariates in neuroimaging data analyses, and he acknowledged individual differences in reacting to different tasks. The paradigms used by Mosso included a baseline/resting segment and revolved around an experimental manipulation where stimuli were matched, while differing in complexity. This builds on a tradition that includes works by Franciscus Cornelius Donders (Donders, 1868; 1969) and is still used to study the neural correlates of specific tasks. In addition to this, Mosso's attention for the signal-to-noise ratio, which is a central topic in contemporary neuroimaging, was remarkable: he minimized artifacts damaging the quality of the recording and removed confounding factors. Mosso's investigations even fueled unsustainable claims. In 1908, a French newspaper reported that numerous people believed that Mosso's devices "would soon fully explain the physiology of the human brain" and lead to new treatments for neurological and mental illnesses (Sandrone et al., 2014, p. 626). A century later, newspapers and social networks are still occasionally packed with misinterpretations, hopes, and hype.

THE BALANCE AFTER MOSSO

We cannot directly prove that the balance could *factually* quantify task-related alterations of cerebral blood flow. A definitive piece of evidence linking increases in blood flow to a detectable increase in brain weight is lacking, and the same is true for the relationship between global and regional blood flow changes and blood volumes in the brain (Krieger et al., 2012; Sandrone et al., 2014). Furthermore, the precise anatomo-functional details of the neurovascular coupling are still elusive (Logothetis, 2008; Iadecola et al., 2017; Drew, 2019; Bright et al., 2020). Despite these limitations, which are still affecting contemporary neuroimaging studies, Mosso's balance can be considered the first *ante litteram* noninvasive "neuroimaging" technique and the conceptual forerunner of neuroimaging (Sandrone et al., 2014; Sandrone et al., 2012).

A modified version of Mosso's balance has been rebuilt at least twice in the last century. In both instances, this happened in the United Kingdom: in 1935 at King's College London and at the University of Reading in 2014. The former failed to confirm Mosso's experiment (Lowe, 1936). A key reason behind this might be the limited knowledge of the details of the original balance and of the experimental paradigms, given the difficult accessibility of the original text, which was written in Italian. But the latest replication, realized after the publication of the 2014 *Brain* paper I authored, which provided an English translation of some of the experiments, was successful. Mosso's balance proved to be "capable of detecting small changes in cerebral blood volume associated with variation in the amount of neural activity taking place in the brain" (Field & Inman, 2014, p. 639). Dimitri Kullmann, editor of *Brain*, commented that "sensory stimulation can indeed lead to a shift in the centre of gravity towards the head," although "some unexpected spontaneous low-frequency oscillations" occurred (Kullmann, 2014, p. 307).

Despite Mosso's and Sherrington's promising reports, research on the relationship between cerebral activity and blood flow ceased *ex abrupto* in 1896. This was mainly due to the influence of Leonard Hill, a member of the Royal College of Surgeons in England, who claimed that no relationship existed between cerebral function and cerebral circulation (Hill, 1896). His ex-cathedra statement remained almost unchallenged for more than three decades, until a *Brain* paper by the American neurophysiologist John Farquhar Fulton on the "vascularity of the human occipital lobe during visual activity" was published (Fulton, 1928). Some years later, the American neuroscientist Seymour Kety and colleagues studied the effect of mental arithmetic on cerebral circulation and metabolism (Kety & Schmidt 1948; Sokoloff et al., 1955). Mosso's name was not included in Fulton nor in Kety's reference lists, but it is about time to recognize Angelo Mosso as a pioneer in the history of neuroimaging.

REFERENCES

Albertotti G, & Mosso A (1878) Osservazioni sui movimenti del cervello di un idiota epilettico. *Giornale della Reale Accademia di Medicina di Torino*, 18: 47–60.

Anonymous (1946) Prof. Angelo Mosso (1846–1910). *Nature*, 157: 689–690.

Bandettini P A (2012) Twenty years of functional MRI: The science and the stories. *Neuroimage*, 62(2): 575–588.

Berger H (1901) *Zur Lehre von der Blutzirkulation in der Schädelhöhle des Menschen namentlich unter dem Einfluss von Medikamenten: Experimentelle Untersuchungen*. Jena, Germany: Gustav Fischer.

Bright M G, Whittaker J R, Driver I D, & Murphy K (2020) Vascular physiology drives functional brain networks. *Neuroimage*, 217: 116907.

Broca P (1879) Sur les températures morbides locales. *Bulletin de L'Académie Nationale de Médecine*, 8: 1331–1347.

Catani M, & Sandrone S (2015) *Brain Renaissance: From Vesalius to Modern Neuroscience*. New York, NY: Oxford University Press.

Chiao J Y, & Cheon B K (2010) The weirdest brains in the world? *Behavioral and Brain Sciences*, 33(2–3): 88–90.

Conti F (2001) Claude Bernard: Primer of the second biomedical revolution. *Nature Reviews Molecular Cell Biology*, 2(9): 703–8.

Costandi M (2016) *Creating a Perfect Brain Storm*. Los Angeles, CA: The Kavli Foundation.

Dearborn G V (1900) Professor Mosso's lectures at the Clark University Decennial. *Science*, 12(295): 312–313.

Di Giulio C, & West J B (2013) Angelo Mosso's experiments at very low barometric pressures. *High Altitude Medicine & Biology*, 14(1): 78–79.

Dolan R J (2008) Neuroimaging of cognition: Past, present, and future. *Neuron*, 60(3): 496–502.

Donders F C (1868) Die *Schnelligkeit psychischer Prozesse. Archiv für Anatomie, Physiologie und Wissenschaftliche Medicin*, 6: 657–681.

Donders F C (1969) On the speed of mental processes. *Acta Psychologica*, 30: 412–431.

Drew P J (2019) Vascular and neural basis of the BOLD signal. *Current Opinion in Neurobiology*, 58: 61–69.

Field D T, & Inman L A (2014) Weighing brain activity with the balance: A contemporary replication of Angelo Mosso's historical experiment. *Brain*, 137(2): 634–639.

Filippi M Ed. (2015) *Oxford Textbook of Neuroimaging*. New York, NY: Oxford University Press.

Foà C (1957) Angelo Mosso. *Scientia Medica Italica*, 5(4): 549–67.

Fulton J F (1928) Observations upon the vascularity of the human occipital lobe during visual activity. *Brain*, 51(3): 310–320.

Gazzaniga M S Ed. (2009) *The Cognitive Neurosciences*. Cambridge, MA: The MIT Press.

Giacomini C, & Mosso A (1876) Esperienze sui movimenti del cervello nell'uomo. *Archivio per le Scienze Mediche*, 1: 245–278

Giulio C D, Daniele F, & Tipton C M (2006) Angelo Mosso and muscular fatigue: 116 years after the first Congress of Physiologists: IUPS commemoration. *Advances in Physiology Education*, 30(2): 51–57.

Henrich J, Heine S J, & Norenzayan A (2010) The weirdest people in the world? *Behavioral Brain Science*, 33(2–3): 61–83.
Hill L (1896) *The Physiology and Pathology of the Cerebral Circulation. An Experimental Research*. London, UK: J & A Churchill.
Iadecola C (2017) The neurovascular unit coming of age: a journey through neurovascular coupling in health and disease. *Neuron*, 96(1): 17–42.
James W (1890) *The Principles of Psychology*. New York, NY: Henry Holt & Company.
Jhaveri M D, Salzman K L, Osborn A G, Vattoth, S, & Gaddikeri, S Eds. (2021) *Diagnostic Imaging: Brain*. Salt Lake City, UT: Elsevier.
Kety S S, & Schmidt C F (1948) The nitrous oxide method for the quantitative determination of cerebral blood flow in man: Theory, procedure and normal values. *Journal of Clinical Investigation*, 27(4): 476–483.
Krieger S N, Streicher M N, Trampel R, & Turner R (2012) Cerebral blood volume changes during brain activation. *Journal of Cerebral Blood Flow & Metabolism*, 32(8): 1618–1631.
Kullmann D (2014) Brain. Editorial. *Brain*, 137(Pt 2): 307.
Logothetis N K (2008) What we can do and what we cannot do with fMRI. *Nature*, 453(7197): 869–878.
Lombard J S (1879) *Experimental Researches on the Regional Temperature of the Head: Under Conditions of Rest, Intellectual Activity, and Emotion*. London, UK: HK Lewis.
Losano G, & Pinotti O (2000) Physiology at the University of Turin from the unification of Italy to the end of the twentieth century. *Vesalius*, 6(2): 114–119.
Lowe M F (1936) The application of the balance to the study of the bodily changes occurring during periods of volitional activity. *British Journal of Psychology. General Section*, 26(3): 245–262.
Mosso A (1870) *Saggio di alcune ricerche fatte intorno all'accrescimento delle ossa*. Neaples, Italy: Tesi di Laurea.
Mosso A (1875) Sopra un nuovo metodo per scrivere i movimenti dei vasi sanguini dell'uomo. *Atti della Reale Accademia delle Scienze di Torino*, 11: 21–81.
Mosso A (1876) Introduzione ad una serie di esperienze sui movimenti del cervello nell'uomo. *Archivio per le Scienze Mediche*, 1: 216–244.
Mosso A (1878) Sul polso negativo e sui rapporti della respirazione addominale et toracica nell'uomo. *Archivio per le Scienze Mediche*, 2: 401–464.
Mosso A (1880) Sulla circolazione del sangue nel cervello dell'uomo. *Atti della Accademia Nazionale dei Lincei, Classe di Scienze Fisiche, Matematiche e Naturali* III: 237–358.
Mosso A (1881) *Concerning the Circulation of the Blood in the Human Brain*. Leipzig, Germany: Verlag von Viet & Company.
Mosso A (1882) Applicazione della bilancia allo studio della circolazione del sangue nell'uomo. *Atti della Reale Accademia delle Scienze di Torino* XVII: 534–535.
Mosso A (1883) *La Paura*. Milan, Italy: Fratelli Treves.
Mosso A (1884a) *La respirazione dell'uomo sulle alte montagne*. Turin, Italy: Celanza e Comp.
Mosso A (1884b) Applicazione della bilancia allo studio della circolazione sanguigna dell'uomo. *Atti della Accademia Nazionale dei Lincei, Classe di Scienze Fisiche, Matematiche e Naturali* XIX: 531–543.
Mosso A (1885) *Una ascensione d'inverno al monte Rosa (13 a 15 febbraio 1885)*. Milan, Italy: Fratelli Treves.
Mosso A (1891) *La Fatica*. Milan, Italy: Fratelli Treves.
Mosso A (1894) *La temperatura del cervello: studi termometrici*. Milan, Italy: Fratelli Treves.
Mosso A (1898) *Fisiologia dell'uomo sulle Alpi: studii fatti sul Monte Rosa*. Milan, Italy: Fratelli Treves.
Mosso A (1900) *La respirazione nelle gallerie e l'azione dell'ossido di carbonio: Analisi e studi fatti per incarico del Ministero dei lavori pubblici nelle gallerie dei Giovi (ferrovie Genova-Novi) e nell'Istituto fisiologico di Torino*. Milan, Italy: Fratelli Treves.
Mosso A (1908) *La democrazia nella religione e nella scienza: studi sull'America*. Milan, Italy: Fratelli Treves.
Mosso A (1909) *L'uomo sulle Alpi: Studi fatti sul Monte Rosa*. Milan, Italy: Fratelli Treves.

Mosso M (1935) *Un cercatore d'ignoto*. Milan, Italy: Baldini & Castoldi.
Nani M (2012) Mosso, Angelo. *Dizionario Biografico degli Italiani*. Volume 77. Rome, Italy: Istituto dell'Enciclopedia italiana.
Nielsen M, Haun D, Kärtner J, & Legare C H (2017) The persistent sampling bias in developmental psychology: A call to action. *Journal of Experimental Child Psychology*, 162: 31–38.
Oliver G (1896) The Croonian lectures: A contribution to the study of the blood and the circulation: Delivered before the Royal College of Physicians of London. *British Medical Journal*, 1(1850): 1433–1437.
Papanicolaou A C Ed. (2017) *The Oxford Handbook of Functional Brain Imaging in Neuropsychology and Cognitive Neurosciences*. New York, NY: Oxford University Press.
Raichle M E, & Shepherd G M Eds. (2014) *Angelo Mosso's Circulation of Blood in the Human Brain*. New York, NY: Oxford University Press.
Roy C S, & Sherrington C S (1890) On the regulation of the blood supply of the brain. *Journal of Physiology*, 11(1–2): 85–108.
Sandrone S, Bacigaluppi M, Galloni M R, & Martino G (2012) Angelo Mosso (1846–1910). *Journal of Neurology*, 259(11): 2513–2514.
Sandrone S, Bacigaluppi M, Galloni M R, Cappa S F, Moro A, Catani M, Filippi M, Monti M M, Perani D, & Martino G (2014) Weighing brain activity with the balance: Angelo Mosso's original manuscripts come to light. *Brain*, 137(Pt 2): 621–633.
Sandrone S (2015) The resting human brain and the predictive potential of Default Mode Network. In S Standring (Ed.), *Gray's Anatomy* (41st edition), Chapter 3.1. London, UK: Elsevier.
Seixas D, & Basto M A (2009) Neuroimaging: Just a collection of brain image files? *Frontiers in Human Neuroscience*, 3: 47.
Sokoloff L, Mangold R, Wechsler R L, Kenney C, & Kety S S (1955) The effect of mental arithmetic on cerebral circulation and metabolism. *Journal of Clinical Investigation*, 34(7, Part 1): 1101–1108.
Various Authors (1912) *Angelo Mosso, la sua vita e le sue opere. In memoriam*. Milan, Italy: Fratelli Treves.
Zago S, Ferrucci R, Marceglia S, & Priori A (2009) The Mosso method for recording brain pulsation: The forerunner of functional neuroimaging. *Neuroimage*, 48(4): 652–626.

CHAPTER 9

The Role of Federico Kiesow in the Development of Experimental Psychology in Europe

STEFANO ZAGO AND LORENZO LORUSSO

For several centuries, psychological questions had been an object of study in philosophy and metaphysics. Only in the 19th century did attempts to analyze psychological issues and try to quantitatively measure them arise. This led to the investigation of psychological aspects in the light of biological knowledge, (i.e., the organization of the nervous system and mental pathology), which made psychology an independent discipline (Mandler, 2011). Europe was at the center of this transformation: It is in Europe that the first laboratories emerged along with the figure of the experimental psychologist, which differed from that of a philosopher (Benjamin, 2000). The birth of psychology as a separate science can be dated back to 1879, when Wilhelm Wundt (1832–1920), opened his Psychological Institute at the University of Leipzig in Germany (Harper, 1950).

At the turn of the 20th century, there was a debate around the foundation of scientific psychology in Italy. This debate included physiologists, neuropsychiatrists, anthropologists, criminologists, and biologists, all of whom were influenced by a positivistic culture (Bongiorno, 2006). They were interested in, or even started to provide data toward, the first experiments on the mind-brain relationship, already pioneered in Germany by Wundt (Sinatra & Monacis, 2010). The Turin scientific environment was one of the first Italian places to welcome these changes, especially the presence of eminent figures from outside Italy, such as the Polish-German experimentalist, but naturalized Italian, Frederick (Federico) Kiesow (1858–1940; Figure 9.1, left). Kiesow trained at the Wundt Institute in Leipzig as an assistant, and then joined the laboratory of the physiologist Angelo Mosso (1846–1910) in Turin, where he established the first Italian psychology laboratory. In 1906, Kiesow founded the Institute of Experimental Psychology, which he directed from 1906 to 1933, and where he remained until his death in 1940. Under his enthusiastic leadership, the

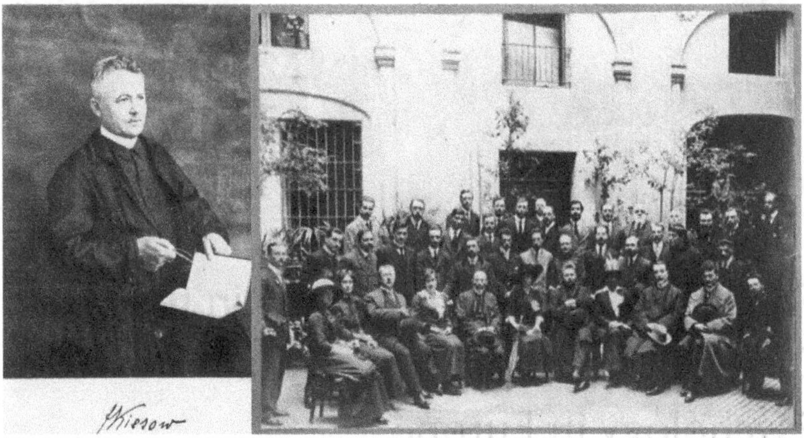

Figure 9.1. Left: Portrait and signature of Federico Kiesow. Kiesow (the fifth seated from the right) at a meeting around 1910s.

Institute acquired a worldwide reputation as a center of experimental psychological research (Ponzo, 1940, 1941, 1942).

Kiesow is a pioneer of experimental psychology in Italy and Europe. He was among the first to hold a chair of Psychology in Italy and further developed Wundt's psychology. With his students, he performed innovative investigations on blood pressure and pulse, taste sensitivity, thermic and tactile points, pain sensations, as well as on geometrical-optical illusions and reaction times, all based on the application of experimental methodology (Kiesow, 1930, 1932). Until at least the 1930s, Kiesow's "Wundtism" shaped the training of the Turin school. He continued to advocate for psychology as a separate and independent discipline from philosophy. His works on psychophysics and psychophysiology gained visibility in Europe from an epistemological point of view, sharing the principle of psychophysical parallelism by enhancing the aspect of "voluntary subjectivism." He studied the "internal" psychic phenomena, those that can be examined together with "environmental" physical-physiological phenomena.

But Kiesow was also influential in the publishing field. He not only translated psychology texts and manuals in German, but he also strengthened international relations with the most renowned European laboratories. Kiesow achieved international accolades for his contributions and even succeeded in the adoption of Italian as the official language for some congresses, including one that took place at Yale University in 1929. He founded the *Archivio Italiano di Psicologia* [Italian Archive of Psychology] in 1919 in collaboration with Agostino Gemelli. After Gemelli had established the *Università del Sacro Cuore* in Milan in 1921, Kiesow became the sole editor of the publication in 1922. In the journal, Kiesow reiterated the concept of causal analysis to explain complex psychic phenomena starting from their ultimate elements. Research on eidetic phenomena can be traced back to this same period, and it was characterized by mnestic traces so vivid as to assume the characteristics of perception and be similar to visual images.

Scientific publishing was flourishing: In the late 19th century, anthropology and biology journals, with several articles on psychology, began to appear in Turin. Among them was the bimonthly *Archivio di Psichiatria, Antropologia Animale e Scienze Criminali* [Archive of Psychiatry, Animal Anthropology and Criminal Sciences], founded in 1880 by Cesare Lombroso (1835–1909), who had published several works on psychology; the *Giornale di Filosofia Scientifica* [Journal of Scientific Philosophy], founded in Turin by Enrico Morselli (1852–1929) in 1881, which contributed to diffusing the evolutionism in Italy thanks to the contributions of Giovanni Canestrini and Filippo De Filippi; and the *Archives Italiennes de Biologie* [Italian Archives of Biology] a periodical founded and directed by Mosso based in Turin (1892–1935), which is still published today.

BIOGRAPHICAL NOTES

Federico Kiesow (Figure 9.1) was born on the 28th of March 1858 in Bruel in Mecklenburg-Schwein, Poland. Due to family economic difficulties and health problems, Kiesow had to work as a private instructor for two noble families. He managed to complete his studies, but he then realized that the development of a pedagogical program was not possible without an in-depth knowledge of psychology. In 1879, he heard of the first psychology laboratory established by Wilhelm Wundt (1832–1920) in Leipzig and, in 1891, he was invited by Wundt to attend courses there. Wundt appreciated the contribution of the new student, and the following year he appointed Kiesow as a voluntary assistant. For his thesis in Philosophy in Leipzig, he developed original techniques to investigate the topographical distribution of taste sensitivity, which are described in the following paragraphs. The thesis was immediately published in the *Philosophische Studien* [Philosophical Studies] (Kiesow, 1894), and, in extended form, in 1896 (Kiesow, 1896). Wundt let Kiesow go to Turin so that he could be exposed to the new graphical methods. In Turin, Kiesow learned how to use the plethysmograph, the ergograph, and the sphygmomanometer, developed in 1876 by the French physiologist Étienne-Jules Marey (1830–1904) and modified, in 1894, by Luigi Corino in Turin. Corino was a technician at the laboratory of the physiologist Angelo Mosso, who later worked on setting up the tools for the Kiesow Psychology Institute (Corallini Vittori, 2006). Mosso obtained the Chair of Physiology in 1879 at the University of Turin, previously occupied by the Dutchman, Jacob Moleschott (1822–1893), who was also a naturalized Italian scientist.

As we have seen in the previous chapter, Angelo Mosso used the sphygmomanometer and the ergograph to record the work of a single muscle, and the plethysmograph in various body parts including arms, feet, and brain (Mosso, 1880; Zago, Ferrucci, Marceglia, & Priori, 2009). Back to Leipzig, together with his fiancée Emma Lough (1871–1951), Kiesow translated Mosso's book, *La paura* [Fear] with Emma Lough (Lough & Kiesow, 1896) and used the sphygmomanometer in various psychophysiological conditions, thus reinforcing Wund's idea of the three-dimensional theory of sentimental states. According to Wundt, these states were based on what constituted the elementary parts of emotions: pleasure/displeasure, tension/relaxation, and excitement/calm.

Upon Mosso's invitation in 1896, Kiesow was appointed as a second assistant and then assistant at the Institute of Physiology of the Faculty of Medicine of the University of Turin. Before moving to Turin, Kiesow married Emma Lough. Mosso allowed Kiesow to establish the first laboratory of experimental psychology and to introduce the working model developed by Wundt in a systematic way. This was possible via Kiesow's pupil, Emilio Pelligrini, whose family gave financial support to purchase valuable research equipment (Corallini Vittori, 2006).

In 1899, Kiesow obtained the position of Free Lecturer in Physiology from the Faculty of Medicine at Turin. In 1901, he was appointed professor in charge of General Experimental Psychology and the uses of new instruments, including the esthesiometer, which assessed the degree of pressure on various body surfaces of the skin. In the academic year 1906–1907, he was appointed full professor of Psychology in Turin: Together with those in Naples and Rome, these were the first three chairs established in 1906 in Italy by the Minister of Education, the neuropsychiatrist Leonardo Bianchi (1848–1927). The other two professorships were occupied by the psychiatrist Sante de Sanctis (1862–1935) in Rome and by the psychiatrist Cesare Colucci (1865–1942) in Naples. In 1910, Kiesow obtained Italian citizenship; in 1911 he organized the first *Congress of the Italian Society of Psychology* in Turin (Figure 9.1, right), and he also served as the president of the Italian Society of Scientific Psychology (Canestrelli, 1962). In 1929, he received an honorary doctorate from Wittenberg College in Springfield, Ohio. Annin, Boring, and Watson (1968) in their list of names of 538 influential psychologists from 1600 to 1967, included Kiesow. Kiesow retired from academic activity in 1933 and was appointed professor emeritus of the Royal University of Turin. He died after a prolonged illness on the 2nd of December 1940, aged 82, in Turin, where he was buried with his wife Emma.

ITALIAN FRIENDS AND COLLEAGUES

In Italy, Kiesow had numerous friends and colleagues from different disciplines. The anthropologist Giuseppe Sergi (1841–1936) contributed to the introduction of psychology in Italian schools and was interested in experimental psychology. The neuropsychiatrist Leonardo Bianchi established the first Italian chairs in experimental psychology in the faculties of literature and philosophy at the universities of Rome, Naples, and Turin (1906). Angelo Mosso, a mentor of Kiesow, introduced him in Turin and allowed him to establish the Laboratory of Experimental Psychology. Sante de Sanctis had a substantial role in the development and diffusion of psychology in Italy between 1800 and 1900 and was one of the first professors of Psychology in Rome. The psychologist Vittorio Benussi (1878–1927), whose first works were on optical-geometric illusions, expanded the study of the perception of form in general and the perception of time. Later, when he occupied the chair of Psychology in Padua (1919), he studied suggestion and hypnosis. The psychiatrist Giulio Cesare Ferrari

(1867–1932) founded, in 1905, the *Rivista di Psicologia Applicata alla Pedagogia ed alla Psicopatologia* [Journal of Psychology Applied to Pedagogy and Psychopathology], progenitor of what would become the *Rivista di Psicologia* [Journal of Psychology]. The neuropsychologist Cesare Colucci (1865–1942) studied language and sensory activities, in particular vision. In 1910, Colucci was also one of the founders of the Italian Society of Psychology, of which he was president in 1935. Father Agostino Gemelli (1878–1959) shared studies with Kiesow on tactile spatial perceptions and participated in the founding of the journal, *Archivio Italiano di Psicologia* [Italian Archive of Psychology] (see Chapter 16 in this volume). Mario Ponzo (1882–1960) was his collaborator for 30 years and conducted histological studies on taste goblets in some aspects of the back of the mouth in studies of perceptual phenomena, besides those on taste and weight, on spatial representations, optical illusions (one of which was given his name), psychomotor processes, and phenomena related to respiratory activity (Ponzo, 1942; see Chapter 17 in this volume). Ponzo left Turin for Rome, succeeding Sante De Sanctis as the chair of Psychology. Another student, also of Mosso, was Zaccaria Treves (1869–1911), who studied fatigue and developed a more sophisticated model of ergographer than Mosso. In Milan, he founded the Civic Laboratory of Pure and Applied Psychology with studies on mental and muscular work of children. Arturo Fontana carried out research on skin sensations and later became involved in dermatology. Another student was Raoul Hahn, an ear, nose, and throat doctor and free lecturer at the University of Turin, who researched the sensitivity of the back of the mouth and taste sensitivity. Emilio Pellegrini was a student of Kiesow who died prematurely and whose family made a donation for the master's laboratories. In his honor, the Institute of Psychology today bears the name of "*Fondazione Enrico Pellegrini*" (Corallini Vittori, 2006). Guido Lerda explored the sensitivity of skin scars. Luigi Agliardi (1876–1952) was the Italian translator of the works of Wilhelm Wundt and conducted research on the sense of temperature. Annibale Pastore (1868–1956), a philosopher who collaborated with Mosso, was interested in fechnerian psychophysics. Luigi Botti, a philosopher from Cremona, analyzed the causes of numerous visual perceptual illusions. Vittorio d'Agostino, also a philosopher, shed light on psychological problems through data taken from overlooked etymological and literary sources. The philosopher and psychologist Luigi Botti collaborated with Kiesow on visual perceptual phenomena with a particular interest in optical illusions and was also a collaborator of Gemelli. The Brescian Leopoldo Chinaglia (1890–1916) made extensive studies of comparative anatomy and physiology and entomology. He then turned toward comparative psychology, entering the laboratory of Kiesow. He devoted his activity to research in the field of thermal, skin, taste sensations and the result of these studies were the positive results around the influence exerted on the appreciation of the weight of objects placed on different parts of the body. Similar research was conducted on the influence exerted by temperature on taste sensitivity. Another close collaborator and friend was Alessandro Gatti (1901–1938), Kiesow's successor to the chair of Psychology in Turin (1933), whose research addressed various areas of psychology (eidetic problems, tactile perception, work psychology, and psychology of peoples) in experimental approach. In 1935 he was appointed director to be appointed director of the Center for Labor Studies in Turin. Angiola Masucco Costa (1902–2001) was the last pupil of Kiesow, who succeeded Gatti, and dealt with experimental psychology by conducting research on visual perception, space-time representation in the blind, and heredity (Kiesow, 1930; Perussia, 2008).

Kiesow often translated his papers into German or commented extensively on the most salient findings in foreign scientific journals. For his pupils he was not only a teacher and scientist but a leader in life (Ponzo, 1941). He took his students with him during international conferences and gave them visibility (Ponzo, 1942).

KIESOW'S INSTRUMENTS

Kiesow used and developed a number of instruments. In Leipzig, under Wundt, he introduced Mosso's plethysmograph, developed in 1875 to study vascular reactions of affective states with the hydrosphygmograph. These were useful to strengthen Wundt's idea of the three dimensional theory of sentimental states. In the laboratory to study skin sensation was adopted the Weber's compass developed by the German Ernst Heinrich Weber (1795–1878) in 1850, but many other instruments were designed by Kiesow himself, such as extensometers. One of the first tools conceived by Kiesow was the von Frey hair extensometer, which consisted of an ebonite rod with brass tweezers at one end, coated internally with layers of cork between which a hair (a woman's hair or horsehair) was attached as a stimulus. Kiesow had to use two devices in the experiments, one acting as a constant or normal stimulus, and the other one with a variable stimulus obtained by cutting the hair in small strands. He built a new instrument that combined the two functions: The end of the rod was equipped with two clamps placed one on top of the other and intersected by a screw that allowed their mutual approach and removal. A third extensometer, the baro and algo esthesiometer, used for the determination of individual pain points, replaced the hairs with the thorns of the robust prickly pear (*Opuntia robusta*). To assess the distribution of the thermal points, Kiesow used a special thermo esthesiometer formed by a hollow metal cylinder with a pointed end and crossed by two glass tubes connected to two containers for hot and cold water (Kiesow, 1928a).

To explore the individual differences of the simple reaction times to tactile, pain, and cutaneous stimuli, Kiesow developed the electro esthesiometer. It consists of two electromagnets, which, when an electric circuit was closed, lowered a lever with a hair of a particular voltage value fixed by pliers. An arm was added to the lever because this allowed contact between a platinum tip and the mercury contained in an ebonite basin. When the hair was lowered to touch the skin, the contact closed another electrical circuit, which set in motion the hands of a chronoscope or chronovisor of Matthias Hipp (1813–1893). This method was used to measure the duration of the interval between the stimulus and the reaction. After the stimulation, the lever was raised by a spring adjusted by a screw. The device was supported by the arm fixed with a vice. The cheat and algo esthesiometer, designed to measure the reaction time to pain stimuli, also was modified with the addition of an electrical circuit. In cases of reaction to thermal sensations, there were shorter and different times: The reactions to cold sensations were faster and with less average variation than those related to heat. Kiesow, in collaboration with Ponzo, built a water drop thermo esthesiometer that was formed by a curved pipette with a rubber pear inserted between two metal sheets. Pressing on the upper foil, a drop of liquid (cold or hot) came out of the pipette beak and at the same time a mercury contact was used to close an electrical circuit connected to Hipp's chronoscope. Later, Kiesow built another thermo esthesiometer to measure the reaction time to heat sensations (Kiesow, 1904a, 1910, 1911, 1912a).

He also invented an instrument to evaluate the taste threshold in the various parts of the oral cavity, which avoided the spread of solutions in the uvula area. It was made of a spoon-shaped glass with a curved handle 16 cm long, and a diameter of 1.5 cm, which was long enough to reach the uvula. The studies showed the levels of insensitivity of both the uvula and other areas, including the anterior and posterior pillars of the pendulous veil, the palatine tonsils, and the anterior face of the epiglottis (Kiesow, 1901a,b). The same algo esthesiometer was used to determine the reaction times to the various taste sensations, but the hair-stimulus was replaced with a brush soaked from time to time with substances of savory taste (Kiesow & Ponzo, 1910).

Studies on Blood Pressure and Pulse

In his early works, Kiesow used the sphygmomanometer of Mosso in different psycho-physiological conditions, paying attention mainly to the emotional aspects. He wrote that: *"changes in blood pressure caused by intellectual activity, or are produced by the excitation of the sense organs, or, again are they to be considered simply as the effects of emotions and the accompanying sensations? According to my experience, it seems that last alternative is the most acceptable"* (Kiesow,1895).

Kiesow added: *"It is necessary to distinguish different types of people. Those whose emotions are readily expressed, show the most distinct changes (blood pressure and pulse), which does not appear in people of calm disposition. In the first case, practice decreases the effect. The individual differences are explainable, not alone by temperament, but also by the different occupations of each person. A mathematician will be less emotional in mental problems which are common to his profession than when not permitted to employ himself this manner"* (Kiesow, 1895). Kiesow concluded that some people are emotionally unresponsive on the blood pressure-pulse test (Kiesow, 1895).

STUDIES ON TASTE

Kiesow investigated the sensations of taste, and he can be considered a pioneer of this study with Bellingeri (see Chapter 3 in this volume). Research on taste sensations was already the subject of his thesis as a student under Wundt in Leipzig and continued for 15 more years in Turin (Kiesow, 1894, 1896; Bartoshuk, 1978). As pointed out by Glaser in his book titled, *The Evolution of Taste Perception*, it is thanks to Kiesow that the perceptions of taste were first depicted geometrically (Kiesow, 1896; Glaser, 1999). This was done in the shape of a circle, on the periphery of which the four basic qualities of sweet, sour, salty, and bitter are located. Kiesow's circle depicts various mixtures, either on the periphery of the circle or in its axes (Glaser, 1999; Figure 9.2).

In his studies, Kiesow demonstrated that the distribution of taste sensitivity lies on the entire dorsal surface of the tongue, the base and inferior part of the tongue, and the hard and soft palate. These topographic researches were conducted together with Raoul Gustavo Hahn, ascertaining that in adults the sensitive areas are present at the level of the posterior wall of the pharynx, the rear face of the epiglottis, and the interior of the larynx. At the same time, it is absent on the anterior and posterior pillars of the pendulous veil, on the palatine tonsils, and the anterior face of the epiglottis. With the German otologist Max Nadoleczny (1874–1940), Kiesow demonstrated individual differences caused by nerve tract lesions or particular forms of otitis with the involvement of the chorda tympani and the taste fibers, the lingual nerve, and the anterior two thirds of the tongue, which is the tract between the anterior end of the foliated region to the tip of the tongue (Kiesow & Nadoleczny, 1900; see also the chapter on Bellingeri in this volume). These studies were completed by histological and chemical methods showing how the taste chalices are present in different parts of the human fetus (palatine tonsils and pillars, oral and nasal side of the soft and hard palate, the two faces of the epiglottis, the larynx, the various portions of the pharynx, the cervical tract of the esophagus, the lower aspect of the tongue, and gustatory chalices on the surface of the human epiglottis) (Kiesow, 1902, 1904b). Kiesow demonstrated that the gustatory surface is reduced in the adult, in particular in the central area of the back of the tongue. This eventually becomes

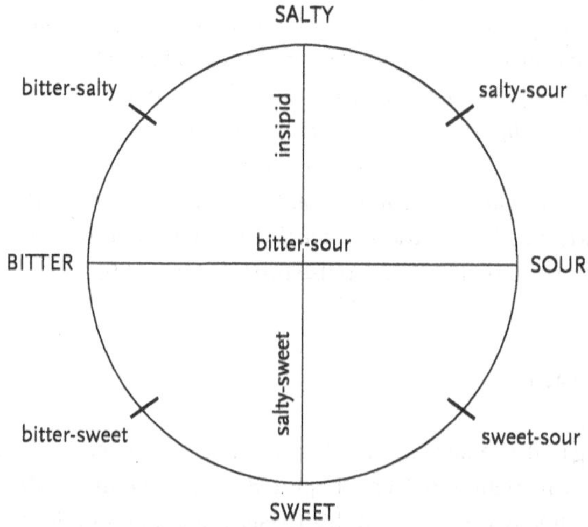

Figure 9.2. Kiesow's circle of taste perception. Adapted from Glaser, 1999.

numb and rarely remains at the level of the hard palate on the edges and or the lower surface of the tongue. He emphasized that the greater extension of the gustatory surface in the child is an ontogenetic repetition of phylogenetic development as a reflex movement, unrelated to the sense of taste and particularly on the inner face of the epiglottis.

With the German researcher Rudolf Höber (1873–1953), Kiesow applied electrochemical studies on the taste of some salts and alkaline substances; in this way he was able to demonstrate that taste sensations are the result of the action of different ions (Höber & Kiesow, 1898). Kiesow also investigated the psycho-physical aspect of the degree of taste sensitivity through the measurement of the taste threshold values in the various areas of the oral cavity (Kiesow, 1894, 1896). He concluded that sweetness is well perceived at the tip of the tongue; bitterness at the base; acidity at the edges; and saltiness is also well perceived at the tip and edges and less at the base of the tongue. Tastes are variously distributed on different parts of the oral cavity, and the normal distribution of sensitivity and individual differences are due to adaptation phenomena. These differences in taste thresholds were investigated in collaboration with Oerwald and showed large functional differences in the reaction of the individual fungiform lingual papillae to various tastes. Kiesow observed that, in childhood, all parts of the tongue perceive sweetness in equal measure except for the tip and edges where sensitivity is more acute. The recognition of four fundamental qualities of taste sensations is owed to the German psychologist, who claimed that alkaline and metallic flavors are the results of a fusion of other sensations. While distinguishing four fundamental qualities of taste sensations, Kiesow believed that all of them were relevant to one sense. He recognized that they occur variously through multiple, very complex, interferences by analyzing them through double sensations, associations, concomitant sensations, consecutive sensations, contrast phenomena, compensation, and mixing. He did not, however, find compensatory phenomena, such as perceptual cancellation for the simultaneous action on the sensitive surfaces of different taste substances to be acting chemically on each other. Kiesow detected phenomena of struggle, fusion, and combination. According to Kiesow, phenomena of contrast were recognizable in the field of taste between the taste of salty and sweet, salty and acid, and sweet and acid; bitterness would remain excluded from the contrasting relationships with other tastes. At that time, psychologists were interested in psychic elements, their quality and number, and Kiesow sketched explanations for complex psychic phenomena such as dreaming. He tackled the problem of oneiric activity related to taste and smell, pointing out that they are not so rare and depend on the subject's interest in this kind of dream (Kiesow, 1929).

THE SPECIFICITY OF SENSATIONS AND COMPLEX PHENOMENA IN THE FIELD OF SKIN PERCEPTIONS

Kiesow explored the action exerted by concomitant tactile, thermal, and pain sensations on the skin; studies in this area had intensified after the research of

Ernst Heinrich Weber (1795–1878). Weber highlighted the problems of sensory qualities related to the doctrine of nerve-specific energies with the psycho-physical law. Kiesow discovered that the constant presence of an area of oral mucosa on the inner surface of the cheek, between the muscles zygomaticus major, triangularis, risorius of Santorini is sensitive to feelings of touch, cold, and heat while appearing insensitive to those of pain caused by mechanical and electrical stimuli (Kiesow, 1926). Kiesow argued that the pain caused by heat, in this analgesic zone of the cheek, was determined by the excitement of organs located more deeply than those of heat sensation and demonstrated the autonomy of different pain sensations (Kiesow, 1910).

Kiesow was involved in studies on the spread, at the skin level, of particular points that were intended to be activated by specific stimuli such as heat, cold, and touch and distributed for these various forms of sense. These investigations were started by the Swedish physiologist Magnus Gustaf Blix (1849–1904) and the German neurologist Alfred Goldscheider (1858–1935). Moreover, the Austrian-German physiologist Maximilian von Frey (1832–1932) discovered skin points that reacted specifically to pain stimuli and supported the independence of pain sensations from other skin sensations, a concept about which Kiesow previously had made numerous contributions regarding the oral cavity. Discoveries also were made in other regions of the oral cavity (palatine tonsils and the median area of the palatine pillars), where tactile skin sensitivity was preserved but pain sensitivity was lacking (Kiesow & Hahn, 1901a). He highlighted the different distributions of tactile and pain points on the skin surface; the different duration of reaction times for the two types of sensations (Kiesow & Ponzo, 1910); the different magnitude of localization errors of tactile and pain sensations (Kiesow, 1933), and the localization of pure skin sensations of touch and pain, as well as of compound tactile and painful impressions (Kiesow, 1905). Kiesow differentiated the impression of touch from the tactile one, such as the punctiform of cold and the more widespread one of heat; he linked the sensation of itching to a particular stimulation of pain endings, tickling approached the tactile one, while a burning sensation was framed as a complex impression. He studied the distribution of specific cutaneous body sensitivity by establishing the parallelism between density of the various tactile points and sensitivity in the various regions of the body, agreeing with Weber's research on the study of the fineness of tactile spatial sense (Kiesow, 1902, 1904a). According to his research, conducted in collaboration with von Frey, the tactile points are arranged close to the emerging points of the hair. In the hair, he identified a suitable organ to receive information on the presence of mechanical stimuli plus their intensity, duration, and extension, especially in those regions of the body without Meissner's organs (von Frey & Kiesow, 1899).

Using his thermo esthesiometer, Kiesow studied the distribution of thermal points, concluding that specific cold points located near the hair are connected with the contraction of its erector muscles. This way, he attributed the lower presence of hot points to the fact that the body is more threatened by cold than heat (Kiesow, 1895, Kiesow & Fontana, 1901). Kiesow also noticed that the tip of the tongue and the red area of the lips possess an extreme tactile sensitivity, and concluded that Ruffini's papillary bows have the same characteristics as the terminal nervous plexuses surrounding the strand of hair. He attributed the functions of receptor organs of cold stimuli, as did von Frey, to the clubs of Krause, and found they were absent, as pain and touch sensations were absent at the lower portion of the uvula, while the heat endings were present (Kiesow, 1904b, 1926, 1933). With von Frey, Kiesow also explored the nature of tactile excitement, demonstrating that deformation of the tactile organ provides the tactile sensation (von Frey & Kiesow, 1899). Moreover, he demonstrated that this depends on a certain negative hydrostatic pressure drop when there is a pressure stimulus or a traction stimulus. These reactions to stimuli, according to Kiesow, depend on the concentration of dissolved substances in the aqueous states of tissues. According to Kiesow, the reaction of the tactile organ is due to the modification of the chemical constitution or osmotic pressure of tissue fluids (von Frey & Kiesov, 1899). This concept was highlighted by Kiesow and the entomologist Leopoldo Chinaglia, who provided explanations as to why cold objects are perceived heavier when heated and hot ones heavier than those at in different temperature. This allowed him to explain the influence of thermal stimuli on the internal pressure of the tissues. By using the extensometer, he demonstrated not only the importance of weight on the tactile surface but also the relative depth at which the excited tactile organ is located in the skin (Kiesow, 1911, 1912a, 1912b).

VISUAL PSYCHIC PROCESSES AND EIDETIC TYPOLOGY

In his essay titled, *Osservazioni sopra il rapporto tra due oggetti visti separatamente con I due occhi* [Observations on the relationship between two objects seen separately with the two eyes], Kiesow captured the psychic dimension (Kiesow, 1920). He did so by studying the visual function as in the case of binocular vision, and specifically of stereoscopic vision, rivalry or competition between fields of vision, and binocular contrast. He adhered to the principle of psychic fusion, or Wundt's concept of creative synthesis. This stated that qualitatively different elements of consciousness can develop new qualities of psychic formation but still retain a degree of independence.

In all cases, the observations were a binocular mixture and under different conditions a pure mixture (principle of fusion), but the rivalry remains when the difference between the two sensations is too large, that is, the principle of independence (Kiesow, 1920). On the rivalry of visual fields and stereoscopic images, the principle of psychic fusion is further confirmed in cases of the dominance of one impression over the other: the latter is only apparently suppressed by consciousness and actually remains to exert its influence on the former by slightly obscuring it (Kiesow, 1925a). This concept of the psychic structure of fusion as a new psychic formation derived from the union of conscious elements, and it aligned Kiesow with Wundt. In describing the gradual genesis of cognitive activity, Wundt affirmed an initial physiological level on which sensations connect to one another, giving rise to perceptions and a subsequent synthesis that merges these connections into a unitary whole. According to Wundt, the notion of space followed the same path because, on a physiological basis, the genesis of the representation of space is given by the formation of the visual field as drawn from eye movement. The eyes, as a result of a "central innervative sensation," move their retinal center and, at the same time, reproduce the points of vision before the displacement. The sensation of the stimulus gives rise to perception and, then, to representation; in turn, it merges with other representations, so that the "spatial representation rests on a gradual fusion of a representation into a series of other representations" (Wundt, 1862).

Kiesow re-studied the Wundtian interpretation of ocular movements in an effort to explain the mechanisms of the so-called optical-geometric illusions. This term was coined in 1855 by the German Johann Joseph Oppel (1815–1894) in relation to phenomena of perceptual deformation. In collaboration with his students Luigi Botti and Mario Ponzo, following the advent of the psychology of form, he provided examples on optical illusions through a systematic analysis of the illusions of Friedrich Sander (1889–1971). Kiesow brought Sander's figure back to Franz Carl Müller-Lyer (1857–1916), in which the two straight lines, even if equal, appear to be of different proportions because of the acute and obtuse angles that close them (Kiesow, 1931). According to Wundt, the illusion was justified by the fact that the eyes were attracted to the segments facing inside the figure, hindering the movement of the same. At the same time, they are facilitated by the outgoing segments of the obtuse angles. Therefore, the first line seems shorter than the second, which needs more muscular effort for the eyes to be able to travel the entire visual pathway. This process was concluded, from the psychological point of view, by a mental mechanism—mediated by the Wundtian concept of the "innervative sensation," which interprets the muscular sensations of greater or lesser effort as signs or transcriptions of the different lengths of the lines. According to Kiesow, the illusion, classified as an error of interpretation, was based on the mechanism of ocular movement and sensations that together with those given by the retinal image (as well as the tactile ones) are linked to this mental mechanism (Kiesow, 1912c, 1924a, 1931). Kiesow concluded, "that neither movements nor sensations will be spoken of but, implicitly admitting them, they will insist, as was already done in part, on particular dynamic mental attitudes in the perceptive act" (Ponzo, 1942). Kiesow was defending his and Wundt's interpretations on illusions, against those of the gestaltic parameters set out by the Czech psychologist Max Wertheimer (1880–1943) in 1912, which were based on an apparent or stroboscopic movement (Phi) concerning the phenomenon of the perceptive persistence of objects (Wertheimer, 1926). Werthemeier's experiences were also developed in the field of chronophotography and film (see the work of the Anglo-American photographer Edward Muybridge [1830–1904]).

Wertheimer studies were also of interest to Kiesow and his close collaborator Ponzo. Sticking to the Wundtian structuralism, Kiesow pointed out that during film screenings the viewer perceives a glossy effect by observing the image of metal objects on the surface of the screen. For viewers who already had the above experience, the vision of the metallic object stimulates the formation of a "positive psychic content," which by associative means joins the complexity represented in front of them by the film (Kiesow, 1928c). The phenomenon is similar to that of stereoscopic photography. This analogy allowed Kiesow to make a connection between stereoscopy and cinema, because, in both cases, the viewer sees something that is not a feature of the individual images. Although it starts from the images, it is born from the psychic synthesis between the current visual stimulus and the memory of other perceptions. He confirmed Ponzo's research, based on the Wundtian concept of creative synthesis as the result of a fusion of distinguishable sensations, finding that these sensations produce a different psychic formation from the individual elements composing it (Kiesow, 1928b). The synthesis implemented by the spectator is realized through two fusion dynamics, such as assimilation, when elements produced by incomplete external stimuli are merged with reproduced elements that have already entered the consciousness a complicated dynamic is activated. A more complex fusion occurs between heterogeneous elements that belong to different sensory fields. Kiesow did not publish the idea on integration between images on the screen and previous experiences on both an individual and collective level, with its social repercussions of cinematographic perception. In 1911, however, Ponzo published a work that sought to demonstrate how certain cinematic images contributed to influencing, if not conditioning, the viewer's daily experience. Similar works were published in 1914 and 1919 by Hugo Münsterberg (1863–1916) and William Moulton Marston (1893–1943).

Ponzo resumed the Wundtian tradition, and this was also possible thanks to the Italian translation of his text on the subject (Wundt, 1912).

Kiesow's eidetism can be identified not only in the study of the visual field, but also in other sensory areas, demonstrating significant individual differences. He came to these conclusions independently, although these had already been described in 1907 by the Austrian otologist Victor Urbantschitsch (1847–1921). He had referred to mnestic images that some subjects keep so active that they assume the characters of perception and are similar to consecutive visual images that arise after the fixation of a luminous chromatic stimulus, but are different from these because they can be evoked at a distance of time (Urbantschitsch, 1907). During the *Groningen Congress* in 1926, the German psychologist, Erich Rudolf Jaensch (1883–1940) set out his theory of personality, based on more or less persistent eidetic images in adult life. Kiesow replied with the *Zur Kritik der Eidetik* [On the critique on eideism], reporting the results of a study on children from 4 to 14 years old with more than a thousand subjects, realized in Turin and in Milan (in collaboration with Gatti, who in the meantime worked at the Catholic University). He compared the true eidetic with the noneidetic, devising the method of graphic reproductions allowing the subjects to provide a graphic representation of their images. Thus, he showed that the non-eidetic visualizes only a few visual impressions presented shortly before in sequence, while the true eidetic continues to see all the individual impressions of the model before his eye with equal hallucinatory clarity and can easily record them (Kiesow, 1924b, 1925b, 1926; Kiesow & Gatti, 1925). Kiesow's contribution to eidetic phenomena gained international recognition (Klüver, 1928).

REACTION TIMES

The physiologists of the 19th century were interested in measuring the speed of the nervous impulse (Wade, 2012). Originally defined as *physiological times*, in 1870 they were called *reaction times by* the physiologist Sigmund Exner (1846–1926). They have been examined by many physiologists, including Johannes Peter Müller (1801–1858), Hermann von Helmholtz (1821–1894), Karl Friedric Wilhelm Ludwig (1816–1895), Emil Du Bois-Reymond (1816–1896), and Ernst Wilhelm von Brücke (1819–1892). In 1849, von Helmholt demonstrated the measurability of conduction by stimulating the frog gastrocnemius nerve at various points and measuring the time between stimulation and contraction with a chronoscope (von Helmholtz, 1850). Kiesow's interest in reaction times was driven by the desire to use suitable means to differentiate one sensory function from another, as in tactile, pain, and cutaneous stimuli. The numerous measurements made by Kiesow demonstrated mutual independence of the various sensations as well as the duration that emerged in the experiments between reactions to pain and reactions to tactile sensations. The reactions to the stimuli applied on the tips of the finger are faster than for equal stimuli on the forearm: this would depend on the greater use of the fingers as touching organs. Kiesow noticed that tactile and acoustic sensations did not always respect the Wundtian law, which postulated that, with the increase of the stimulus intensity, the duration of the reactions first decreases and then remain constant with subsequent increases. The reaction times to various taste sensations are rather long compared to the stimuli of bitterness (Kiesow, 1903a; Kiesow & Ponzo 1910). Reactions to thermal sensations instead had shorter times: reactions to cold sensations were faster and with smaller average variations than those related to heat (Kiesow, 1903b). Kiesow also tried to determine nerve conduction velocity in the psychic nerve, which had already been attempted by von Helmholtz. For this purpose, he was acting on single tactile points and measured the reaction time to stimuli placed at different distances from the root of the upper and lower limbs. He concluded that, with the instruments available at the time, measuring the difference in the speed of the propagation current between the motor nerve and the sensory nerve in humans was an uncertain process (Kiesow, 1903c, 1904c). Kiesow even noticed the presence of a third form of reaction that he called "indifferent." This is characteristic of the mental attitude of a subject who does not pay attention to the expected impression (sensory reaction) nor to the consequent movement to be made (muscular reaction), but rather to another predetermined sensory one. The reaction times of the latter have an intermediate duration between the other two forms of reaction. The identification of a mental attitude as a condition of choice of the various forms of reaction signals Kiesow's interest in psychic processes. For example, he recorded delay in reaction time to taste sensations motivated by the longer time they take to reach consciousness. According to the different mental attitudes, dependent on particular forms of adaptation of the subject to the task, or according to particular situations the specific differences between the motor type (fast), the sensory type (slow), and the mixed type, the different kinds of disposition, as Kiesow states, were due to personal experiences (Kiesow, 1904d).

EPISTEMOLOGICAL ASPECTS

For over 30 years, the Wundtian speculative rigor was mitigated by (and receptive of) the teachings from Mosso, in whose laboratory Kiesow learned how to do sensory recordings (Ponzo, 1942). Kiesow had to give up the structuralist categories of Wundt to adhere to the theory of form or Gestalt. But the idea that the maximum gestalt postulated, according to which the whole is more than the sum of the parts, was nothing more than the re-edition of the Wundtian thesis for which, " every perception can be broken down into elementary sensations, but it is never equal to the simple sum of the latter." It was thus not possible to refer to a concept of atomism or, as far as theoretical-conscious reflections were concerned, to the associative system of mental chemistry of the empirical tradition of the British philosopher John Stuart Mill (1803–1873). These associative systems are realized in terms of regularity and constancy, allowing for decomposition and recomposition. In accordance with the Wundtian tripartite theory of feelings, sensations and will, it is possible according to Kiesow to isolate and analyze the basic elements, elementary feelings and sensations.

Kiesow concluded that *"like any other positive science, also our discipline must have as a guide the rule according to which an overall fact is understood only by analyzing it [. . .]. Such an analysis makes us know not only the composition of a complex, but also the laws, according to which it was formed [. . .]"* (Kiesow, 1929). A confirmation of this epistemological approach concerns the pain sensations: pain is distinct, depending on whether it is addressed from the scientific perspective as a sensation or from a daily life viewpoint as an affective state. Following the concept of the psychic element, and applying Mosso's plethysmograph, Kiesow noticed considerable individual differences in the vasal reactions of affective states. He opposed the epigenetic thesis of Georg Theodor Ziehen (1862–1950), a theorist of associationism in psychology. Moreover, he disagreed with the German philosopher and psychologist Carl Stumpff (1878–1936). Stumpf was close to the traditional empiricism of the American psychologist philosopher, of Irish origin, William James (1842–1910) who considered emotions as authentic sensory phenomena arising from peripheral excitement and from a central or peripheral addition to specific sensations. In 1928, during the inauguration of the new laboratory of Experimental Psychology at Wittenberg College in Springfield, Ohio, Kiesow mentioned that he demonstrated the independence of feelings from sensations: "the nature of feeling and that of sensation are essentially different from each other" (Kiesow, 1929). In his approaches, Kiesow misunderstood the Gestaltists, believing that: "the Gestalten of the representations built from the sensations, formed, that is, through a secondary process completely absent in the

Gestaltic perspective, where the Gestalt is instead an immediate datum of the perceptual experience" (Luccio, 1994).

CONCLUSIONS

Kiesow further developed Wundtian psychology by founding an experimental psychology laboratory and encouraged the debate between physiology and psychology of perception during a critical period of Italian positivism. His psycho-physiological research, in contrast to William James's and Gestalt's antielementism, functionalism, behaviorism, and psychoanalysis, received international appreciation. Still, by the 1920s the Wundtian model had been abandoned in Europe, and Kiesow's research seemed outdated. Although he has been blamed for ineffective efforts to give theoretical depth to the rigorous experimental work, his contribution to the development of Italian scientific psychology is beyond any doubt. Kiesow and his students reinforced the study of psychology as an autonomous discipline, through its biological and physiological aspects. His school on experimental psychology enriched the cultural climate of Turin, which could, in turn, consolidate its role in Europe.

REFERENCES

Annin E L, Boring E G & Watson R I (1968) Important psychologists, 1600–1967. *Journal of History of Behavioural Sciences*, 4: 303–315.

Bartoshuk L M (1978) History of taste research. In E C Carterette & M P Friedman (Eds.), *Handbook of Perception* (Volume via. Tasting and Smelling). New York, San Francisco, London: Academic Press.

Benjamin Jr L T (2000). The psychology laboratory at the turn of the 20th century. *American Psychologist*, 55: 318.

Bongiorno V (2006) The "project of experimental psychology" developed in Italy by neurophysiologist and psychiatrist. *Physis*, 43: 387–405.

Canestrelli L (1962) The Italian Society of Scientific Psychology (S.I.P.S.). Its history, structure and present role. *Applied Psychology*, 11: 23–35.

Corallini Vittori A G (Ed.) (2006) *Nel labirinto della Psicologia Sperimentale. La strumentazione del '900: catalogo (sui generis)*. Torino: Edizioni Angolo Manzoni.

Glaser D (1999) The Evolution of Taste Perception. In A Corti (Ed.), *Low-Calorie Sweeteners: Present and Future*. Basel: Karger.

Harper R S (1950) The first psychological laboratory. *Isis*, 41: 158–161.

Höber R & Kiesov F (1898) Ein einfacher Apparat zur Bestimmung der Empfindlichkeit von Temperaturpunkten. *Zeitschrift für Physiologische Chemie* 82: 172–174.

Kiesow F (1894) *Beiträge zur physiologischen Psychologie des Geschmackssinnes.* Philosophische Studien, 10: 329–368; 523–561.

Kiesow F (1895) Expériences avec le sphygmomanomètre de Mosso sur les changements de la pression du sang, chez l'homme, produits par les excitations psychiques. *Archives Italiennes de Biologie*, 23: 198–211.

Kiesow F (1896) *Beiträge zur physiologischen Psychologie des Geschmackssinnes. Philosophische Studien*, 12: 255–276; 464–473.

Kiesow F & Hahn R (1901a) Beobachtungen über die Empfindlichkeit der binteren Theile des Mundraumes für Tast-, Schmerz-, Temperatur-, und Geschmacksreize. *Zeitschhrift für Psychologie und Physiologie, der Sinnesorgane* 26: 383–417.

Kiesow F, & Hahn R (1901b) Sulla sensibilità gustativa di alcune parti della retrobocca e dell'epiglottide. *Giornale della Reale Accademia di Medicina, di Torino* 7: 497–502.
Kiesow F, & Fontana A (1901) Sulla distribuzione dei peli come organi tattili sulla superfice del corpo umano. *Rendiconti Reale Accademia dei Lincei,* 10: 24–31.
Kiesow F (1902) Ueber Verteilung und Empffindlichkeit der Tastpunkte. *Philosophische Studien* 19: 260–309.
Kiesow F (1903a) Zur Frage nach der Fortpflanzungsgeschwindigkeit der Erregung im sensiblen Nerven des Menschen. *Zeitschrift für Psychologie und Physiologie,* 33: 444–452.
Kiesow F (1903b) Contributo allo studio del tempo di reazione delle sensazioni gustative. *Rendiconti della Reale Accademia dei Lincei,* 12: 27–39.
Kiesow F (1903c) Ein Beitrag zur Frage nach den Reaktionszeiten der Geschmacksempfindungen. *Zeitschrift für Psychologie und Physiologie der Sinneorgane,* 33: 453–461.
Kiesow F (1904a) Ueber die einfachen Reaktionszzeiten der taktilien Belastungsemfindungen. *Zeitschrift für Psychologie und Physiologie der Sinneorgane,* 35: 8–49.
Kiesow F (1904b) Ueber die Tastempfindlichkeit der Körperoberfläche für punktuelle mechanische Reize. *Zeitschrift für Psychologie und Physiologie der Sinneorgane,* 35: 234–251.
Kiesow F (1904c) Nochmals Zur Frage nach der Fortpflanzungsgeschwindigkeit der Erregung im sensiblen Nerven des Menschen. *Zeitschrift für Psychologie und Physiologie der Sinneorgane,* 34: 132–133.
Kiesow F (1904d) Zur Kenntnis der Nervenendigungen in den Papillen der Zungenspitze. *Zeitschrift für Psychologie und Physiologie der Sinneorgane,* 35: 252–259.
Kiesow F (1905) Ueber die mittlere Schwelle des Tastpunktes bei Application mechanischer Reize. *Atti del V congresso internazionale di psicologia,* Roma.
Kiesow F (1910) Beobachtungen über die Reaktionszeiten der schmerzhaften Stichempfindung *Archiv für die gesamte Psychologie,* 18: 265–304.
Kiesow F & Ponzo M (1910) Beobachtungen über die Reaktionszeiten der Temperaturempfindungen. *Archiv für die gesamte Psychologie* 16: 376–396.
Kiesow F (1911) Ueber die Versuche von E. H. Weber und M. Szabadföldi, nach welchen einer Hautstelle aufliegende Gegenstände von gleicher Grösse nicht gleich schwer empfunden werden, wenn ihre Temperaturen gewisse Unterschiede aufweisen. *Archiv für die gesamte Psychologie Archiv für die gesamte Psychologie,* 22: 50–104.
Kiesow F (1912a) Della causa per la quale oggetti freddi posti sulla pelle vengono percepiti più pesanti di quando sono riscaldati. *Rivista di Psicologia,* 8: 181–199.
Kiesow F (1912b) Ein Aesthesiometer für die Bestimmung der Reaktionszeiten der einfachen Wärmeempfindung. *Zeitschrift für Biologische Technik und Methodik,* 2: 23–32.
Kiesow F (1912c) Demonstration einiger optischer Täuschungen. *Ber. d. V.Kong.f. exper. Psychol. Berlin, S* 162–163.
Kiesow F (1920) Osservazioni sopra il rapporto tra due oggetti visti separatamente con due occhi. *Archivio Italiano di Psicologia.* I: 3–38; III: 239–290.
Kiesow F (1924a) Di una illusione ottico-geometrica. *Archivio Italiano di Psicologia,* 3: 180–184.
Kiesow F (1924b) Si verificano nei bambini e nei fanciulli immagini consecutive contrarie? Contributo allo studio dei fenomeni eidetici. *Archivio Italiano di Psicologia,* 3: 121–132.
Kiesow F, & Gatti A (1925) Nuove osservazioni sui fenomeni eidetici. *Archivio Italiano di Psicologia,* 4: 79–84.
Kiesow F (1925a) Di un fenomeno ottico. *Archivio Italiano di Psicologia,* 4: 77–78.
Kiesow F (1925b) Zur Kritik der Eidetik, Arch für die gesamate Psychologie. LIII, reprinted. In *Proceeding and Papers of the VIII Congress of Psychology,* Groningen, 1926.

Kiesow F (1926) Ueber die Empfindungsqualitäten der Uvula. *Archiv für die gesamte Psychologie Archiv für die gesamte Psychologie*, 56: 452–462.
Kiesow F (1928a) The Problem of the Condition of Arousal of the Pure Sensation of Cutaneous Pain. *The Journal of General Psychology*, 1:2, 199–212.
Kiesow F (1928b) Il principio della sintesi creatrice di G. Wundt e la teoria della forma. *Archivio Italiano di Psicologia*, 7: 78–79.
Kiesow F (1928c) Del lucido metallico in immagini cinematografiche. *Archivio Italiano di Psicologia*, 6: 225–229.
Kiesow F (1929) Sulla frequenza dei sogni gustativi ed olfattivi. *Archivio Italiano di Psicologia*, 7: 226–231.
Kiesow F (1930) F. Kiesow. In C. Murchinson (Ed.), *A History of Psychology in Autobiography* (Vol. 1), pp. 163–190. Worcester, MA: Clark University Press; Russel & Russel/ Atheneum.
Kiesow F (1931) L'illusione di Sander. *Archivio italiano di psicologia*, 9: 284–299.
Kiesow F (1932) In memoria di Guglielmo Wundt. *Archivio Italiano di Psicologia*, 10: 3–23.
Kiesow F (1933) Sulla localizzazione di sensazioni cutanee pure di tatto e di dolore, nonché di impressioni tattili e dolorose composte. *Archivio Italiano di psicologia*, 10: 201–244.
Kiesow F, & Nadoleczny M (1900) Sulla fisiologia della corda del timpano. *Archivio Italiano di Otologia, Rinologia e Laringologia*, 9–10: 297–304.
Klüver H (1928) Studies on the eidetic type and on eidetic imagery. *The Psychological Bulletin*, 25: 69–104.
Lough E, & Kiesow F (1896) *Fear*. Translated from the Fifth Edition of *La Paura* by Angelo Mosso. London, New York, Bombay: Longmans, Green and Co.
Luccio R (1994) L'inizio del dibattito sulla psicologia della Gestalt in Italia.[The beginning of the debate on the psychology of Gestalt in Italy]. In P Legrenzi & R Luccio, (Eds.), *Immagini della psicologia*. [Images of psychology], pp. 143–146. Bologna: Il Mulino.
Mandler G (2011) *A History of Modern Experimental Psychology. From James and Wundt to Cognitive Science*. New York: MIT Press.
Mosso A (1880) Sulla circolazione del sangue nel cervello dell'uomo. Atti della R. *Accademia dei Lincei*, 3: 237–358.
Perussia F (2008) Note sui periodici della ricerca scientifica in psicologia all'Università di Torino, su Federico Kiesow e sull'Archivio Italiano di Psicologia. *Giornale di Psicologia*, 2: 277–291.
Ponzo M (1940) Federico Kiesow (1858–1940). *Rivista di Psicologia*, 36: 173–174.
Ponzo M (1941) Obituary Federico Kiesow (1858–1940) (1858–1940). *Psychological Review*, 48: 268–269.
Ponzo M (1942) Vite di psicologi, pagine di psicologia. Federico Kiesow (1858–1940) *Archivio di Psicologia, Neurologia, Psichiatria e Psicoterapia*, 3: 3–30.
Sinatra M, & Monacis L (2010) The influence of the Leipzig Institutes on the School of Turin. *Physis*, 47: 173–198.
Urbantschitsch V (1907) *Über subjektive optische Anschauunssbilder*. Leipzig und Wien: Deuticke.
von Helmholtz H (1850) Note sur la vitesse de propagation de l'agent nerveux dans les nerfs rachidiens. *Comptes rendus des seances de l'Academie des Science de Paris:* 30: 204–206.
von Frey M, & Kiesow F (1899) Ueber die Funktion der Tastkörperchen. *Zeitschhrift für Psychologie und Physiologie*, 20: 126–163.
Wade EP (2012) Reactions times: connected histories in Germany, Italy, and United States. *Physis*, 48: 15–37.
Wertheimer M (1926) Experimentelle Studien über das Sehen von Bewengungen. *Zeitschrift für Psychologie* 61: 161–265.

Wundt W (1862) *Beiträge zur Theorie der Sinneswarhnemung*. Leipzig und Heidelberg: Winter.
Wundt W (1912) *Elemente der Völkerpsychologie. Grundlinien einer psychologischen Entwicklungsgeschichte der Menschheit.* Leipzig: Kröner.
Zago S, Ferrucci R, Marceglia S, & Priori A (2009) The Mosso's method for recording brain pulsation: The forerunner of functional neuroimaging. *Neuroimage*, 48: 652–656.

CHAPTER 10

Camillo Negro

Neurologist, Neuroscientist, Science Communicator, and Mentor

ADRIANO CHIÒ AND ANDREA CALVO

Camillo Negro (1861–1927; Figure 10.1) is considered one of the most representative Italian neurologists of the era between the 19th and the 20th century. He was the founder of the Neurological School in Turin and a Professor of Neurology in the same university; his chair of Neurology was the first in Italy to be separated from the Chair of Psychiatry.

TRAINING AND EARLY YEARS: FROM BIELLA TO HEIDELBERG

Camillo Negro was born in Biella, a small town approximately 60 kilometers from Turin, on the 6th of June 1861, less than three months after the proclamation of the unified Kingdom of Italy. Biella was an industrial city, mostly engaged in wool tissue production, with a strong relationship with wool producers in Australia and the United Kingdom, and permeated by a quasi-Protestant attitude toward work. Negro attended the high school in Biella, and then he moved to Turin to attend the Faculty of Medicine, at that time one of the most prestigious in Italy and one of the few with a complete six-year study cycle. In 1880, he was admitted, after a public examination, to the *Reale Collegio delle Province* [Royal College of Provinces], an institution established in 1729 by Viktor Amadeus II, King of Sardinia-Piedmont, which hosted the one hundred most valuable alumni from all the provinces of the Kingdom to attend the University of Turin on a scholarship (Ormezzano, 1891).

During his graduate years, Negro attended not only the Human Anatomy Institute directed by Carlo Giacomini as an intern, but also the Institute of Medicine led by Camillo Bozzolo (1882; Roasenda, 1927). From the academic year 1882 to 1883, he

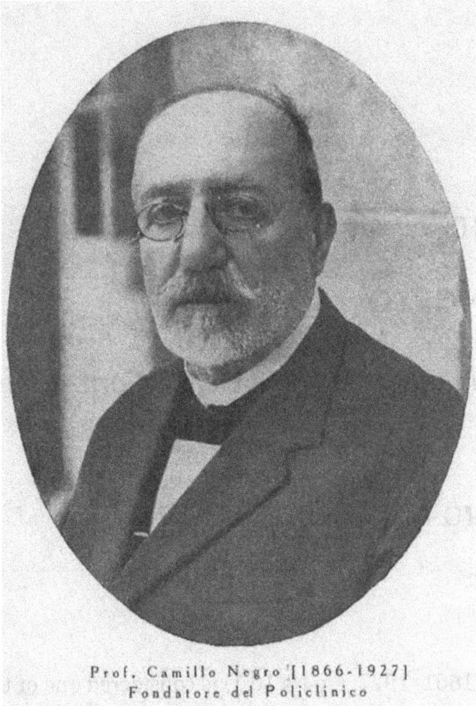

Figure 10.1. Portrait of Camillo Negro. Courtesy of Adriano Chiò.

was working, as an intern first, then as a fellow, at the Laboratory of Physiology directed by Angelo Mosso. During this period, Negro explored the peripheral nervous system. He also published a paper, with the results of his MD dissertation, on the effects of hydrochloric acid on sensitive and motor nerves (Negro, 1884). A summary of Negro's research also was read by Mosso at the Royal Academy of Sciences of Turin. In addition to this, Negro performed some naïve observations concerning the human body's reactions to altitude and fatigue (Negro, 1885; Negro & Antoniotti, 1885), which was an area of preeminent interest for Mosso, a pioneer in the study of altitude physiology.

On the 21st of November 1884, Negro received his MD degree and, shortly after, he moved to Heidelberg, Germany, where he remained until December 1887. In Heidelberg, he worked with Wilhelm Heinrich Erb and Wilhelm Kühne, Professor of Neurology and Professor of Physiology, respectively, at the local University. Heidelberg, which is Germany's oldest university and one of the oldest surviving universities, was an ideal place to improve his research skills, especially in the area of electrophysiology under the guidance of Professor Erb. The results of his research stay in Heidelberg, which were published in 1888 and 1889 (Negro, 1888; Negro, 1889), dealt with the effect of unipolar currents on electric excitability of the brain.

CAMILLO NEGRO, THE NEUROLOGIST

Camillo Negro returned to Turin in 1888. Professor Camillo Bozzolo asked him to deliver a series of formal lectures at the Faculty of Medicine to the fifth and sixth-year medical students on the electrodiagnosis and the electrotherapy of nervous system disorders. He also started a private practice as a neurologist in Turin and in his hometown, Biella. In 1889, he was among those who advocated the establishment of the "King Humbert I" *Policlinico Generale of di Torino,* a multispecialty outpatient clinic with particular provisions for those people who could not afford private medical consultations (Piccardi, 1929). Until the 1930s, the Policlinico remained one of the most prestigious medical institutions of the city, and it was the location of several academic departments of the University of Turin. Besides the relatively young Negro, two already established physicians were among the founders: Carlo Forlanini, pulmonologist, and Giuseppe Gradenigo, otolaryngologist.

Negro also became a consultant neurologist at the hospital annexed to the *Piccola Casa della Divina Provvidenza* [Small House of Divine Providence], best known as *Cottolengo*, a landmark religious charity institution. In the following two decades, he was very active both as a clinical neurologist and as a researcher. As a neurologist, Negro had a particular interest in the study of neurological signs and symptoms, but also continued his research on neurophysiology. A fascinating document of this period is his publication of a journal (titled *Rivista Iconografica della Sezione Malattie Nervose del Policlinico Generale di Torino* [Iconographic Journal of the Nervous Diseases Section of the General Polyclinic of Turin], 1897–1901) reporting remarkable clinical cases he had the opportunity to diagnose at the Policlinico Generale di Torino. In 1892, the Italian Ministry of Education appointed Camillo Negro as a lecturer for neuropathology at the University of Turin. In 1904, upon request of Cesare Lombroso, at that time professor of Psychiatry and Legal Medicine at the University of Torino, Negro obtained the professorship for neuropathology, and in 1911 he became a full professor of neuropathology (in modern terms, neurology) within the same University. In 1907 he was one of the founders of the *Società Italiana di Neurologia* [Italian Society of Neurology], which is still active today. Camillo Negro died aged 66, on the 16th of October 1927, because of stomach cancer. He was survived by his wife and four children.

CAMILLO NEGRO, THE NEUROSCIENTIST

During 30 years of research activity, Negro published more than one hundred papers, mostly in Italian or French. His most remarkable achievements were in the area of neurological semiotics. In 1901, with the collaboration of Zaccaria Treves, formerly an assistant in Mosso's laboratory, Negro published the first-ever description of cogwheel rigidity in Parkinson's disease using a pneumatic ergograph (Figure 10.2) (Negro & Treves, 1901). Today, cogwheel rigidity is still called Negro's sign or Negro's phenomenon after him (Ghiglione et al., 2005). In 1907, Negro described the bulbo-palpebral event in peripheral palsy of the facial nerve, that is, in the upward gaze, the ocular bulb seems to rotate higher on the side of the palsy (Negro,

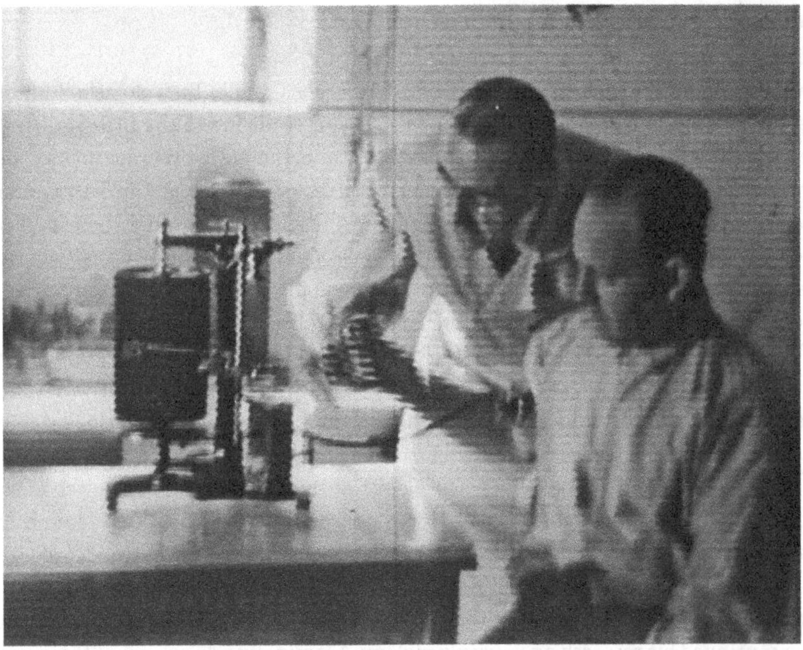

Figure 10.2. The ergograph used by Camillo Negro for the original description of the cogwheel sign. Still photo from Fedele Negro films on the treatment of Parkinson' disease with atropa belladonna, in the 1930s (Courtesy of Museo Nazionale del Cinema, Torino, via Adriano Chiò).

1907). Finally, he was the first who described the meso-rotuleus sign associated with the pyramidal deficit. After World War I, he investigated patients affected by lethargic encephalitis. This condition was first described by the Austrian neurologist and psychiatrist Constantin von Economo in 1917 (von Economo, 1917), especially the clinical characteristics of the parkinsonian syndrome (Negro, 1921; Negro, 1922; Negro & Negro, 1922). Negro's interest in lethargic encephalitis was subsequently carried on by his son, Fedele Negro, a neurologist himself (Negro, 1938).

Negro's interest in clinical neurology is perhaps best pointed out by the manual of neurology he published in 1912 (*Patologia e Clinica del Sistema Nervoso*), which he dedicated to Camillo Bozzolo and Wilhelm Erb, his mentors. The book originated from a series of lectures he gave to the medical students. In essence, these were not based on a systematic description of neurology, but rather on the presentation and in-depth discussion of clinical cases. Only a small portion of each lesson was devoted to theoretical issues. A significant exception to this is the detailed discussion of the basic function of the system in the first two chapters. In the section titled *The Theory of Neurons,* he specifically supported the doctrine proposed by Santiago Ramón y Cajal and refused the syncytial theory, supported by Camillo Golgi, both Nobel Laureates for Medicine and Physiology in 1906 (Mazzarello, 2006). According to Negro, neurons are independent units, which do not establish anastomosis at the protoplasm or the axonal level. All neurites or axons end with arborizations, which have connections by contiguity or contact, but never by continuity. He also reinforced this notion with original drawings.

His experimental research was mainly related to the localization of motor centers, in particular in the cerebellum, using various types of electrical stimulations (Negro & Roasenda, 1907), and to the excitability of peripheral nerves (Negro, 1915). Negro also realized pivotal studies on neuromuscular plaques. He published several reports on the histology of the plaques using a modified hematoxylin method, also assessing the effect of tetanism on the motor terminals.

CAMILLO NEGRO, THE SCIENTIFIC COMMUNICATOR

Besides the electrophysiological studies, a significant interest of Camillo Negro was teaching and disseminating clinical neurology. In September 1906, he founded the monthly journal, *Rivista Neuropatologica. Periodico per i Medici pratici* [Neuropathological Journal. A Periodical for Practitioners], which was published until 1911 and then, after an interruption of three years, for about a year, in 1914, with a small change to the title, becoming *Rivista Neurologica. Periodico per i Medici Pratici* [Neurology Journal. A Periodical for Practitioners]. In the preface to the first issue, he wrote: "This periodical aims to provide practitioners, in particular those who live far away from academic centers, the more recent acquisitions of clinical neurology. Several high-level Italian periodicals are dealing with neurological topics, but their interests are mainly related to the scientific aspects of nervous diseases; on the other hand, medical journals are more interested in reporting rare or curious clinical cases, which are of interest for the specialists more than for the generalists (Negro, Preface, *Rivista Neuropatologica*, vol. I, 1906).

Similarly, Negro is still renowned for his movie (*Neuropatologia*) on neurological and psychiatric cases (Chiò et al., 2016). The original purpose of this movie was mainly educational, to offer materials to "small Universities, where there is a shortage of patients, to have movie reproduction of principal signs and true characteristics of nervous diseases" (F.E.Z. 1908; Chiò et al., 2016). Camillo Negro purposefully selected the patients to be filmed to show students and physicians neurological signs and movement disorders, which are not easily understood with photographic images (Roasenda, 1957). The movie in its original form included 24 "scenes" organized from the presentation of clinical signs (eye movement, facial paresis, deep tendon reflexes) to that of neurological syndromes (ataxias, hemiplegias, Parkinson's disease, Huntington's chorea) and psychiatric disorders (mainly hysterias). Interestingly, in several scenes, Camillo Negro and his assistant, Giuseppe Roasenda, are also filmed while actively participating in the examination of patients and often interacting with them (Chiò et al., 2016).

The filming took place from 1906 to early 1908, and Negro was helped by Roberto Omegna, a camera operator, who authored a large number of scientific documentaries in the following years. The movie was shown in preview in Torino, at the Royal Academy of Medicine, on the 17th of February 1908, and officially at the first meeting of the Italian Neurology Society, on the 11th of April 1908. *Neuropathology* was used by Camillo Negro on several occasions after 1908. In some instances, he changed the order of the scenes or even added new ones according to the audience and the context (Roasenda, 1928).

The interest of Camillo Negro in filmography was not limited to *Neuropatologia*. In 1915, when Italy declared war on the Austrian Empire, Negro was appointed as a consultant neurologist for the 1st Italian Army. He filmed several cases of "war neurology," including muscular disorders, war wounds, and subjects affected by mental disorders, instances that we now would call post-traumatic stress disorder. These recordings are probably the most impressive ones among the whole corpus of preserved films.

Camillo Negro was not the first neurologist to film neurological patients. We still have precious movies made by the Romanian neurologist Gheorghe Marinescu, who filmed patients with hemiplegia and ataxias in Bucharest in 1899 (Buda et al., 2009). Arthur Van Gehuchten filmed several patients at the Catholic University of Leuven, Belgium, in 1907, and used frames from his films as iconographic material for his scientific publications (Aubert et al., 2002). In the United Kingdom, Major Arthur Hurst filmed patients with war neurosis (mostly intractable movement disorders) in 1917–1918 (Jones, 2012).

Negro was the first one, however, to organize the cases into a logical sequence and to use it on several public occasions. Moreover, differently from the other films of this period, *Neuropatologia* has a particular artistic value for the quality of the images and the richness of details (Chiò et al., 2016; Dagna & Gianetto, 2013).

CAMILLO NEGRO, THE MENTOR

His tutoring activities also show Camillo Negro's interest in teaching and research. Among the numerous students supervised by Negro, Carlo Angela, Mario Gozzano, and Luisa Levi should be mentioned.

Carlo Angela (1875–1949) obtained his MD degree in 1899 and was an assistant of Camillo Negro. He authored several scientific publications, including a monograph on affective lability as a consequence of cerebrovascular lesions (Angela, 1913) and a paper on sensibility and cardiac disturbances in Friedreich's disease (Angela, 1914). Angela was an active antifascist and during the 1930s became the director of a nursing home a few miles from Turin, where, during World War II he offered a safe place to stay to numerous antifascists and Jews. In August 2001, he was awarded the medal recognizing him as a Righteous Among the Nations.

Mario Gozzano (1898–1986) received his MD degree in 1922 and became an internal fellow at Negro's Institute of Neuropathology while also attending the Institute of Physiology, then directed by professor Amedeo Herlitzka. During this period, he mostly investigated experimental physiology before moving to the University of Rome, where he became an assistant to Professor Giovanni Mingazzini at the Institute of Nervous and Mental Disorders. He was appointed professor of neurology at the universities of Cagliari, Bologna, and, finally, at the Sapienza University in Rome (Mazza et al., 2002). He completed pivotal works on the electrophysiology of the cerebral cortex and electroencephalography. His *Trattato delle*

Malattie Nervose, first edited in 1946, remained the most relevant Italian textbook of neurology for decades.

Luisa Levi (1898–1983) was the sister of the antifascist writer Carlo Levi, the author of the masterpiece, *Cristo si è fermato a Eboli* [Christ stopped at Eboli]. She obtained her MD in 1920 in Turin with a thesis on "the slow endocarditis," but soon after her graduation she was admitted as an internal fellow at Camillo Negro's Institute of Neuropathology. During her practice, she published several papers on hemifacial spasm and encephalitic parkinsonism (Levi, 1922; Levi, 1923). After Negro's death, her interest shifted toward childhood neuropsychiatric disorders, and in 1955 she obtained a professorship in childhood and adolescent psychiatry. She authored the first Italian treatise on sex education (*L'educazione sessuale: orientamenti per i genitori*, Levi, 1962).

HIS LEGACY

Camillo Negro was a keen clinician, who paid particular attention to neurological signs and symptoms, and a reputable researcher, especially in the areas of electrophysiology and movement disorders. He strongly supported the dignity of neurology as an independent science, at a time when neurology and psychiatry were still combined as a single teaching subject in Italian universities. In this respect also Negro was a precursor when we consider that neurology and psychiatry were separated only in 1976, some 49 years after his death. The most important legacy of Professor Negro, however, remains his passion for teaching and for what we would define today as public engagement activities with a general audience, as witnessed by the periodical he edited for physicians and by the movies he filmed. Once again, Negro was, undeniably, a forerunner of the modern communication of scientific discoveries to a lay audience. Interestingly, in the Italian landscape of science communication, the best-known key player is Piero Angela, son of Carlo Angela, who is one of the scholars mentioned earlier, for whom Camillo Negro served as a mentor.

REFERENCES

Angela C (1913) *Il riso ed il pianto spasmodico nelle lesioni cerebrali d'origine vascolare*. Torino: Lattes.

Angela C (1914) I disturbi della sensibilità ed i disturbi cardiaci nella malattia di Friedreich. *Rivista Neurologica*, 1: 67–80.

Aubert G (2002) Arthur van Gehuchten takes neurology to the movies. *Neurology*, 59 (10): 1612–1618.

Buda O, Arsene D, Ceausu M, Dermengiu D, & Curca G C (2009) Georges Marinesco and the early research in neuropathology. *Neurology*, 72(1): 88–91.

Chiò A, Gianetto C, & Dagna S (2016) Professor Camillo Negro's neuropathological films. *Journal of the History of the Neurosciences*, 25(1): 39–50.

Dagna S, & Gianetto C (2013) Volti senza maschera: una nuova edizione dei filmati neuropatologici di Camillo Negro. *Immagine*, 6(1): 16–31.

F.E.Z. (1908) I progressi della scienza. La Nevropatologia nella Cinematografia. *Gazzetta del Popolo*, 17 febbraio 1908.

Ghiglione P, Mutani R, Chiò A (2005) Cogwheel rigidity. *Archives of Neurology*, 62(5): 828–830.
Jones E (2012) War Neuroses and Arthur Hurst: A pioneering medical film about the treatment of psychiatric battle casualties. *Journal of the History of Medicine and Allied Sciences*, 67(3): 345–373.
Levi L (1922) *Sugli emispasmi facciali di origine nervosa periferica*. Milano: Pensiero medico.
Levi L (1923). *Sopra un caso di parkinsonismo encefalitico con disturbi mentali*. Pensiero medico.
Levi L. (1962) *L'educazione sessuale: orientamenti per i genitori*. Roma: Editori Riuniti.
Mazza S, Pavone A, & Niedermeyer E (2002) Mario Gozzano: The work of an EEG pioneer. *Clinical Electroencephalography*, 33(4): 155–159.
Mazzarello P (2006) *Il Nobel dimenticato. La vita e la scienza di Camillo Golgi*. Torino: Bollati Boringhieri.
Negro C (1884) De l'action que l'acide chlorhydrique dilué exerces sur la sensibilité et la motilité des nerfs. *Archives Italiennes de Biologie*, 6(6): 357–365.
Negro C (1885) Un po' di fisiologia a 1200 metri sul livello del mare. In A Paschetto (Ed.), *Atti dell'Associazione Prealpina Biellese*, 19–22. Biella: Tipografia Amosso.
Negro C (1888) Les courant unipolaires induits appliqués à l'étude de l'excitabilité du cerveau. *Archives Italiennes de Biologie*, 9: 48.
Negro C (1888) Sur les terminations nerveuses motrices. *Archives Italiennes de Biologie*, 9(1): 49–51.
Negro C (1889) Les courants unipolaires dans l'étude de l'excitabilité électrique du cerveau. *Archives Italiennes de Biologie*, 11: 212–225.
Negro C (1889–1890). La terminazione nervosa motrice dei muscoli striati; nota prima (nuovo metodo di colorazione). *Archives Italiennes de Biologie*, 25: 1889–1890.
Negro C (1890) Nuovo metodo di colorazione della terminazione nervosa motrice dei muscoli striati. *Bollettino dei Musei di Zoologia e Anatomia Comparata della Regia Università di Torino*, 5(76): 35–38.
Negro C (1907) Di un fenomeno che si verifica durante la rotazione massima verso l'alto del bulbo oculare nei casi di paralisi del corrispondente muscolo frontale. *Rivista di Neuropatologia*, 2(1–2): 129–138, 161–167.
Negro C (1908) Sui risultati di ricerche sperimentali sull'azione fisiologica che esercitano sui nervi motori della rana le scariche elettriche di piccolo potenziale, ottenute da un polo unico di coppie voltaiche. *Archivi di Psichiatria e Neuropatologia*, 29(8): 563–577.
Negro C (1915) Ricerche sperimentali di elettrofisiologia sull'azione che esercitano sui nervi motori della rana le scariche elettriche a basso potenziale ottenute a circuito aperto dai singoli poli di copie voltaiche. *Atti della Reale Accademia dei Lincei*, serie V, 10(14): 632–669.
Negro C (1918) L'emploi de la poudre bleue de tournesol dans l'étude topographique des sudations locales de la peau. *Archives Italiennnes de Biologie*, 68(2): 131–134.
Negro C (1921) Osservazioni sulla sindrome Parkinsoniana dell'encefalite letargica. *Minerva Medica*, 1(1): 45–50.
Negro C (1922) Sul fenomeno della troclea dentata nella malattia di Parkinson e nel parkinsonismo dell'encefalite epidemica. *Rivista di Patologia Nervosa e Mentale*, 27(3): 269–275.
Negro C, & Antoniotti F (1885) Termometria del corpo umano normale nella fatica. In A Paschetto (Ed.), *Atti dell'Associazione Prealpina Biellese*, 41–47. Biella: Tipografia Amosso.
Negro C, & Negro F (1922) Annotazioni cliniche relative al parkinsonismo postencefalitico. *Pensiero Medico*, 38–39(1): 669–681.
Negro C, & Roasenda G (1907) Risultati di esperienze sulla eccitabilità del cervelletto alle correnti elettriche unipolari. *Archivi di Psichiatria e Neuropatologia*, 28(2): 125–132.
Negro C, & Roasenda G (1909) Risultati di una IV serie di ricerche sperimentali sulla fisiologia del cervelletto. *Rivista di Neuropatologia*, 3(1): 13–19.

Negro C, & Treves Z (1901) Physiopathologie de la contraction musculaire volontaire (maladie de Parkinson). *Archives Italiennes de Biologie*, 26(2): 121–123.
Negro F (1938) *Trattamento delle sindromi parkinsoniane postencefalitiche con le radici di atropa belladonna*. Torino: I.T.E.R.
Ormezzano G (1891) *Cenni storici sul regio collegio Carlo Alberto per gli studenti delle provincie in Torino e sulle varie fondazioni al medesimo annesse*. Torino: Tipografia Editrice G. Candeletti.
Piccardi G (1929) *Policlinico generale di Torino 'Re Umberto I'*. Torino: Tipografia Editrice Minerva.
Roasenda G (1927) Camillo Negro. *Minerva Medica*, 7(32): 1237–1241.
Roasenda G (1957) *La neuropatologia e la psichaitria all'Università di Torino nella prima metà del secolo XX*. Torino: Tipografia Bellone.
von Economo K (1917) Encephalitis lethargica. *Wiener klinische Wochenschrift*, 30(6): 581–585.

CHAPTER 11

Brief Happy Military-Neurophysiological Stint of Mario Camis in Wartime Turin

GIOVANNI BERLUCCHI

Mario Camis (Venice, 1878 – Bologna, 1946) spent in Turin, during and in the aftermath of World War I, a brief period of his wandering and troubled life that turned out to be very important for Italian neuroscience.

An ardent patriot, after Italy entered the war in 1915, he returned from Argentina to enroll in the army as a medical captain. To be able to do this, he gave up the professorship of physiology at the University of La Plata to which he had been appointed by the Argentinian government just two years earlier. After working for some time in field hospitals, he was put in charge of evaluating potential airplane pilots for fitness for flying and air combat in the Psycho-physiological Office of Military Aviation in Turin. Since its foundation, in the summer of 1917, the Office was housed in the University Institute of Physiology. Professor Amedeo Herlitzka (1872–1949) headed the Institute as well as the Office. He was one of the many disciples of the eminent physiologist Angelo Mosso (1846–1910) and had succeeded him as the chair of Physiology at the University of Turin. In addition to the Turin Psycho-physiological Office, attitudinal psychophysical evaluations of candidate aviators also were carried out in a laboratory set up at the Supreme Military Command by Agostino Gemelli (more about him later) and in two other psychophysiological offices. The first of these offices was located in Rome and headed by the physiologist Alberto Aggazzotti (1877–1963), a pupil of Mosso and Herlitzka; the second office was located in Naples and led by the pathologist Gino Galeotti (1867–1921). The support that physiology could then offer to aviation was chiefly based on the studies performed by Mosso in the laboratories at the Col d'Olen and the "Capanna Margherita" on Mount Rosa on life functions at high altitudes. In Herlitzka's words, Mosso's results on the physiology of mountaineers could be advantageously applied, *mutatis mutandis*, to the physiology of aviators (Herlitzka, 1923). Mosso, however, had been a firm believer in the theoretical and practical usefulness of a continuous interaction between physiology and psychology, and with that aim in mind he had attracted Wundt's disciple Frederick Kiesow (1858–1940) to the University of Turin. As implied by the "psycho-physiological" adjective in the name of the Aviation Office, psychology and physiology could both contribute to the Office's practical purposes, particularly concerning the impact of emotionality on aviation ability. Herlitzka held Camis in esteem and appointed him deputy director of the Psycho-physiological Office. Camis was in charge of investigating emotionality in military-pilot candidates. He occupied this position with the degree of major until almost the end of 1919.

A "BORN PHYSIOLOGIST"

When in Turin, Camis had no official position at an Italian university. Still, he was already well-known internationally as an established researcher and scholar who had been asked by John Newport Langley (1852–1925), the Cambridge professor of physiology, to edit the English translation of Luigi Luciani's *Fisiologia dell'Uomo* [Physiology of Man]. Born in 1878 in Venice to upper-middle-class Jewish parents from Verona, Camis studied medicine at the universities of Bologna and Rome. Camis obtained his degree from the latter University with a thesis supervised by Luciani himself. Camis became academically related to Mosso through Vittorio Aducco (1860–1937), Mosso's oldest pupil, collaborator, and a regular experimental subject in Mosso's famous studies on fatigue (Mosso, 1904). Aducco had left Turin to take up the chair of Physiology first at the University of Siena (1891), and then at the University of Pisa (1894), where Camis joined him in 1902 as an assistant in the Institute of Physiology, which was then located in the Medical School, near the Santa Chiara Hospital. Aducco thought highly of Camis, whom he regarded as a "born physiologist"; and despite the difference in age and academic rank, a real friendship developed (Pupilli, 1941, 1947). Yet Camis needed more intellectual stimulation than Pisa could offer, and in 1907 he took an extended sabbatical to work in physiological laboratories in England, first in Cambridge and then in Liverpool. In Cambridge, he collaborated with Joseph Barcroft (1872–1947) in pioneering research on the respiratory functions of the blood and, later, in the organization of the 1911 British scientific expedition to Mosso's laboratories on Mount Rosa for the study of high-altitude physiology. Barcroft and Camis joined the expedition both as scientists and as experimental subjects (Barcroft, Camis et al., 1915). In Liverpool, Camis met the man whom he always regarded as his true maestro in science and life: Charles Scott Sherrington, the Father of Neurophysiology, who would win the Nobel Prize in 1932. Camis brought back Sherrington's ideas and techniques from Liverpool to Pisa, and he did research work on the vestibular system and the cerebellum. But not for long, because, once again, his restless nature took him far away from Italy. As already mentioned, in 1913 he was granted a professorship of physiology at the University of La Plata in Argentina, which he gave up in 1915 to join the Italian army in the war effort. We shall see how his ending up in Herlitzka's psycho-physiological office made a small, but noteworthy, addition to the history of neuroscience in Turin.

REACTION TIMES AND EMOTIONALITY IN ASPIRING AVIATORS

Camis screened the aspiring aviators based on their resilience toward an emotional perturbation induced by unexpectedly startling stimuli, such as a nearby explosion of a petard or the sudden release of a strong hissing air jet at the neck or a forearm. He assessed simple reaction times to visual and acoustic signals, and choice reaction times to visual cues, before and just after the startling experience. Reaction times had been imported to Turin by Kiesow, and Herlitzka had been a keen adopter of this method among the physiologists (Herlitzka, 1908). Camis's results were published in a research paper in the *Giornale di Medicina Militare* [Journal of Military Medicine] in January 1919, and reported, almost verbatim, in his book on the mechanism of the emotions in the same year (Camis, 1919a, 1919b). The results indicated that the emotional perturbation systematically increased the mean time of simple reactions by about 17% with visual stimuli and about 15% with acoustic stimuli. Continuous graphic plots of reaction time showed that the return to pre-perturbation values of the speed of reaction varied considerably among individuals, presumably as a function of their constitutional resilience. For the assessment of choice reaction time, Camis used the Herlitzka apparatus consisting of four light sources spatially arranged as the main cardinal points around a fifth central light source (Figure 11.1 and Figure 11.2). Subjects had to quickly move a lever, in a spatially compatible manner, in response to the lighting of each of the four peripheral sources, and to refrain from responding to the lighting of the central source.

Emotional perturbation did not influence the number of errors and, surprisingly, decreased choice reaction time in the majority of subjects. Based on these results, Camis suggested that the emotional perturbation interfered negatively with the speed of simple psycho-motor reactions, while, on the contrary, it tended to facilitate higher psychical functions such as choice and decision. He also mentioned that the ability to refrain from responding to the central light source of the Herlitzka apparatus in the choice reaction time experiment could be taken as a measure of the capacity for inhibition, but he did not provide data to corroborate this. For the practical purposes of the selection of aviation personnel at the psycho-physiological office, the paper proposed the following classification: "good" if the emotional reaction time increase in the simple task was equal to or smaller than 10%; "mediocre" if the increase was between 10% and 25%; and "inept" if the increase was more than 25%. In the words of an American commentator, "(a)lthough these limits are somewhat arbitrary their choice is colored by the fact that patients whose hardships had rendered their nervous condition clearly pathological showed the greatest effect" (Johnson, 1923).

THE BOOK ON EMOTIONS

Camis's experience with the evaluation of emotionality led him to write a book on emotions. He completed the book in July 1919, and it was published in the same year by the Fratelli Bocca, a historical publishing house based in Turin. Its title (*The*

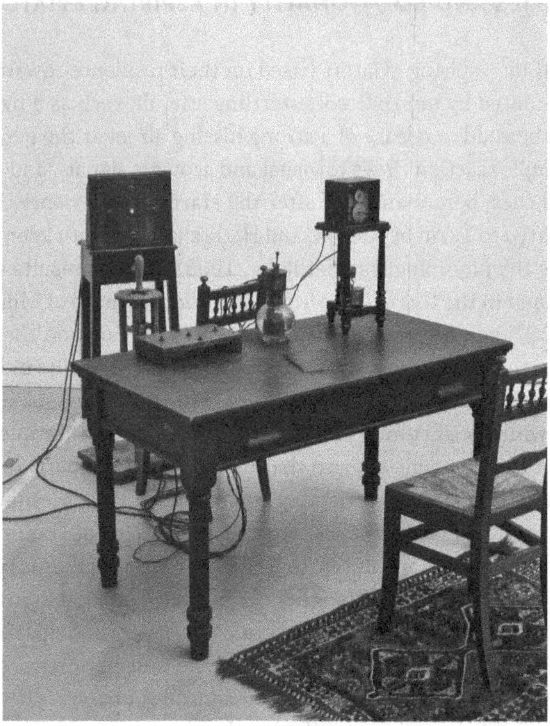

Figure 11.1. Herlitzka's original apparatus for testing choice reaction times is preserved at the Sistema Museale d'Ateneo, ASTUT, Archivio Scientifico e Tecnologico dell'Università di Torino. Herlitzka described it in his book *Fisiologia ed Aviazione* (1923), p. 131–132. Subjects were to move a lever in one of the four cardinal directions in response to the appearance on the screen of a light at one of the four cardinal points in a spatially compatible manner (right for right, left for left, forward for top, backward for bottom). Reaction times were measured with the Hipp chronoscope and response accuracy was checked with electrical circuits closed by the final position of the lever. When a central light appeared, subjects had to refrain from responding, using their capacity for inhibition. The photograph is available at the website http://www.grandeguerra.unito.it/items/show/635 and is reproduced here by permission of ASTUT, Archivio Scientifico e Tecnologico dell'Università di Torino.

Mechanism of the Emotions) is the same as the one Mosso had given to his 1899 conference at the decennial celebration of Clark University in Worcester, Massachusetts, while its subtitle (*History—Critique – Experiments*) synthesizes the structure of the narrative. Throughout Camis's life, Sherrington was his guiding light and his scientific inspiration; this strong influence is apparent as well in Camis's book on emotions. In 1900, Sherrington had published experiments to refute the peripheral or physiological or somatic theory of emotions, ascribed by him to James, Lange, and Sergi (Sherrington, 1900a, 1900b). William James, the Harvard physiologist–psychologist–philosopher, and the Danish neuropsychiatrist Carl Lange had independently put forward the hypothesis that the subjective component of emotions is caused directly not by external emotion-laden stimuli, but by the bodily responses to

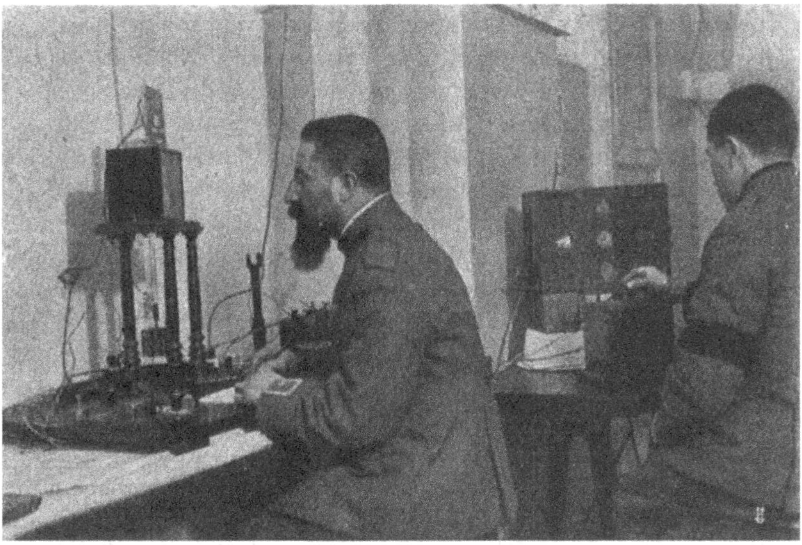

Figure 11.2. The photograph shows Mario Camis testing an aspirant pilot with the Herlitzka's apparatus for choice reaction times at the Ufficio Psico - Fisiologico dell'Aviazione - Sezione di Torino. Camis, sitting in front of the Hipp chronoscope, delivers the stimuli, checks the accuracy of the response and records the response time. (From p. 148 in Herlitzka A., L'arruolamento dei piloti dell'aria, in Le Vie d'Italia, III (2): 137–145, 1919).

such stimuli. Without vasomotor responses–according to Lange–and more generally without vascular, visceral, and motor responses–according to James–the psychical process of emotion would not exist. Sherrington had added the name of Giuseppe Sergi, professor of anthropology at the University of Rome, to those of James and Lange. In fact, Sergi had supported their theory by arguing that emotional stimuli act on the medulla oblongata, producing cardiac, vascular, and respiratory effects as well as effects upon the abdominal and pelvic viscera. Sherrington, instead, found that expressions of emotions, such as joy, anger, fear, and disgust, persisted in the cephalic region of dogs deprived of visceral sensations and vascular reactions in most other parts of their bodies, in obvious contrast with the James-Lange-Sergi theory. It may be of interest to historians of Turin neuroscience that in his paper in the *Proceedings of the Royal Society of London,* Sherrington mentions an experiment that he carried out "in the laboratory of my friend Professor Mosso of Turin," presumably in 1899. This must have occurred on the occasion of his meetings with Mosso in preparation for the fifth International Congress of Physiologists, which was to take place in 1901 in Turin, with Sherrington as Anglo-American Secretary. In a dog with a complete disconnection between the vasomotor center and the spinal cord, there was an increase in blood pressure, despite a heart frequency decrease, when the dog heard the noise of the stimulator used in the past on the conscious animal for demarcating sensitive from anesthetic skin areas with painful stimulations. Sherrington attributed those effects to an emotion engendered in the dog by an acoustic stimulus that in its experience had been associated with pain. More specifically, he attributed the heart frequency decrease to a vagal action and the blood pressure increase to an increase in respiratory frequency, both effects being caused by the brain memory of the painful experience, independent of any feedback from viscera or blood vessels. Based on Sherrington's report of that single experiment, Dror (1999) wrote that Sherrington "discovered" emotions in Turin. Yet, this seems doubtful, because he must have known James's *Principles of Psychology* independent of Mosso and his most important experiments on emotions in dogs were performed in Liverpool.

In his book, Camis discussed the theories of James, Lange (whom he cited with the initials F. A. rather than C., presumably in mistaken reference to the neo-Kantian philosopher Friedrich Albert Lange), and Sergi in the light of the theoretical considerations of the concept of emotion by many authors of those times, including Mosso and Kiesow, and based on empirical results from animal experiments, such as those of Sherrington, Cannon, and others, as well as from his psycho-physiological tests of aspiring pilots. He concluded that the mechanism of the emotion must be conceived as the result of two factors: the sensory or representational cerebral reaction to the exciting stimulus, and its cortical elaboration, whether conscious or unconscious, aimed at the protection of the organism. The visceral functional changes associated with the second factor may contribute to the psychical process but are not its primary cause. A benevolent reviewer of the book (Carrara, 1922) wrote that Camis's reaction time results had provided impressive, if not decisive, evidence that the origin of emotional states must be sought centrally rather than peripherally, that is in the brain rather than in the body. Yet, by modern standards, the reaction time data presented by Camis were insufficient to draw any definite conclusion. Nevertheless, Camis's book on the emotions had the merit of putting together much of the physiological and psychological information available at the time, including reflections on the emotional behavior and experiences of actors on the stage, such as the Diderot paradox according to which the best actors must be completely unemotional and its devastating critique by Binet (1896), only partially shared by Camis.

A CONSPICUOUS OMISSION

The extensive bibliography of Camis's book contains 182 references in four languages (Italian, English, French, and German) and contributions from not only physiology and psychology, but also from psychiatry and the humanities. But there was a conspicuous and surprising omission in it. In 1909, a man who was specializing in psychology in Turin with Kiesow published a thorough description of the theories and experiments on the physiology, psychology, and philosophy of emotions in the *Rivista di Filosofia Neoscolastica* [Journal of Neoscholastic Philosophy]. In this journal, admittedly, one would not expect to find a paper titled *The Somatic Theory of Emotion*. The author of that paper was the Franciscan friar Agostino (formerly Edoardo) Gemelli, the future founder of the Catholic University in Milan and a dominant figure in Italian psychology for many decades. Gemelli and Camis were born in the same year, 1878, and their lives shared several significant events and vicissitudes. Both had graduated in Medicine, and both had been trained in science by Nobel Prize winners in physiology or medicine, Gemelli by Golgi in Pavia (Cosmacini, 1985) and Camis by Sherrington in Liverpool (Berlucchi, 2008; Berlucchi & Moruzzi, 2017). As a medical student, Gemelli had been an atheist and a Marxist socialist, but shortly after graduating, he converted to Catholicism and entered the Franciscan order. Camis belonged to a Jewish family of ancient Sephardic lineage and, after the death of his wife in 1930, he also converted to Catholicism and became a Dominican friar. The different paths and destinies of their lives, tragic in the case of Camis (Moruzzi, 1948; Cosmacini, 1985; Gondola & Ferrari, 2012; Berlucchi & Moruzzi, 2017), are told elsewhere. For the purposes of the present chapter, it is appropriate to suppose that Gemelli and Camis must have interacted in some way during the Great War, when both were involved in the testing of aspiring pilots. Camis's neglect of Gemelli's paper on emotions is therefore surprising, all the more so because in that paper Gemelli claimed to have repeated and confirmed Sherrington's experiments on dogs and cats, presumably in a laboratory that he kept at the Sant'Antonio convent in Milan (Cosmacini, 1985). However, he never reported those results in detail in specific publications, while in that period he published several research papers on the anatomy and physiology of the hypophysis. Neither Camis's book nor Gemelli's paper appear to have left enduring traces worthy of note in the modern literature on emotion. Both of them, however, attest to the intellectual stature of two fascinating characters of early 20th-century science in Italy.

ELECTRICAL RECORDINGS FROM THE CEREBELLUM OF DOGS

Camis was, by nature and by training, an experimental physiologist, a phrase which, at that time, meant someone who performs experiments on animals. Upon his return from England to Pisa in 1910, he started intensive experimental work in the newly built Institute of Physiology in via San Zeno, which, decades later, became the theater of the neurophysiological research guided by his pupil Giuseppe Moruzzi. In Pisa, Camis studied the anatomical relations between the labyrinth and the cerebellum by tracing the central degeneration of fibers of the VIIIth cranial nerve after the destruction of the semicircular canals in dogs and cats. In the footsteps of Stefani, Luciani, and Sherrington, he believed that the cerebellum was the reflex center for the impulses arising from the vestibular or nonacoustic labyrinth. His histological findings suggested that the vestibular projections to the cerebellum were predominantly directed at the cerebellar nuclei and to a lesser degree to the cerebellar cortex. In a fit of restlessness, he abandoned this research subject in 1913 when he moved to the University of La Plata, in Argentina. While in Turin, he profited from the hospitality of Professor Herlitzka at the Institute of Physiology for resuming his interest in the relations between labyrinth and cerebellum, as investigated with a new method.

He employed the large model of the Einthoven's string galvanometer developed by the Edelman firm in Munich to record the electrical responses of the cerebellar cortex and nuclei to mechanical, electrical, and natural stimulations of the semicircular canals. At the Turin Institute, Herlitzka and Gayda used the string galvanometer for obtaining electrical measures of the heat produced by non-nervous organs such as the heart and the salivary glands, and the apparatus was made available to Camis. Camis's experiments were carried out in the summer of 1919, and the results were published at the end of that same year in Volume 1 of the newly founded *Archivio di Scienze Biologiche*, the official journal of the Italian Society for Experimental Biology. Camis's affiliation in the paper refers to the Institute of Physiology of Turin, headed by Professor A. Herlitzka, and the paper ends on a note of thanks to Herlitzka himself for allowing the author to use his laboratory and for giving him help and advice. In dogs under "AEC" narcosis (meaning presumably atropine-ether-chloroform), Camis exposed a median region of the cerebellar cortex in the region of the lobuli simplex and ansiformis; he also exposed the bony semicircular canals in the *rocca petrosa* of one side through a personally developed occipital approach. Mechanical stimulation consisted in the repeated scraping of the bony canals, while electrical stimulation of the canals was both faradic and single-shock. Natural vestibular stimulation was carried out by a 90- or 180-degree rotation of the prone horizontal animal to bring it in a vertical head-up position or a supine horizontal position. The effectiveness of stimulations was assessed based on the appearance of nystagmus during the stimulation, which was the case with mechanical and single-shock but not faradic or rotating stimulation. No electrical responses were ever recorded from the cerebellar cortex. In contrast, short or long-lasting monophasic, biphasic, or multiphasic responses were obtained when the cerebellar cortex was removed and the recording electrodes were brought in the vicinity of the cerebellar nuclei in both vermis and hemispheres, one in the fastigial nucleus and the other in the dentate nucleus. Faradic stimulation was ineffective, whereas a single-shock stimulation induced both nystagmus and a monophasic electrical response from the nuclei. When present, electrical cerebellar responses were stronger on the side of the stimulated labyrinth than on the other side. Camis's work on the cerebellum in Turin was of some historical importance because it was the second attempt, after the Beck and Bikeles (1912) study on curarized dogs, to record cerebellar "action currents," that is electrical activity presumably related to function. Also, because Beck and Bikeles (1912) had limited their observations to cerebellar vermal responses elicited by stimulations of the anterior and posterior limb nerves and the vagus nerve, Camis's effort provided the first-ever, if tentative, physiological demonstration of the influence of the vestibular labyrinth on cerebellar electrogenesis. Unlike Caton and Beck, however, who were eventually credited for discovering the spontaneous electrical activity of the cerebral cortex before Berger's electroencephalogram and for being pioneers of the evoked potentials (Brazier, 1959), Camis's work on the evoked electrical activity of the cerebellum received scanty recognition in the international literature. At that time, ideas about the functioning of the cerebellum were under the influence of the articulate, but mistaken belief of Horsley and Clarke (1908) that the cerebellar cortex was electrically unexcitable, insofar as its stimulation produced no motor effects (Dow & Moruzzi, 1958). Camis's attempt to attribute to the cerebellar nuclei, but not to the cerebellar cortex, a role in the vestibular reflexes was undoubtedly misguided by that mistaken belief. He cannot be blamed for trying to begin to analyze anatomo-functional relations that would be understood only many years later, with the benefit of a detailed knowledge of the neuronal machinery and architecture of the cerebellum (Eccles et al., 1967; Ito, 1984).

EPILOGUE

Camis probably had a very good time in Turin. He was working for his beloved country in a war and, at the same time, he could do research. He was with his wife Beatrice Cagli, also Jewish, whom he married in 1916, and their marriage, though childless, was a happy one (Berlucchi & Moruzzi, 2017; Figure 11.3). From an academic perspective, the time spent by Camis in Turin was of great importance for neuroscience: not so much for what he accomplished there in research, though the results were valuable, but primarily because of the opportunity to restart his academic career in Italy. Beginning in October 1919, he moved to the University of Parma, where he became a full professor of Physiology in 1925 as the successor of Alberto Aggazzotti, who had directed the Aviation Psycho-Physiological Office in Rome. As attested to by various publications (Pupilli, 1941, 1949; Moruzzi, 1948; Gondola & Ferrari, 2012; Berlucchi & Moruzzi, 2017), in Parma, Camis exerted a

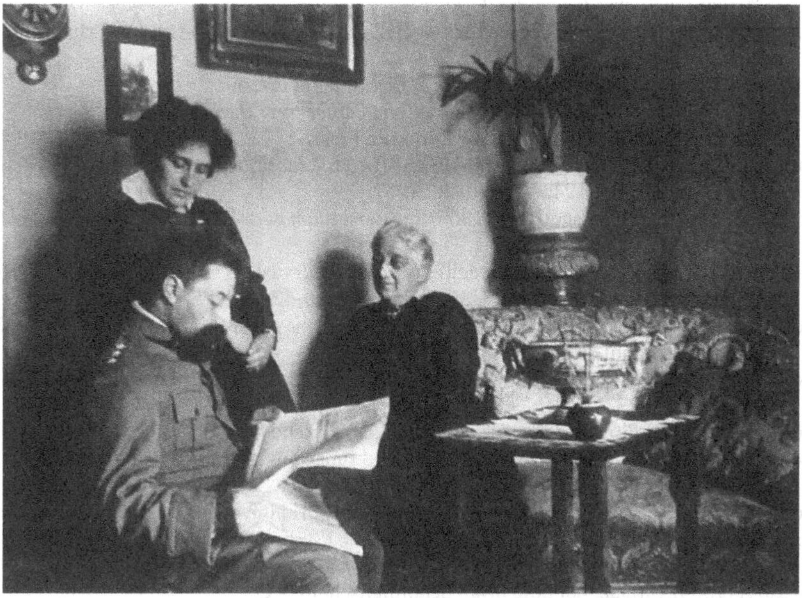

Figure 11.3. Medical officer Captain Mario Camis with his wife Beatrice Cagli and his mother Elisabetta Rava during the Great War (courtesy of Vasco Senatore Gondola, Caprino Veronese).

strong influence on the development of physiology and biochemistry. One of his great merits was instructing the young Giuseppe Moruzzi in the Sherringtonian methods for studying the nervous system and for launching him on a career as a world-class neurophysiologist. All those interested in the history of neuroscience in Italy know how much Italian neuroscientists owe to Moruzzi. But they should also be aware of the fortunate circumstances that, through Herlitzka and Turin, brought Camis back to Italy and allowed him to give Moruzzi to neuroscience.

REFERENCES

Barcroft J, Camis M, Mathison C G, Roberts F, & Ryffel J H (1915) Report of the Monte Rosa Expedition of 1911. *Philosophical Transactions of the Royal Society of London. Series B*, 206: 49–102.

Beck A, & Bikeles G (1912) Versuche über die sensorische Funktion des Kleinhirnmittelstücks (Vermis). *Pflüger's Archiv für Physiologie*, 143: 296–302.

Berlucchi G (2008) British roots of Italian neurophysiology in the early 20th century. *Current Biology*, 18: R51–R56.

Berlucchi G, & Moruzzi P (2017) Mario Camis—the forgotten physiologist who introduced Giuseppe Moruzzi to neurophysiology. *pH*, 2: 2–26.

Binet A (1896) Réflexions sur le paradoxe de Diderot. *L'année psychologique*, 3: 279–295.

Brazier M A B (1984) Pioneers in the discovery of evoked potentials. *Electroencephalography and Clinical Neurophysiology*, 59: 2–8.

Camis M (1919a) Un mezzo per giudicare il grado di sensibilità agli stimoli emozionali. *Giornale di Medicina Militare*, 67: 188–196.

Camis M (1919b) *Il meccanismo delle emozioni. Storia—Critica—Esperimenti.* Torino: Fratelli Bocca.

Camis M (1919c) Le correnti d'azione nel cervelletto per eccitamento del labirinto. *Archivio di Scienze Biologiche*, 1: 92–119.

Carrara M (1922) A. Camis—Il meccanismo delle emozioni. Storia, critica, riferimenti. *Scientia*, 31: 167–169.

Cosmacini G (1985) *Gemelli. Il Machiavelli di Dio*. Milano: Rizzoli.

Dow R S, & Moruzzi G (1958) *The Physiology and Pathology of the Cerebellum.* Minneapolis: The University of Minnesota Press.

Dror O E (1999) The affect of experiment: The turn to emotions in Anglo-American physiology, 1900–1940. *Isis*, 90: 205–237.

Eccles J C, Ito M, & Szentágothai J (1967) *The Cerebellum as a Neuronal Machine.* New York: Springer-Verlag.

Gemelli A (1909) La teoria somatica dell'emozione: osservazioni critiche e ricerche. *Rivista di Filosofia Neoscolastica*, 1: 77–96; 241–268; 461–474; 570–590.

Gondola V S, & Ferrari G (Eds.) (2012) *Mario Camis: uomo di scienza e di fede (1878–1946).* Verona: Edizioni Stimmgraf.

Herlitzka A (1908) Ricerche cronografiche sui movimenti volontari bilaterali. *Archivio di Fisiologia*, 5: 277–284.

Herlitzka A (1923) *Fisiologia ed aviazione*. Bologna: Zanichelli.

Horsley V, & Clarke R H (1908) The structure and functions of the cerebellum examined by a new method. *Brain*, 31: 45–85.

Ito M (1984) *The Cerebellum and Neural Control*. New York: Raven Press.

Johnson H M (1923) Reaction-time measurements. *Psychological Bulletin*, 20: 562–589.

Moruzzi G (1948) Mario Camis (1878–1946). *Archivio di Scienze Biologiche*, 32:159–163.

Mosso A (1904) *Fatigue*. London: Swan Schonnenschein & Co.

Pupilli G C (1941) *Di P.Alberto: il fisiologo.* Bollettino di S.Domenico. Anno XXII. Fasc.di luglio-agosto. Bergamo: Società Editrice Alessandro.

Pupilli G C (1949) Mario Camis. In: Il contributo veronese alle scienze mediche. *Il Fracastoro*, 42: 147–156.
Sherrington C S (1900a) Experiments on the value of vascular and visceral factors for the genesis of emotion. *Proceedings of the Royal Society of London*, 66: 390–403.
Sherrington C S (1900b) Experimentation on emotion. *Nature*, 62: 328–331.

CHAPTER 12

Seeing the History of Neuroscience in Turin through the Lenses of Its Instruments/Part 2

MARCO R. GALLONI

During the 19th century, anatomy and physiology progressively became distinct disciplines. Yet, they closely interacted to capture the complexity of the brain with constructive collaborations that transcended the respective boundaries. For example, the anatomist Carlo Giacomini (1840–1898) often worked with the physiologist Angelo Mosso (1846–1910). Mosso was a brilliant student and became very skilled in handling the physiological instruments. After graduation, he worked in Leipzig, within the laboratories of Carl Ludwig (1816–1895), and later in Paris, where he met Claude Bernard (1813–1878) and Étienne-Jules Marey (1830–1904). Mosso became an expert in the use of Ludwig's kymograph (Ludwig, 1847), which is a clockwork-driven tool for the continuous time-recording of biological phenomena (Figure 12.1), and Marey's tympanum, which was a sensible pneumatic capsule by which even minimal movements could be recorded (Marey, 1885). As we have seen in Chapter 8, the first original apparatus invented by Mosso was the plethysmograph, which could measure the slow changes in volume of the forearm because of variations in blood supply caused by contraction or relaxation of smooth muscle cells in the media layer of local arteries (Mosso, 1875). These movements are under the control of the autonomic nervous system, so these measures give evidence of the effects exerted on the blood flow by emotional states and variations of cerebral and respiratory activities.

More generally, the collaboration between Mosso and Giacomini revolved around the pulsation of the cerebral vessels, the so-called "brain movements" (Giacomini et al., 1876): After cranial traumas, openings in the bones of the skulls of a man and a woman could be noticed. Through these openings, which were covered only by the skin, the membrane of a tympanum of Marey could be pushed against the

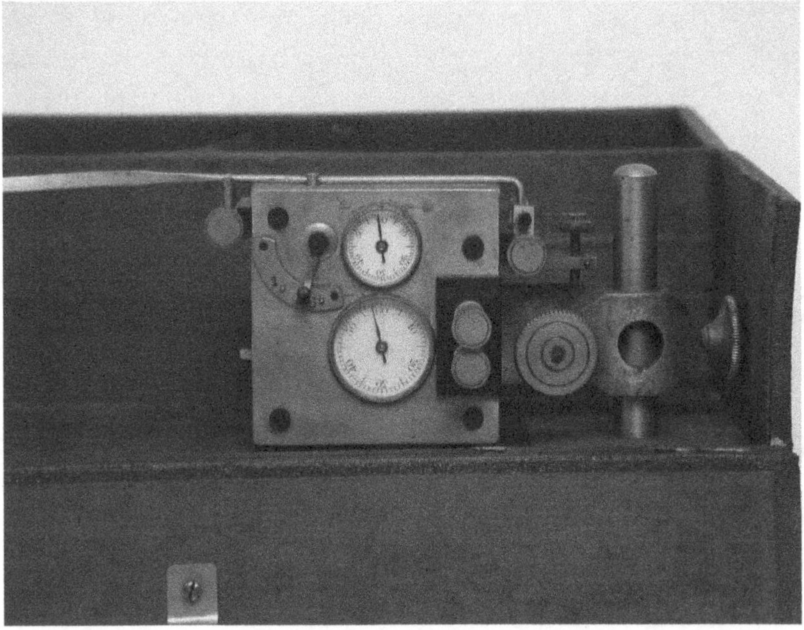

Figure 12.1. The chronograph invented by the Swiss watchmaker James Jaquet was made in Paris by G. Boulitte: It is a stopwatch with a stylus that writes a time-base line on the kymograph paper to evaluate the duration of recorded physiological events. Courtesy of Marco Galloni.

meninx and, via a hydro-pneumatic system, the movements of this membrane were transmitted to the membrane of another tympanum connected to a pen writing on the paper of a kymograph. This way, the pulsation of the cerebral vessels was recorded, and this was an essential step in exploring the relationship between mental activity and cerebral circulation.

By exploiting a similar "human" experimental model, Mosso tried to quantify another parameter related to brain function: the variations of temperature (Mosso, 1894). For this purpose, he used very long thermometers that guaranteed an accuracy of more than one thousandth of centigrade degree. Another important instrument invented by Mosso was the ergograph, which was used to measure muscular exertion and fatigue, using the flexor of the second phalanx of the middle finger of the hand. While the forearm was kept fixed, the middle finger performed flexures and lifted a weight at any contraction via a string and a pulley. At each contraction, the movements of the weight were recorded with a kymograph. The results differed from one individual to another given that they depended on the various components of fatigue, including the psychological and emotional ones. For a better understanding of the nervous component of fatigue, Mosso also introduced the ponometer, an instrument similar to the ergograph, but which could disconnect the weight from the muscle at the very end of the contraction, so that the muscle was released from the weight during the relaxation phase.

As we have seen in Chapter 8, probably the most important instrument invented by Mosso for neurological research was the "human circulation balance" (Mosso, 1884), a forerunner of the modern techniques for neuroimaging (Sandrone et al., 2012). This was an oscillating bed working as a scale for the fine measure of the distribution of blood throughout the entire human body. A patient lying on this bed could oscillate, pivoting on his center of gravity, mainly in response to the respiratory movements, so that correlations between respiration and circulation could be identified through the simultaneous record of the blood flow to a foot, obtained with a plethysmograph. Mosso tried to study the relationship between the distribution of the blood to the brain and various types of stimulation, in the attempt to correlate cerebral activity and energy supply.

Approximately 20 years before the experiments that Mosso performed with the "human circulation balance," Vitige Tirelli (1866–1941) was born in Carpi, a *comune* not too far from Modena. He obtained his degree in medicine in Bologna and later, in Pavia, became one of the pupils of Camillo Golgi (1843–1926). As a psychiatrist and a pathologist, he then joined the old mental hospital of Collegno, near Turin. Tirelli's name is mostly attached to the use of photography as a documentation of altered behaviors: in a 20-year time frame spanning from 1890 to 1910, he produced hundreds of pictures of patients, in an attempt to show the most significant aspects of the various pathologies (Bruni, 1971). These pictures must be considered "snapshots," because their scientific value largely depended on the spontaneity of the images. This was made possible only at the beginning of the 1880s thanks to the introduction of relatively highly sensible dry photographic plates, such as the "Lumière" used by Tirelli.

Upon his arrival in Turin, Tirelli found a very lively scientific environment, with the School of Pathology directed by Giulio Bizzozero and Benedetto Morpurgo (1861–1944) Professor of Morbid Anatomy. The excellence in histology was confirmed in 1885, when Giovanni Martinotti (1857–1928) translated into Italian, and widely integrated with original observations, the manual of microscopic techniques written in Berlin by Karl Friedlander (1847–1887) (Friedlander, 1885). The pathology laboratory in Collegno had a renowned tradition of scientific quality; here, Tirelli had the opportunity to combine observations on both the macro- and microscopic levels of dead patients, so he could realize several photomicrographies with methods that appear rather outdated (Martinotti & Tirelli, 1899). For instance, the light source was then an Auer burner fed with gas directly produced in the laboratory, because electricity was not yet widely distributed in Turin at the end of the 19th century. Furthermore, the disadvantaged position of the building did not permit to capture sunbeams with a heliostat. Nevertheless, the pictures taken with a Zeiss microscope of neurons stained with the Golgi's "black reaction" are apparent even at high magnifications.

Despite the good quality and the clinical significance of Tirelli's pictures, the inadequacy of still photography to depict some of the behaviors caused by mental diseases was evident, but a new media appeared on stage. The first public presentation of cinematography took place in Paris at the end of 1895, when the brothers Auguste (1862–1954) and Louis (1864–1948) Lumière could show short sequences of moving pictures. This was the beginning of new technology and, even more, of a novel art. Yet the roots of the movie camera must be traced back to the physiology laboratory of Jules Marey (1830–1904) in Paris where, among other research topics, the movements of humans and animals were studied with dynamic photographic methods. Thanks to the pivotal contribution of the French inventor Georges Demeny (1850–1917), new cameras able to take pictures in sequence, with short time intervals, were devised. This technique is called chronophotography and allows the recording of fast movements in a series of different pictures. Those researchers were very close to the invention of cinematography; however, their aim was not the reproduction of the living image of life, but the fine analysis of the motion.

When cinematography grew up as an industry, in the first decade of the 20th century, Turin, which still hosts the National Museum of Cinema, became the capital of silent movies, both from the technical and the artistic point of view. In 1908, the clinical neurologist Camillo Negro (1861–1927) asked Roberto Omegna (1876–1948), an accomplished cinematographer, to help him in filming clinical cases of neurological disorders in the mental hospitals. Today, this is not only a documentation of pathological conditions; above all, it is a touching witness of the extremely poor life of those patients. And the high pictorial quality of these moving pictures is a rather surprising example of the perfection of the crank-driven cameras, made mainly of wood, which were used at that time. A historian of the scientific cinematography (Arnold, 1994) wrote that the sequence in which Negro himself is shown performing the successful treatment of an acute onset of hysteria can also be considered an archetypal example of a specific dramatic language. Nowadays, these images look quite naïve; for example, because of the poor recitation of the lady acting as a patient or the fabric-made scenery. A second and important part of this film was shot during the First World War and shows soldiers in a hospital deeply affected by shell shock. This was a completely new psychiatric disorder caused by the unbearable conditions of life in the trenches, with men exposed to the extreme violence of the battle carried out with the power of modern technological weapons.

The First World War produced more than 15 million deaths and many more wounded and amputees; among them, a high number of men suffered from head injuries, because this often was the most exposed part of the body in the trenches. It is less known that, during the first year of the war, Italian soldiers did not have iron helmets; only after the experience of shrapnel bombs and aviation attacks from the sky an urgent need for head protection became evident. The solution was the purchase of the Adrian helmet, which was already in use within the French army. Nevertheless, a high number of nonlethal head wounds, about 50% of the total, were treated in the first-line infirmaries and the war hospitals, even in the case of loss of cerebral matter. Surprisingly, the majority of these patients at the time experienced only minor functional problems from the cognitive point of view (Fasiani, 1916). These results contrasted sharply with the very negative approach of surgeons to abdominal wounds: Lacking any effective antibiotic therapy, these were left without any treatment, relying only on the natural and possibly fortunate resources of the patient. The observations of the neurologists were in contrast with the old and classic phrenology, introduced by Franz Joseph Gall (1758–1828) at the end of the 18h century, which already had been criticized by Rolando. Still, it had not been replaced by a more complete and satisfactory theory (Brugia, 1923). Therefore, the vast majority of surgeons who had to face the unprecedented number of wounds on all the fronts of the war were quite surprised by the results of operations carried out on profoundly injured heads of soldiers. Indeed, the clinical outcome often was more positive than expected, and many maimed veterans could return to civilian life and resume their previous jobs, despite the brain damage they had experienced.

Giuseppe Levi (1872–1965) was a military surgeon during World War I and afterward became Professor of Human Anatomy in Turin in 1919. He was a pioneer of the techniques of in-vitro tissue culture and realized, within a laboratory, a particular glass room to ensure better sterility, necessary for this research. Because of the shallow rate of growth of cultured cells, direct observation through the microscope was not sufficient, and stop-motion cinematography was needed, as this technique allows the virtual acceleration of slow movements. To organize all the equipment, Levi contacted the LUCE Institute, which was the national institution for educational cinema, founded in 1925 in Rome, in which the aforementioned Roberto Omegna was leading the scientific laboratory. The camera that was installed on the microscope was the German Askania Z 35mm movie camera, linked to a time-lapse timer, which could shoot one frame per minute. The first results were published in 1934 (Levi, 1934), and then neurons became the main subject of Levi's research about the in-vitro growth and differentiation (Levi et al., 1937). As you will read in the next chapters, the excellence of the scientific work accomplished by Giuseppe Levi and the impact of his mentoring is evidenced by the extraordinary result of three Nobel Prize winners coming from the Anatomy School of Turin: Salvador Luria in 1969, Renato Dulbecco in 1975, and Rita Levi-Montalcini in 1986.

REFERENCES

Arnold J M (1994) La grammaire cinématographique: une invention des scientifiques. In A Martinet (Ed.), *Le cinéma et la science*. Paris: CNRS Editions.

Brugia R (1923) *La irrealtà dei centri nervosi*. Bologna: Cappelli.

Bruni B (1971) *Un atlante inedito di psichiatria clinica di Vitige Tirelli*. Milano: U. Hoepli.

Fasiani G M (1916) Sopra alcuni casi di ferite da arma da fuoco del capo. *Giornale della R. Accademia di Medicina di Torino, anno LXXIX*, vol. 22: 278–294.

Friedlander C, & Martinotti G (1885) *La tecnica microscopica applicata alla clinica e all'anatomia patologica*. Torino: U.T.E.

Giacomini C, & Mosso A (1876) Esperienze sui movimenti del cervello nell'uomo. *Archivio per le Scienze Mediche*, vol. I: 245–278.

Levi G (1934) Explantation, besonders die Struktur und die biologischen Eigenschaften der in vitrogezuchteten Zellen und Gewebe. *Ergebnisse Anat. Und Entwicklungs Geschichte*, 31: 125–707.

Levi G, & Meyer H (1937) Die Struktur der lebenden Neuronen. Die Frage der Praexistenz der Neurofibrillen. *Anat. Anz.*, 83: 401–422.

Ludwig C (1847) Beiträge zur Kenntniss des Einflusses der Respirationsbewegungen auf den Blutlauf im Aortensysteme. *Archiv für Anatomie, Physiologie, und wissenschaftliche Medicin*, n. 4: 242–302.

Marey E J (1885) *La méthode graphique dans les sciences expérimentales et principalement en physiologie et en médecine. Deuxième tirage augmenté d'un supplément sur le développement de la méthode graphique par la photographie*. Paris: G. Masson.
Martinotti C, & Tirelli V (1899) La microfotografia applicata allo studio della struttura della cellula nei gangli spinali (con 5 tavole) *Annali di freniatria e scienze affini*, vol. IX: 229–272.
Mosso A (1875) Sopra un nuovo metodo per scrivere i movimenti dei vasi sanguigni nell'uomo. *Atti della Reale Accademia delle Scienze di Torino*, vol. IX: 21–81.
Mosso A (1884) Applicazione della bilancia allo studio della circolazione sanguigna dell'uomo. *Atti della Reale Accademia dei Lincei—Memorie della Classe di Scienze Fisiche, Matematiche e Naturali*, vol. XIX: 534–535.
Mosso A (1894) *La temperatura del cervello. Studi termometrici*. Milano: Treves.
Sandrone S, Bacigaluppi M, Galloni M R, & Martino G (2012) Angelo Mosso (1846–1910). *Journal of Neurology*, 259 (11): 2513–2514.

CHAPTER 13

Giulio Bizzozero and Aldo Perroncito

Reform and Regeneration

ARIANE DRÖSCHER

INTRODUCTION

During the postunification period, Giulio Bizzozero (1846–1901) was the central figure of the modernization of biomedical studies in Turin, and perhaps in Italy. He grew up when Italian science and medicine first suffered from political and scientific isolation. Then, after the unification in 1861, he saw the country going through a period of profound institutional and theoretical transformation, to which he actively contributed.

The reformist politicians and scientists built their hopes on the new generation of scholars who graduated in the 1860s. A selected group of them received scholarships to study abroad. This was a chance for them to learn new theories, techniques, and institutional settings before returning to Italy with a Chair, laboratories, and funds. Bizzozero was one of these and did not disappoint expectations. In Turin, he brought Italian pathology and cytology back to international standards. Moreover, he founded modern research and teaching facilities, and established a highly successful research school. He also championed several public-health-related values. For all these merits, he is remembered as the "Italian Virchow" (Cappelletti, 1968). The following paragraphs will trace his role in the tormented process that transformed Turin into the most prominent Italian medical faculty of the 1880s.

Bizzozero's scientific investigations did not focus on the nervous system. Only two of his numerous publications dealt with neurohistology. Shortly after he settled in Turin, he coauthored a report with Camillo Golgi (1843–1926; Bizzozero & Golgi, 1873). One year later, he coauthored with Cesare Lombroso (1835–1909) a brief note on the relationship between the structure of the cerebellum and the "median occipital fossa" of the skull of a 22-year-old madman (Bizzozero & Lombroso, 1874). The study of this median fossa, an anatomical abnormality, was of pivotal importance for Lombroso's conception of atavism and the anatomical basis of criminality (Pancaldi, 1991, 142–145). Yet, Bizzozero never followed up on this research line. However, an analysis of his treatises shows that he was well-briefed on the state of the art in neurohistology and neuropathology, especially about Golgi's breakthrough works (Bentivoglio, 2002). Bizzozero's relationship with Golgi was, in fact, more than just professional. Golgi's wife, Lina Aletti, was the daughter of Bizzozero's sister Maddalena. Still, another member of this family, whose significant contributions to neuroscience will be shortly analyzed, was Aldo Perroncito (1882–1929), Maddalena's grandson and hence nephew and grandnephew to Golgi and Bizzozero (Mazzarello, 1999, 181).

BIZZOZERO'S ROLE IN THE MODERNIZATION OF TURIN'S MEDICAL FACULTY

Giulio Bizzozero (Figure 13.1) was born on the 20th of March 1846. He was the son of a manufacturer in Varese, a city in Northern Italy, close to the Swiss border. After attending the classical grammar school in Milan, he enrolled in the medical course of the University of Pavia, which, until 1860, was part of the Habsburg Empire. He

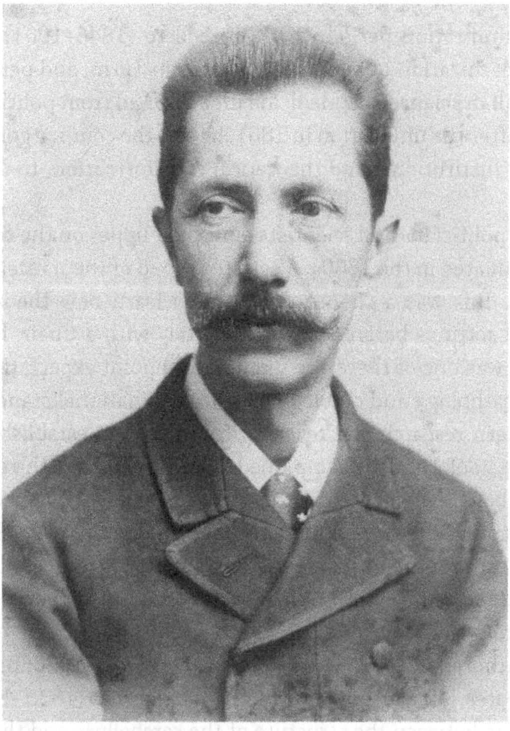

Figure 13.1. Portrait of Giulio Bizzozero.
Credits: Università di Pavia. Courtesy of Valentina Cani and Paolo Mazzarello.

came into close contact with long-standing local as well as German and Austrian microscopic, anatomical, and medical traditions. He trained in cytology, histology, and other recent developments that were, due to the isolation after the failed 1848 revolts, almost unknown across the universities of the peninsula (Dröscher, 1996). He soon stood out for his skills in microscopy, in anatomical preparations and observation, as well as for his intellectual autonomy. Even before obtaining his medical degree, he published seven papers: The first one, on the fine anatomy of bones, was published in 1862, when Bizzozero was 16 years old. Of deep empiricist conviction, he took any theory as a working hypothesis rather than as an unquestionable truth (Gravela, 1989; Dröscher, 2002b). As a student, he challenged his masters. For instance, he disproved Paolo Mantegazza's (1831–1910) intimate conviction of the spontaneous generation of cells, and, a few years later, he corrected Rudolf Virchow's (1821–1902) idea about the origin of connective tissue tumors (Franceschini, 1962). Notwithstanding the critique, Mantegazza continued to support him, and Virchow stayed on cordial terms with him. Virchow published some of his papers in Bizzozero's journal and paid a three-day-visit to Turin in March of 1883 (Andree, 2002, 2017).

In 1865, the 19-year-old Bizzozero supplied Mantegazza, who had moved to Rome as a deputy in the national parliament. In 1866, Bizzozero enrolled as a volunteer military physician in the Third War of Independence against Austria. The following year, he received a scholarship from the Italian government, and passed a year of advanced training as "Virchow's ablest pupil" (Anon, 1946) in the institutes of Berlin and of histologist Heinrich Frey (1822–1890) in Zurich. Back to Pavia, and supported by the Italian Minister of education, in 1869, he became the official supply teacher for General Pathology, and, the following year, lecturer in Histology. Yet the medical faculty of Pavia deemed him too young for a tenured position. Disappointed by this, but aware of his skills, he decided to leave Lombardy and moved to Turin.

The situation in Turin, however, was challenging too. On the one hand, the city was gaining back its international prestige and undergoing industrial and financial expansion. After the suppression of the 1848 revolts, the political liberals, as well as the economic elite, undertook considerable efforts to transform the authoritarian Kingdom of Piedmont into the last stronghold of independence and liberalism on the Italian peninsula. Cavour's regime invested in scientific, cultural, and intellectual reforms, guided by a double-faced desire: internally, of being in a leadership position to shape the future kingdom; externally, to be recognized in such a prestigious role by other European nations and compete with them. Among other things, Piedmont opened its doors to the refugees of the other Italian states and modernized its institutions, including the university. In 1861, Turin became the first capital of the unified Italian kingdom. At first, this realized an ambitious vision, but it was followed by violent dismay when the capital was moved first to Florence and finally to Rome. Still convinced of its leadership role, a consortium of state, provincial, and communal bodies raised funds to create new chairs, attract innovative teachers, and improve education. Empiricism, progress, and science became central ideologies. Turin, according to the famous statement of philosopher Norberto

Bobbio (1909–2004), "was in the last years of the century the most positivistic city in Italy" (Bobbio, 1996, 62).

The medical faculty, however, resisted any attempt to change and reform. In the 1870s, the preunification local medical elites still held power. One of the implications was their ability to recruit professors from the centuries-old doctoral collegium—a local stronghold that helped them avoid any external intrusion. Bizzozero's arrival in Turin in 1872 was therefore much more than just the appointment of a young outsider. It marked the decisive move in the struggle for power between the traditionalists and the liberals. Bizzozero was the face of this battle. Besides his charisma and his qualifications, he was politically skilled, ready to fight for his professional and scientific beliefs, and able to develop far-sighted strategies.

Upon his arrival, he had to face many obstacles. His few supporters in these initial years were the Italian-Flemish clinician Giuseppe Timermans (1824–1873), the Dutch materialist Jakob Moleschott (1822–1893), who had been directly appointed to the chair of Physiology by the minister against the will of the faculty, and some colleagues from the Faculty of Natural Sciences. When Timermans suddenly died at the age of 49, the counsel of the faculty tried to dismiss Bizzozero because his teaching neglected "clinical propaedeutic, semiotics and systematology." Yet the 28-year-old Bizzozero defended his reasons and resisted the strident debate (Montaldo, 2002, 105). This episode probably marks the turning point in the history of academic medicine in Turin. The traditionalists were still there, but they became ever less influential. Bizzozero stayed in Turin for the rest of his life and transformed the Piedmontese institution into the most important center of scientific medicine in Italy. He realized his reforms: He introduced experimental science and practical teaching, re-established an international prestige, and attracted students from the whole country.

In 1876 and 1877, due to his perseverance and his political talent, he finally managed to obtain funds from the ministry and the consortium to finance a laboratory, an assistant, and a technician. Yet it was not until 1881 that he headed a proper academic institution. Indeed, from the early 1880s onward, Turin saw the establishment of several new institutes and the incremental improvement of the existing ones. Among these was the Cabinet of General Pathology. Within the Cabinet, he organized the scientific activity into working groups composed of a professor, an assistant, and 10 students, which was a model similar to the one he had experienced in Virchow's laboratory in Berlin. It proved to be so successful that it was adopted in other Italian universities.

Giulio Bizzozero's Modernization of Medical Research

Doing experimental work in Turin in the 1870s was challenging. Many people within the medical faculty, especially those who embraced a more traditionalist view, did not consider laboratory work to be a proper occupation for a "good" physician. Along with their Italian colleagues of that period, they were still convinced that long-term practical and clinical experience was the unique appropriate competence for a future university professor. Whoever aspired to have an academic career, had, therefore, to climb the hospital hierarchies. Personalities such as Bizzozero were just the opposite of that ideal, and one of the reasons why he had left Pavia had been the refusal to be granted a proper laboratory. In Turin, in his position as rector, Timermans gave his guarantee to provide research facilities. Yet, upon Timermans's all too premature death in May 1873, Bizzozero lost the rooms he had occupied in the anatomical institute. When his colleague and ally, the naturalist Michele Lessona (1823–1894), became rector, Bizzozero reported to him what had happened:

"During the first year (1873) of my professorship in Turin, the laboratory was, thanks to the attentive practices of the university rector prof. Timermans, temporarily installed inside the anatomical institute. Concerning the rooms, at the beginning of the second year, instead of improving the situation, they took away any possibility of official existence, when my egregious colleague and then dean of the faculty, professor Malinverni, threw me and my collections out with a more or less polite letter of [date not discernible]. Regarding the equipment, I was forced to pay by myself everything that had been bought and conserved in the laboratory, but still not paid by the funds of the institute. In this curious course of things, I had no better choice than to retreat with some of my most willing students into one of the rooms of my private home. It is exactly from this <u>private</u> laboratory that some of the works published by my students during that period come from." (Letter of Bizzozero to Lessona, January 30, 1878; cit. from Montaldo 2002, 105; Bizzozero's underlining; my translation).

Things changed when national tenders replaced the local appointments. The minister nominated the members of the commission, and the new Education Law, the *Legge Casati*, provided for recruitment with no distinction regarding the geographical origin of the candidates and an emphasis on high research qualification. These regulations left no chance for hospital physicians and practicing doctors, and paved the way for the appointment of experimental physicians. Between 1874 and 1886, a crucial process rejuvenation, actively campaigned for by Bizzozero, took place at the Medical Faculty of Turin. Young and promising scholars replaced the old (and mostly local) generation, and they soon founded notable schools. Shortly after Bizzozero's establishment, it was the turn of Carlo Giacomini (1874, Human Anatomy), Cesare Lombroso (1876, Forensic Medicine), Luigi Pagliani (1878, Sanitation), Camillo Bozzolo (1878, Propedeutic Clinics), Angelo Mosso (1880, Physiology), Enrico Morselli (1881, Psychiatry), Piero Giacosa (1882, Pharmacology), Edoardo Perroncito (1885, Parasitology), and Pio Foà (1886, Morbid Anatomy) (Dröscher, 2002a, 371–398).

The excellence of Bizzozero's research was, therefore, much more than a contribution to scientific progress. By publishing research papers that gained international praise, he proved his doubters wrong and established a new medical philosophy in Turin (and Italy). His research mainly followed in the footsteps of Virchow's *Cellularpathologie* (1859), on cells as the origin and cause of normal and pathological phenomena (Dröscher 1998). About 60 papers were of anatomical nature, mainly about normal and pathological connective tissue, hematology, and general cytology.

Bizzozero's first important contributions concerned connective tissue. In 1864, when he was 18 years old, he gave the first description of small dense nodules between the cells of the squamous epithelium. Hitherto these structures had been considered as intercellular bridges, whereas Bizzozero discovered they functioned as points of cell-to-cell adhesion. They were later termed "nodes of Bizzozero" and, since 1920, described as "desmosomes" (Waschke, 2008). But it was not until the advent of electron microscopy that his view found conclusive acceptance. In 1865, he published a brief note, *Sulla neoformazione del tessuto connettivo* [On the new formation of connective tissue], providing the first histological description of loose connective tissue. The following year, he experimentally injured connective tissue and described the cellular process of wound healing, revealing the essential role of wandering or amoeboid cells, discovered three years earlier by Friedrich Daniel von Recklinghausen (1833–1910). By doing so, he went beyond Virchow's concept of *Bildungszellen* [embryonic cells], because he demonstrated that the cells he called *cellule semoventi* originate from the lymphatic system, migrate into the tissue, and there start to proliferate to form the granulation tissue and even blood capillaries. "Based on these facts, I think I can conclude that the mobile cell represents the embryonic element of connective tissues" (Bizzozero 1905 [1866], I, 125). At the beginning of the 20th century, this line of research was taken up by Russian-American histologist Alexander Maximov (1874–1928), who connected the "polyblasts" with his concepts of blood stem cells (Franceschini, 1962). In 1872, Bizzozero resumed his research into connective tissue, showing that epitheliomas, the tumors of the epithelium, derive from epithelial tissue proper, hence representing homologous formations. In the same year, he published a paper that related all known types of neoplasm to their respective tissues of origin, thus confuting Virchow's idea of the exclusive role of connective tissue in oncogenesis.

In 1872, he also published *Saggio di studio sulla cosidetta endogenesi del pus* [Essay on the so-called endogenesis of the pus], which represents the first clear description of a process known today as phagocytosis. Bizzozero experimentally induced inflammation in the anterior chamber of the eye and then followed the steps of the process. He observed that the pus did not form spontaneously inside bigger cells, as even Virchow assumed, but rather that the big and contractile cells (*cellule cellulifere,* [celluliferous cells]) actively absorbed and devoured them. In this way, Bizzozero interpreted the contractile cells as "unicellular organs of re-absorption" (Bizzozero, 1905 [1872], I, 296–308). However, he did not stress the general importance of his observation for the subject of immunology. In 1873, he reported to the Royal Medical Society of Turin that he had injected China ink into the subcutaneous of rabbits, finding the ink granules two to three days later in the reticular cells of the lymph nodes, thus concluding that this devouring process might stop some infections. Unfortunately, the report did not find a proper audience, and neither he nor any of his students further explored this research area. In 1882, Elie Metchnikoff (1845–1916) described the process in the larvae of starfishes, applied the term phagocytosis, and developed a general microbiological theory of self-defense of the organism against external agents.

Bizzozero's most celebrated contribution was his pioneering studies in hematology, in particular, the discovery of hematopoiesis, platelets, and thrombosis. Aged 19, he began to investigate the histology of the bone marrow. The traditional view held bone marrow to constitute the "excrement" or the nutritional "matrix" of the bone (Mazzarello et al., 2001). Bizzozero, instead, distinguished red, gelatinous, and yellow marrow. Three years later, he documented the role of the bone marrow in the process of hematopoiesis. Unaware of Ernst Neumann's (1834–1918) similar studies, published four weeks earlier, Bizzozero noted a particular kind of nucleated red blood cell in the bone marrow. He interpreted these nucleated cells as precursors of the (non-nucleated) erythrocytes of the circulating blood and elaborated a concept of erythropoiesis, the process of differentiation of red blood cells. Unlike Neumann, however, Bizzozero extended his perspective and recognized the bone marrow to be also the site of the production of white blood cells. Yet, Neumann linked his discovery to the discussion of blood stem cells. In 1869, Bizzozero had also noted megakaryocytes, the precursor cells of thrombocytes, but ignored their function. Finally, in 1879, he developed a chromo-cytometer, an instrument for counting the number of cells as well as quantifying the content of hemoglobin in the blood. He also applied it the following year to investigate, with Golgi, the variations of hemoglobin content in the blood under certain pathological conditions and during a blood transfusion.

A few years later, in 1881–1882, Bizzozero made his most famous discovery: the platelets. Max Schultze (1825–1874), Georges Hayem (1841–1933), William Osler (1849–1919), and others had described them some years earlier, but given that platelets were few, tiny, transparent, irregular in shape, and anuclear, they regarded them as products of degeneration of blood cells or the unnatural clotting of blood materials (Dianzani, 1994; Ribatti & Crivellato, 2007). Bizzozero described the *piastrine* in flowing conditions in the vessels of the mesentery of living mammals, and concluded they represented a constitutive element of circulating blood, unrelated to red and white blood cells (Bizzozero, 1882, 275). Observing the behavior of platelets and their alterations during injuries, he first noted that the platelets agglomerate and fuse together to form granular masses with leucocytes and long fibrin filaments. In 1891, he developed the first "flow chamber" for platelet counting in circulating blood using a microscope slide, strips of blotting paper, and a piece of thread (Brewer, 2006, 256). He was, therefore, able to observe blood drops immediately after their release on an object slide. Moreover, putting into the chamber a small piece of twisted thread, which had been frayed at both ends, he observed that the platelets adhered to the thread and after a while covered it with thick layers (de Gaetano & Cerletti, 2002). He identified them as "new centres for coagulation" (Bizzozero, 1882, 292). Even more astonishing, when he exerted with a needle a slight pressure on the point of the artery wall, he could observe in vivo the building of a thrombus.

From 1879 onward, Bizzozero also published studies on infectious diseases. From 1883 onward, he devoted part of his laboratory to their investigation. Bizzozero's most important discovery in this field, however, remained unknown for a long time, and he did not realize its main significance himself (Figura & Bianciardi, 2002). Between 1888 and 1893, he carried out a series of studies on the gastric and intestinal glands of healthy dogs. He reported that he observed an abundance of elegant *spirilla*, extremely fine, about 3–8 μm long and with three to seven spiral turns, scattered in the lumen of the gland of the pylorus and in the epithelium of the stomach. He also described some of them forming a cavity within the cell. Yet Bizzozero was particularly keen to stress that these spirilla appeared in healthy animals, whereas today *Helicobacter pylori* are known to cause gastritis and ulcers.

After 1890, Bizzozero's eyesight was impaired by a serious form of choroiditis, preventing him from continuing his microscopical investigations. He devoted himself to theoretical considerations, overcoming his profound reticence over the formulation of theories. The most important of his reflections concerned the histological significance of the mitotic activity of cells. The phases of cell and nuclear division had been documented in their main outlines in the late 1870s and 1880s by Eduard Strasburger (1844–1912), Walther Flemming (1843–1905), Eduard van Beneden (1846–1910), and others. Bizzozero became interested in exploring the relationship between the number of mitotic figures and the processes of normal and pathological tissue regeneration, following up previous studies on the presence of karyokinetic figures around inflamed foci (1885) and on his new technique for the quantification of the mitotic activity of various tissues (1886). Having accumulated an abundance of observations and histological experiences, he felt authorized to develop generalizations. In 1894, during the XI International Medical Congress in Rome, he put forward a new classification of tissues, based on the capacity of their cells to reproduce and regenerate. He distinguished three groups: firstly, the cells of "labile" tissues (e.g., lymph gland, bone marrow), which continue to multiply throughout their lives, old cells giving way to a steady replacement. Secondly, the cells of "stable" tissues (e.g., smooth muscle, bones), which multiply until they have reached a certain degree of specificity, but can regenerate under certain pathological conditions. Thirdly, the cells of "perennial" tissues (e.g., nervous system, striated muscles) that lose any capacity to divide and regenerate after the postembryonic period). Much later, some cancer and stem cell researchers took up this general distinction naming them renewing, expanding, and static cells (e.g., Marshak et al., 2001).

This was Bizzozero's last scientific contribution. On the 8th of April 1901, he fell ill with acute double pulmonary pleurisy, and died a few days later at the age of 55.

Bizzozero's Legacy

Through his school, Bizzozero decisively influenced the epistemology of medical research in Turin and part of Italy for decades (Dröscher, 1996, 67–74; Dianzani, 2002; Margreth, 2002). He was the hero of the positivistic science for which Turin's liberal circles had wished. His research was a combination of mastery of microscopical techniques, use of an innovative device and new methods, observational skills, and an extremely meticulous and scrupulous procedure. Yet his approach was limited to morphology. Moreover, he often failed to explore in depth his numerous lines of research and to draw theoretical conclusions. As a consequence, some of his achievements vanished into oblivion, and some were rediscovered and appreciated only decades later. However, his charismatic personality, his passionate promotion of scientific medicine and public health (Dröscher, 2013), coupled with his ability to explore new frontiers, and the international attention his results aroused, transformed him into a role model in the eyes of the younger generation of Italian physicians and experimental biologists.

Even during the difficult initial years in Pavia and Turin, numerous students flocked to his laboratory, many of them from other universities. From 1878 until his death, besides his official course of general pathology, he offered free classes in clinical microscopy and in histology. In 1879, he published a successful *Manual of Clinical Microscopy* (Bizzozero, 1879), which went through five editions and was translated into German (1883) and French (1888). Intended to help physicians in their medical diagnoses, it distinguished itself from similar treatises by its clear exposition and its focus on practical applications. In 1876, he founded the journal *Archivio per le Scienze Mediche*, modeled on Virchow's *Archiv für pathologische Anatomie und Physiologie*, to propagate, in Italy and abroad, the results of the new positivistic medical research. From the late 1870s on, Bizzozero made use of his growing political influence to promote many of his students to academic positions. By 1895, nine of his students had become professors of general pathology: in Bologna (1878), Pavia (1879), Padua (1882), Siena (1885), Parma (1887), Modena (1888), Sassari (1889), Genoa (1890), and Ferrara (1895) (Dröscher, 2012).

ALDO PERRONCITO AND THE REGENERATION OF PERIPHERAL NERVE FIBERS

Aldo Perroncito's research on the regeneration of peripheral nerve fibers was carried out in Golgi's laboratory after Bizzozero's death. But it traces an investigative path running from Bizzozero to Perroncito, to Giuseppe Levi and, finally, to Rita Levi-Montalcini.

When Bizzozero left Pavia for Turin, he left behind his first group of collaborators, among them the surgeon Edoardo Bassini (1844–1924), the ophthalmologist Nicolò Manfredi (1836–1916), and the future Nobel Laureate Camillo Golgi (1843–1926), but they all remained in close contact. The relationship with Golgi was particularly strong. They embodied almost opposite personalities: Bizzozero was perceptive, determinate, and eloquent; Golgi was prudent, hesitant, and uncommunicative. Nonetheless, both shared profound mutual respect, common intents, and a scientific philosophy, mainly based on meticulous fact-checking, microscopy, and morphological explanations. In 1877, Golgi married Bizzozero's niece, Evangelina Aletti. Both families spent their holidays together in the countryside of Varese (Golgi, 1901). They frequently exchanged their results and views, with Bizzozero usually on the encouraging and advising side, not hesitating to reprove Golgi when he thought that his preparations were not executed with sufficient rigor. It is therefore understandable that Golgi was alarmed when Bizzozero manifested his skepticism regarding the studies on nerve regeneration done in Pavia.

In 1873, Bizzozero published a short note in the Viennese *Medizinische Jahrbücher* on the consequences of experimental sectioning of nerves with Golgi (Bizzozero & Golgi, 1873). Although they focused on the degenerative processes taking place in the muscle tissue, the paper shows that both were acquainted with the surgical procedures and the microscopic facts of nerve sectioning. After this joint paper, Bizzozero focused on other topics, whereas Golgi became one of the protagonists of neurohistological debate. Golgi owed a great part of his celebrity and scientific success to the "black reaction," a technique he had developed in 1873 when he was a head physician in a hospice near Pavia. The great advantage of the method is that it finely blackens entire nerve cells with all their hitherto invisible extensions, and that it stains only a limited number of cells in the mass of nervous tissue treated. Golgi's method finally started to unravel the brain's complex organization. It took a surprisingly long time for the international community to realize the importance of the technique, yet this gave Golgi and, from 1879 onward, his numerous students in Pavia the time to publish groundbreaking reports. They developed several modifications of the method, applying these to other fields and making numerous discoveries (Pannese, 1996). Unfortunately for Golgi, international recognition came along with the rise of Santiago Ramón y Cajal (1852–1934). The Spanish neuroscientist had learned about Golgi's method in the late 1880s. He himself soon became a master and innovator, and used his own modifications to disprove Golgi's theory of the brain as a continuous network of anastomosed cells. Unlike Golgi, he was eloquent and knew how to attract the attention of an international audience. Though they shared the Nobel Prize in 1906, Golgi and Cajal became lifelong rivals, whose claims over priority clashed on several issues.

One of the discoveries contested between Pavia and Madrid concerned the regeneration of peripheral nerves. It was already known that limbs and muscles could recover their functionality after nerves were cut. Around the turn of the century, the research shifted to the cytological aspects. Staining techniques were of fundamental importance to approach the cellular dimension of inquiry. The first two who took up the research field in Pavia were Golgi's favorite pupil Giovanni Marenghi (1868–1903) in 1897 and Francesco Purpura (1873–1943) in 1901. In the experiments for a habilitation thesis, Marenghi was not able to see (regrown) cylinder axes within the scar, and he concluded that the recovery of the functionality was not due to an anatomical restoration of the severed nerve. Still, other structures took over the lost functions. Bizzozero criticized the lack of sufficient proof and told Golgi he wanted to repeat the experiments himself (Mazzarello, 1999, 308). His skepticism certainly did not originate from a limited quantity of data, given that Marenghi carried out 127 experiments. It soon became evident that the missing proof of nerve fibers in the scar tissue was due to methodological inadequacy. Indeed, a few years later, applying the black reaction, Purpura observed that a few days after the cut, the anatomical continuity of the nerve was re-established, and the regenerative process always proceeded in one direction: from the proximal stump of the severed fiber toward the peripheral one (Purpura, 1901).

The third scholar to venture forth on the subject was Aldo Perroncito (Figure 13.2). Bizzozero and Golgi knew him very well. His father Edoardo Perroncito (1847–1936) was professor of parasitology at the Veterinary University of Turin and husband of Arminia Aletti, Bizzozero's niece and Golgi's sister-in-law. Born in Turin, Aldo enrolled in the University of Pavia and became a member of Golgi's household and

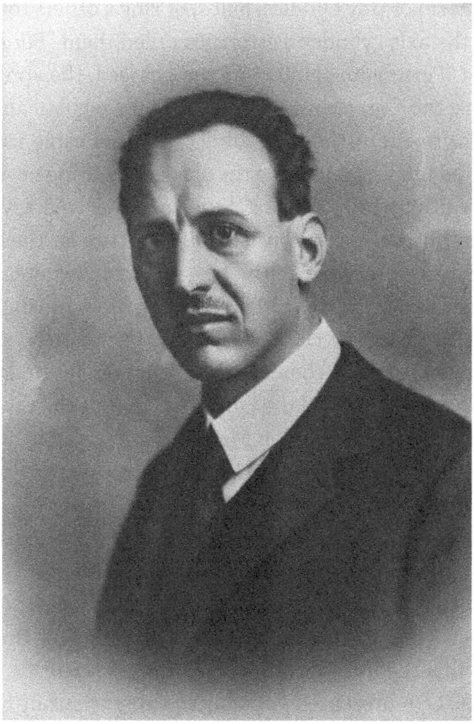

Figure 13.2. Portrait of Aldo Perroncito.
Credits: Università di Pavia. Courtesy of Valentina Cani and Paolo Mazzarello.

laboratory staff (Mazzarello, 1999, 264, 273). Aged 19, he published his first paper on nerve endings (Cani & Berzero, 2015). In 1905, Perroncito graduated with a thesis on nerve regeneration. He published his findings in Italian, French, and German in several brief notes and papers (Perroncito, 1905a,1905b, 1905c, 1905d, 1906a, 1906b, 1907a, 1907b, 1907d, 1908b, 1909) and two more voluminous treatises with a series of colored illustrations (1907c, 1908a). As with most of Golgi's students, Perroncito worked with modifications of the black reaction. Purpura's work had been a contribution of considerable originality. Silver nitrate, however, could not penetrate those nerve cell types that possess a myelin sheath, whereas Ramón y Cajal's refined "photographic method" of 1903 could. Encouraged by this, Perroncito set out to focus his attention on the (myelinated) peripheral nerves, known to have regenerative properties. At the end of his three-year project, he provided the first systematic and detailed account of the morphogenetic kinetics of the neuroregenerative process (Mazzarello et al., 2004).

Perroncito demonstrated that the regenerative process of the sciatic nerve fiber started very quickly, about two hours after the cut. The severed portion (sometimes the portion immediately above) of the proximal stump bloated and degenerated. Perroncito then saw numerous tiny ramifying fibrils growing out of the fiber beneath the swollen part, initially in an amoeboid manner and into various directions.

Some ended in the form of tiny bundles, bulbs, or rings; others formed characteristic structures around the axis cylinder. Perroncito called them "*Elica nervosa*" [nervous helix], later termed "Perroncito spirals." As time passed, the sprouts moved toward and crossed the necrotic area, became increasingly regular and seemingly coordinated. The fibrils grew into the same direction, then came together in bundles, traversed the scar and finally, grew along the old degenerating nerve axes of the distal stump. These descriptions proved to be decisive and solved several controversies. Nerve fiber regeneration definitely consisted of a reaction of the severed fiber itself. The process originated exclusively at the proximal side, whereas the distal stump underwent a degenerative process. Initially fanning, the growing fibers assumed an evermore targeted direction the closer they came to the distal part, providing important evidence for an extrinsic chemotropic attraction. Perroncito received several prizes for his achievement: in 1906 the Quaglino Prize of the town council of Pavia, in 1907 the Warren Prize of the Boston Medical School, and in 1910 the Lallemand Prize of the Paris *Académie des Sciences*. Nevertheless, his contribution was soon almost forgotten, overshadowed by others.

Being apparently neutral observational data, Perroncito's results concealed two very delicate questions for Golgi's school: its implications for the neuron controversy and inaugurating yet another battle with the school of Madrid. Perroncito was extremely careful not to contrast his work with Golgi's theory of the diffuse nervous network. This theory, which damaged Golgi's scientific reputation (Jones, 1999; Shepherd, 1991), represented probably the only scientific taboo in Golgi's laboratory (Mazzarello, 2011, 65). In the first years of the 20th century, the debate between neuronists and reticularists rekindled, and the reason was the supposed polygenist origin of regenerated nerve fibers. The polygenist theory, sustained by Albrecht Bethe (1872–1954) and others, saw new fibers formed from the coalescence of linear chains of Schwann cells, which later linked up with the fibers of the central stump. Perroncito's results were decisive proof to confirm the monogenist origin. Yet, demonstrating that only that part of the fiber linked to the cell body gave way to the regeneration process likewise spoke in favor of Cajal's neuron theory. Perroncito denied that and made:

> "a precise declaration, which corresponds to a factual ascertainment. If affirming the polygenist theory of the regeneration of nerves is equivalent to denying the neuron doctrine, affirming the monogenist theory does not imply the admission of that theory. The origin of the new fibres via germination of the central stumps of the old severed fibres is in equal measure explainable applying the neuron theory as it is admitting Golgi's diffuse nervous network, which is a precise anatomical fact." (Perroncito 1907b, 702)

Although Perroncito's argument was logically correct, the conscious or unconscious restriction the taboo imposed on all Golgians ultimately prevented the researchers of the Pavia school from translating the morphological findings into valuable neurophysiological research hypotheses. Ramón y Cajal did not have such problems. One of the reasons his descriptions of nerve regeneration and degeneration gained constant attention and praise was that they became part of his neurotrophic and neuroplastic theories. Notwithstanding all their shortcomings (Stahnisch, 2009), both emerged as particularly stimulating for future research.

It did not make things easier for Perroncito that the Romanian school of Gheorghe Marinescu (1864–1938) and, most of all, Cajal and his collaborator Jorge F. Tello (1880–1958) obtained—almost contemporaneously, but independently—very similar results (Cajal, 1905, 1908, 1913–1914; De Felipe & Jones, 1991). Instead of being happy over this confirmation, it meant yet another stage in the long-term and long-distance competition with Madrid. Like Golgi, the Spanish neurohistologist also worked with the steady awareness of being scooped (De Felipe & Jones, 1991, 6). Initially, he maintained he had priority over Perroncito (Jones, 1999, 175–176). A mutual exchange of subtle jibes followed, disguised as apparent demonstrations of admiration and respect, yet questioning priority and correctness (e.g., Cajal, [1914] 1991, 20, 158; Perroncito, 1906b, 459; 1907c, 358–359). Finally, in his groundbreaking book, *Estudios sobre la degeneración y regeneración del sistema nervioso* (1913–1914), Cajal not only accepted Perroncito's priority, but suggested the following:

> In honour of its discoverer, or at least of the investigator who first carefully studied it, we have called this curious phenomenon of the multiple production of the nervous branches the phenomenon or apparatus of Perroncito. (Cajal [1913] 1991, 20–21)

The subtle reservation it contained was more explicit in the footnote:

> In reality the phenomenon of Perroncito in its late stages was observed at nearly the same time by him, by ourselves, and by Marinesco; but we must recognize that it is the studies of the Italian investigator that brought out the initial phases and the mechanisms. (Cajal [1913] 1991, 20–21)

Taking into account present-day historical accounts, the winner of the tussle over nerve regeneration is Cajal, whereas Perroncito's publications are rarely cited (Vikhanski, 2001; Stahnisch, 2016). After 1909, Perroncito abandoned the field, but not Golgi's laboratory, serving as an assistant until 1914, except for a year of scholarship he spent between Berlin and Paris. In 1915, he was appointed professor of General Pathology in Cagliari, and in 1922 became Golgi's successor in Pavia. He died prematurely on the 22nd of January 1929 of a tuberculosis infection he had caught in the laboratory (Veratti, 1929). Nevertheless, the topic did not fall into complete oblivion.

Two further implications of Perroncito's work are worth mentioning. The first regards its practical usefulness. Perroncito dedicated ample space in his two treatises and a special paper to the clinical aspects (Perroncito, 1907c, 1907d, 1908a). These were resumed in 1910, by another of Golgi's students, Giovanni Verga (1879–1923), who began to investigate how these findings could be transferred to the field of surgery (Verga, 1910a, 1910b; Mazzarello & Pascual, 2014). The second implication concerns how the growing nerve fibers find their target. The increasing directness of the regenerating fibers provided fine evidence for the idea of a positive chemotactic effect of nerves on the axes cylinder. It would be Giuseppe Levi, a pioneer of cell culturing, who would take up this challenge in Turin and transport it to a new level (Dröscher, 2018). In 1927, Perroncito published in Turin a long entry for Pio Foà's manual of morbid anatomy, in which he dealt with the studies on nerve regeneration together with those of cell and tissue culturing (Perroncito, 1927). The same year that Levi wrote Perroncito's necrology, praising his technical skills and clear mind (Levi, 1929a), he started his research on the neurotropism of in vitro nerve cells (Levi, 1929b). This new approach culminated in Levi and Hertha Meyer's joint paper on the extrinsic factors of nerve growth in cultured spinal ganglions (Levi & Meyer, 1945) inspiring, among others, Rita-Levi Montalcini.

REFERENCES

Andree C (2002) La correspondance entre Giulio Bizzozero et Rudolf Virchow. In *Convegno per il centenario della morte di Giulio Bizzozero, 14–15 maggio 2001*, 51–56. Varese: Accademia di Medicina di Torino.

Andree C (Ed.) (2017) *Rudolf Virchow: Sämtliche Werke*. Hildesheim—Zürich—New York: Georg Olms Verlag, Band 1.6, Abt. I (Medizin).

Anon. (1946) Giulio Bizzozero (1846–1901). *Nature*, 157: 331–332.

Bentivoglio M (2002) Il tessuto nervoso nelle lezioni di Giulio Bizzozero. In *Convegno per il centenario della morte di Giulio Bizzozero, 14–15 maggio 2001*, 137–140. Varese: Accademia di Medicina di Torino.

Bizzozero G (1879) *Manuale di microscopia clinica. Con aggiunte riguardanti l'uso del microscopio nella medicina legale*. Milano: Fr. Vallardi Editore (2nd edition, 1882; 5th edition, 1901).

Bizzozero G (1882) Ueber einen neuen Formbestandtheil des Blutes und dessen Rolle bei der Thrombose und der Blutgerinnung. Untersuchungen. *Archiv für pathologische Anatomie und Physiologie und für klinische Medicin*, 90: 261–332. [On a new blood particle and its role in thrombosis and blood coagulation] (1982). Eugen A. Beck (Trans.). Bern: Verlag Hans Huber.

Bizzozero G (1905) *Le opere scientifiche di Giulio Bizzozero. Introduzione del prof. Camillo Golgi*. 2 vols. Milano: U. Hoepli.

Bizzozero G, & Golgi C (1873) Ueber die Veränderungen des Muskelgewebes nach Nervendurchschneidung. *Medizinische Jahrbücher (Wien)*: 125–127.

Bizzozero G, & Lombroso C (1874) Sui rapporti del cervelletto colla fossa occipitale mediana. *Nota. Archivio per l'Antropologia e l'Etnologia*, 3: 23–25.

Bobbio, N (1996) *De senectute ed altri scritti autobiografici, a cura di Pietro Polito*. Torino: Einaudi.

Brewer D B (2006) Max Schultze (1865), G. Bizzozero (1882) and the discovery of the platelet. *British Journal of Haematology*, 133: 251–258.

Cajal S Ramón y (1905) Sobre la degeneración y regeneración de los nervios. *Boletín del Instituto de Sueroterapia Alfonso*, XIII(1): 113–119.

Cajal S Ramón y (1908) *Studien ueber Nervenregeneration, übersetzt v. J. Bresler*. Leipzig: Barth.

Cajal S Ramón y (1913–1914) *Estudios sobre la degeneración y regeneración del sistema nervioso*. 2 volumes. Madrid: Imprenta de Hijos de Nicolás Moya.

Cani V, & Berzero A (2015) Perroncito, Aldo. In: *Dizionario Biografico degli Italiani* (vol. 82: 31–43). Roma: Treccani.

Cappelletti V (1968) Bizzozero, Giulio. In *Dizionario Biografico degli Italiani* (vol. 10: 747–751). Roma: Treccani.

De Felipe J, & Jones E G (Eds.) (1991) *Cajal's Degeneration and Regeneration of the Nervous System*. Raoul M. May (Trans.). New York and Oxford: Oxford University Press.
De Gaetano G, & Cerletti C (2002) Platelet adhesion and aggregation and fibrin formation in flowing blood: A historical contribution by Giulio Bizzozero. *Platelets*, 13(2): 85–89.
Dianzani M U (1994) Bizzozero and the discovery of platelets. *American Journal of Nephrology*, 14: 330–336.
Dianzani M U (2002) Le scuole di Giulio Bizzozero. In *Convegno per il centenario della morte di Giulio Bizzozero, 14–15 maggio 2001*, 151–159. Varese: Accademia di Medicina di Torino.
Dröscher A (1996) *Die Zellbiologie in Italien im 19. Jahrhundert*. Leipzig: Barth Verlag.
Dröscher A (1998) La "Cellularpathologie" di Rudolf Virchow e il rinnovamento della medicina italiana nella seconda metà dell'Ottocento. *Annali dell'Istituto Storico Italo-Germanico in Trento*, 24: 87–112.
Dröscher A (2002a) *Le Facoltà Medico-Chirurgiche Italiane (1860–1915). Repertorio delle cattedre e degli stabilimenti annessi, dei docenti, dei liberi docenti e di tutto il personale scientifico*. Bologna: CLUEB.
Dröscher A (2002b) Giulio Bizzozero e Rudolf Virchow: due vite per la patologia cellulare. In *Convegno per il centenario della morte di Giulio Bizzozero, 14–15 maggio 2001*, 39–49. Varese: Accademia di Medicina di Torino.
Dröscher A (2012) "Fallaci sistemi forestieri": I docenti italiani di fronte alla riforma della medicina. In A Ferraresi & E Signori (Eds.), *Le Università e l'Unità d'Italia (1848–1870)*, 217–231. Bologna: CLUEB.
Dröscher A (2013) Bizzozero, Giulio. In *Encyclopedia of the Life Sciences*. Chichester: John Wiley & Sons. www.els.net/WileyCDA/ElsArticle/refId-a0025073.html
Dröscher A (2018) Senescenza, rigenerazione e immortalità: Giuseppe Levi e il fenomeno vitale. *Medicina nei secoli*, 30(1): 105–126.
Figura N, & Bianciardi L (2002) Helicobacters were discovered in Italy in 1892: An episode in the scientific life of an eclectic pathologist, Giulio Bizzozero. In B Marshall (Ed.), *Helicobacter Pioneers: Firsthand Accounts from the Scientists Who Discovered Helicobacters*, 1–13. Victoria, Australia: Blackwell Science Asia.
Franceschini P (1962) La conoscenza dei tessuti connettivi nelle ricerche di Giulio Bizzozero. *Physis*, 4: 227–267.
Golgi C (1901) Giulio Bizzozero. *Archivio per le Scienze Mediche*, 25: 205–234.
Gravela E (1989) *Giulio Bizzozero*. Torino: Allemandi.
Jones EG (1999) Golgi, Cajal and the neurodoctrine. *Journal of the History of the Neurosciences*, 8(2): 170–178.
Levi G (1929a) Aldo Perroncito. *Monitore Zoologico Italiano*, 40: 30–31.
Levi G (1929b) Il contributo portato dal metodo della coltivazione in vitro alla conoscenza della struttura del tessuto nervoso. *Monitore Zoologico Italiano*, 40: 302–313.
Levi G, & Meyer H (1945) Reactive, regressive and regenerative processes of neurons cultivated in vitro and injured by micromanipulator. *Journal of Experimental Zoology*, 99: 141–181.
Margreth A (2002) Allievi di Bizzozero a Torino, in cattedra a Ferrara, Modena e Padova tra Ottocento e Novecento. In *Convegno per il centenario della morte di Giulio Bizzozero, 14-15 maggio 2001*, 161–173. Varese: Accademia di Medicina di Torino.
Marshak D R, Gottlieb D, & Gardner R L (2001) Introduction: Stem Cell Biology. *Stem Cell Biology* 40: 1–16.
Mazzarello P (1999) *The Hidden Structure: A Scientific Biography of Camillo Golgi*. Oxford: Oxford University Press.
Mazzarello P (2011) The rise and fall of Golgi's school. *Brain Research Reviews*, 66: 54–67.
Mazzarello P, Calligaro A L, & Calligaro A (2001) Giulio Bizzozero: A pioneer of cell biology. *Nature Reviews Molecular Cell Biology*, 2: 776–784.
Mazzarello P, Calligaro A, Patrini C, & Vannini V (2004) La rigenerazione del nervo periferico: il contributo della scuola pavese. *Neurological Sciences*, 25: 423–425.

Mazzarello P, & Pascual J M (2014) Giovanni Verga, un pioniere della chirurgia del nervo periferico. In F Zucca, A Baretta, & M P Milani (Eds.), *Divulgatori di conoscenza, di idee, e di metodi: I docenti dell'Università di Pavia raccontati attraverso le loro carte*, 57–79. Milano: Edizioni Unicopli.
Montaldo S (2002) L'arrivo di Giulio Bizzozero a Torino: Strategie accademiche nella fondazione del Positivismo subalpino. In *Convegno per il centenario della morte di Giulio Bizzozero, 14–15 maggio 2001*, 95–109. Varese: Accademia di Medicina di Torino.
Pancaldi G (1991) *Darwin in Italy: Science Across Cultural Frontiers* (Ruey Brodine Morelli, trans.). Bloomington: Indiana University Press.
Pannese E (1996) The black reaction. *Brain Research Bulletin*, 41(6): 343–349.
Perroncito A (1905a) Sulla questione della rigenerazione autogena delle fibre nervose: Nota preventiva. *Bollettino della Società Medico-Chirurgica di Pavia*, 20: 360–363.
Perroncito A (1905b) Sur la question de la régénération autogène des fibres nerveuses. Note préventive. *Archives Italiennes de Biologie*, 44: 289–291.
Perroncito A (1905c) La rigenerazione delle fibre nervose. *Archivio per le Scienze Mediche*, 29: 597–606.
Perroncito A (1905d) La régénération des fibres nerveuses. *Archives Italiennes de Biologie*, 44: 352–360.
Perroncito A (1906a) La rigenerazione delle fibre nervose: III Nota preventiva. *Bollettino della Società Medico-Chirurgica di Pavia*, 21: 94–105.
Perroncito A (1906b) La rigenerazione delle fibre nervose: III Nota preventiva. *Archivio per le scienze mediche*, 30: 453–462.
Perroncito A (1907a) La régénération des fibres nerveuses: IIIe note préventive. *Archives Italiennes de Biologie*, 46: 273–282.
Perroncito A (1907b) La rigenerazione dei nervi dal punto di vista anatomico. *R. Istituto Lombardo di Scienze e Lettere, Rendiconti s. II*, 50: 701–705.
Perroncito A (1907c) Die Regeneration der Nerven. Beiträge zur pathologischen Anatomie und zur allgemeinen. *Pathologie*, 42: 354–446.
Perroncito A (1907d) Il ripristino funzionale nel territorio dei nervi lesi in rapporto con la questione anatomica della rigenerazione. *Rendiconti del R. Istituto Lombardo di Scienze e Lettere s. II*, 50: 920–922.
Perroncito A (1908a) La rigenerazione dei nervi. *Memorie del R. Istituto Lombardo di Scienze e Lettere*, 20(11): 293–370.
Perroncito A (1908b) Sulla rigenerazione dei nervi. (Risposta ad Albrecht Bethe). *Bollettino della Società Medico-Chirurgica di Pavia*, 23: 237–247.
Perroncito A (1909) Gli elementi cellulari nel processo di degenerazione dei nervi. *Bollettino della Società Medico-Chirurgica di Pavia*, 24: 108–117.
Perroncito A (1927) Rigenerazione e trapianti, con appendice sui risultati delle culture dei tessuti. In Foà P (Ed.), *Trattato di Anatomia patologica*, 3–148. Torino: UTET.
Purpura F (1901) Contributo allo studio della rigenerazione dei nervi periferici in alcuni mammiferi. *Bollettino della Società Medico-Chirurgica di Pavia*, 23: 1–61.
Ribatti D, & Crivellato E (2007) Giulio Bizzozero and the discovery of platelets. *Leukemia Research*, 31(10): 1339–1341.
Shepherd G M (1991) *Foundations of the Neuron Doctrine*. Oxford: Oxford University Press.
Stahnisch F W (2009) Transforming the lab: Technological and societal concerns in the pursuit of de- and regeneration in the German morphological neurosciences, 1910–1930. *Medicine Studies*, 1: 41–54.
Stahnisch F W (2016) From "nerve fiber regeneration" to "functional changes" in the human brain: On the paradigm-shifting work of experimental physiologist Albrecht Bethe (1872–1954) in Frankfurt am Main. *Frontiers in Systems Neuroscience*, 10(6): 1–16.

Veratti E (1929) La vita e l'opera scientifica di Aldo Perroncito. Commemorazione fatta nella Clinica medica di Pavia alla trigesima della sua morte. *Bollettino della Società Medico-Chirurgica di Pavia*, 44: 149–169.
Verga G (1910a) Sui fatti rigenerativi che si svolgono in alcune cicatrici nervose operate. *Bollettino della Società Medico-Chirurgica di Pavia*, 25: 16–21.
Verga G (1910b) *Le basi anatomiche della chirurgia dei nervi periferici*. Milano: Casa Editrice Vallardi.
Vikhanski L (2001) *In Search of the Lost Cord: Solving the Mystery of Spinal Cord Regeneration*. Washington DC: Dana Press and John Henry Press.
Waschke J (2008) The desmosome and pemphigus. *Histochemistry and Cell Biology*, 130(1): 21–54.

CHAPTER 14

Ernesto Lugaro

The Founder of the Turin Neurological School

DAVIDE SCHIFFER

The story of Ernesto Lugaro begins in the Psychiatric Clinic of San Salvi in Florence when Professor Eugenio Tanzi was called to lead it (Figure 14.1). Tanzi was born in Trieste in 1836 and, as a citizen of the Austro-Hungarian empire, he studied in Padua and Graz, where he graduated in Medicine in 1880. He was an irredentist and, for political reasons, he had to emigrate to Italy, where he became a coworker of Professor Tamburini at the San Lazzaro Psychiatric Hospital of Reggio Emilia. He then attended the psychiatric clinics in Genoa (from 1884) and Turin (1891) and became Professor of Psychiatry at the University of Cagliari. The following year Tanzi moved to Palermo and, finally, to Florence, where he succeeded Tamburini himself who, in the meantime, had moved from Reggio Emilia. He then became director of the San Salvi Clinic. Ernesto Lugaro followed Tanzi from Palermo to Florence.

Tanzi was a fervid supporter of the neuron theory of Santiago Ramón y Cajal against that of the diffuse neuronal net of Camillo Golgi. As a psychiatrist, he was also a keen supporter of Kraepelin, Professor of Psychiatry in München, who was an organicist to the bitter end, applying to Psychiatry the descriptive and the pathologic method and gaining international consensus. Tanzi was convinced that experience causes a real modification of the nervous tissue. His idea was that "neuronal waves" were responsible for the neuron growth through recurrent stimuli. Practically, he was a forerunner of the synapse description of Sherrington in 1897. Together with Tamburini and Morselli, he founded the *Journal of Nervous and Mental Diseases*, which was the most prestigious Italian journal in the field of Neuropsychiatry.

Ernesto Lugaro, born in Palermo in 1870, joined Tanzi's team in Florence, where he became editor (with Tanzi) and then director of the journal mentioned earlier. As a professor of Psychiatry, he moved to Sassari and Messina and, finally, to Turin in 1911. In Turin, he succeeded Lombroso and, in 1927, he was appointed as a professor

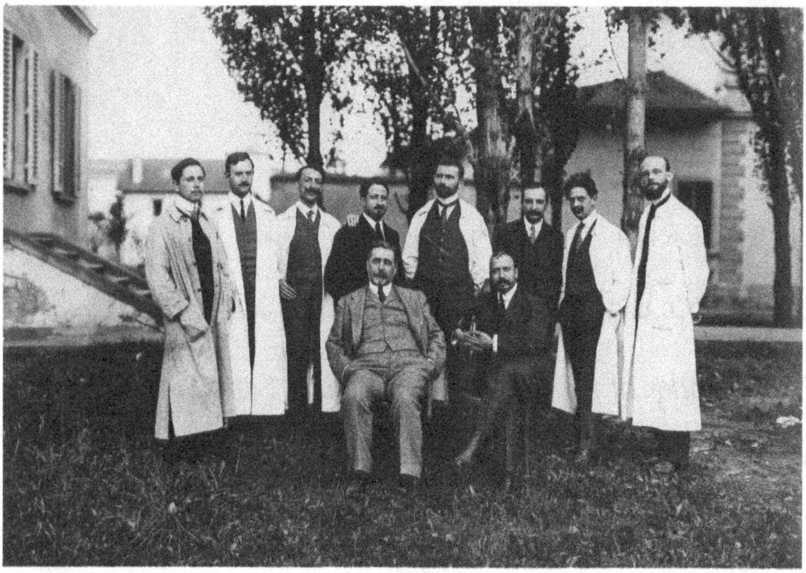

Figure 14.1. Medical staff at the San Salvi Psychiatric Hospital in Florence, 1911. Seated: director Eugenio Tanzi (left) and his assistant Ernesto Lugaro (right).
Credits: Aspi-Archivio storico della psicologia italiana, Università degli di Milano-Bicocca, Archivio Alfredo Coppola. Courtesy of Paola Zocchi.

of Neuropathology, which had just been officially recognized as an autonomous discipline thanks to Camillo Negro's work. In 1935, when Neurology and Psychiatry merged, he became professor of the Clinic of Nervous and Mental Diseases.

Talking about the scientific production of Lugaro means understanding why Neurology and Psychiatry merged. Despite the dominance of Dilthey's ideas on *Geisteswissenschaften* and *Naturwissenschaften*, it was the right time to recognize that both disciplines had a common biological basis. This was also Lugaro's perspective. He began his career as a neuropathology student and, after learning how to use Golgi's technique, he became a researcher in the field of neuronal death and axonal regeneration. In 1906 he coined the expression "Neuronal Plasticity," in complete agreement with the theory of the neuron of Ramon y Cajal and against that of the diffuse net of Golgi. In 1894, when he was in Palermo with Professor Mondino, he wrote two papers on the fine structure of the cerebellum by using Golgi's technique. Besides the cells of Golgi and Cajal, he described a previously unknown cell type, located in the granular layer and sometimes occurring along with Purkinje cells. He called these "intermediary cells." They were recognized as Lugaro's cells, despite the opposite opinion of Cajal, but finally confirmed later (Palay & Chan-Palay, 1974; Dieudonnè, 2001) as inhibitory interneurons using GABA and glycine as neurotransmitters and as recipients of serotoninergic input to the cerebellum (Lugaro, 1899; Lugaro, 1904).

While in Palermo, Lugaro was fascinated by a lecture given by Tanzi, who believed that the nervous system was an aggregation of neurons located at a distance from one another, and that "neuronal waves" during learning stimulated the growth of neurons, thereby reducing the distance between them. This was the first impression of what Sherrington later would describe as synapses. According to Berlucchi (2002), Tanzi was the first to speak about neuron plasticity, a concept he extended to psychiatric plasticity (1893). Still, Lugaro was the first to exploit Tanzi's ideas to introduce the term *plasticity* to memory and learning (before Minea who, in 1909, had already used the term for peripheral regeneration). He thought that, during development, new connections took place among neurons and neurons adapted their morphological and chemical-physical properties to explain psychic plasticity. The transmission among neurons was, in his opinion, a matter of chemistry and energy (Lugaro, 1899, 1904). The emerging problem was the difference between neuronal conduction and transmission. Berlucchi (2002) mentioned the sentence from Sherrington (1925): "Lugaro has proposed restricting the term 'conduction' to intracellular propagation of the excited state, and the employment of the term 'transmission' for intercellular transference of the excited state."

For him, the concept of synaptic plasticity was based on the studies by Ramon y Cajal, of whom he was a scientific admiror. Cajal's demonstrations convinced him that learning, and any form of experience, induces new connections among neurons in the central nervous system, and that neurons are capable of adaptation to the environment. More or less, the neuronal plasticity concept is today the same, especially after Kandel demonstrated that synapses could increase or decrease in number and size according to learning and experience. Not only neuron plasticity was a deduction in the years 1898–1909; Lugaro even presumed the chemical nature of synaptic transmission. The concept of plasticity also was used by Lugaro when referring to the mind, given the possibility of nervous path modifications under the influence of the external world. Lugaro's genius becomes more evident when we remember that Cajal's discovery took place in 1894, and Sherrington's one, from whom we got the name of synapses, in 1897.

Berlucchi (2002) wrote that Lugaro was really responsible for introducing the term plasticity into the neurosciences, because, as suggested by Jones (2000), it was the Romanian Ioan Minea who first used the terms in his 1909 thesis, but referring, as mentioned, to regeneration in the peripheral nervous system. It was thanks to Lugaro (1906) that definitions such as "psychic plasticity", "plasticity of the neurons", and "plasticity of the neurofibrils" were introduced. Lugaro followed Tanzi's original synaptic hypothesis of learning and memory, believing that the chemotropic activities of prenatal organization of the nervous system continue later, allowing new interneuronal connections at the base of psychic plasticity or of damage repair.

A strong believer in Cajal's neuron theory, Lugaro was very active in the search for the mechanisms allowed the crossing of interneuronal space. Two possibilities were anticipated: either the undulation waves passed from one neuron to another or it was a matter of physical-chemical stimuli between the two neurons. He considered the latter hypothesis to be the most probable one, given that a process of energy transformation repeated itself in the successive passages of the stimulus to other neurons. He established a real difference between "conduction" and "transmission," and this was recognized by Sherrington (1925). Lugaro even foresaw the phenomena of facilitation and inhibition chemically conceived.

Berlucchi and Buchtel (2009) dedicated an entire paper to the development of the concept of neuronal plasticity and quoted many authors who followed Tanzi's and Lugaro's opinions on the subject. Besides a long passage from the paper of Lugaro of 1898, James, Meyer, Schiefferdecker, Lashley, Herrick, and Hebb were quoted. They said that Hebb himself, responsible for the theory of cell assemblies, acknowledged the false credit given him for initiating the concept of changes at the synaptic level and they reproduced a letter where Hebb credited Tanzi for the idea.

Lugaro was a real neuropathologist; at least, he started his career as such. He was interested in glia cells, which he believed not only exerted nutritive and mechanical functions, but also protective and antipoisonous ones, and that they were endowed with secretory chemotactic influences on axonal growth during development that became detrimental to neurons in the case of glial tumors (1907). Lugaro was also active in the field of pathology of the nervous system. For example, he described "glial death," which he later called "clasmatodendrosis," described in the brain swelling of Reichert. His activity was also dedicated to experimental demonstrations of theoretical concepts; for example, that synaptic modifiability could be due to changes in the volume of the soma or dendrites of neurons (Lugaro, 1898).

Other subjects of interest were central pain and myelinic and amyelinic fibers in posterior roots, the structure of Cornus Ammoni, the descending root of the trigeminal nerve, the nucleus dentatus, and so on. When many years later I became the director of the Department of Neurosciences, University of Turin, that is, the same institute as Lugaro, I had the opportunity to examine his large collection of histological sections and to save them from destruction. I remember, not without emotion, his histological sections with neurons as black cockroaches by Golgi's black reaction and the *Treponema pallidum* in syphilitic granulomas demonstrated by special staining that brought me back to Leverkühn of "Doctor Faustus" by Thomas Mann.

As it always happens when one wants to interpret several neuropsychic processes with one idea, Lugaro issued hypotheses that turned out to be wrong: for example, the idea that affective phenomena were supported by intracellular mechanisms and intellective phenomena by interactions between afferents to the dendrites and somata of cortical pyramidal cells (Lugaro, 1899) or that analytic and synthetic psychic processes utilized the same cerebral pathways, but with opposite directions of conduction (Lugaro, 1894).

Lugaro also dedicated himself to animal experimentation, but without achieving results equal to those on nervous transmission. As a man of remarkable culture, he wrote articles on various topics not only of neuropathology and psychiatry, but also of psychoanalysis and philosophy (Visintini, 1940).

For the students and for those who came after him in the study of the nervous system, not only in Italy, but throughout Europe, the main work of Lugaro was recognized in the *Treatise of Mental Diseases*, in collaboration with Eugenio Tanzi (Figure 14.2). It was published in 1913, and then in 1916 and 1922. It was based

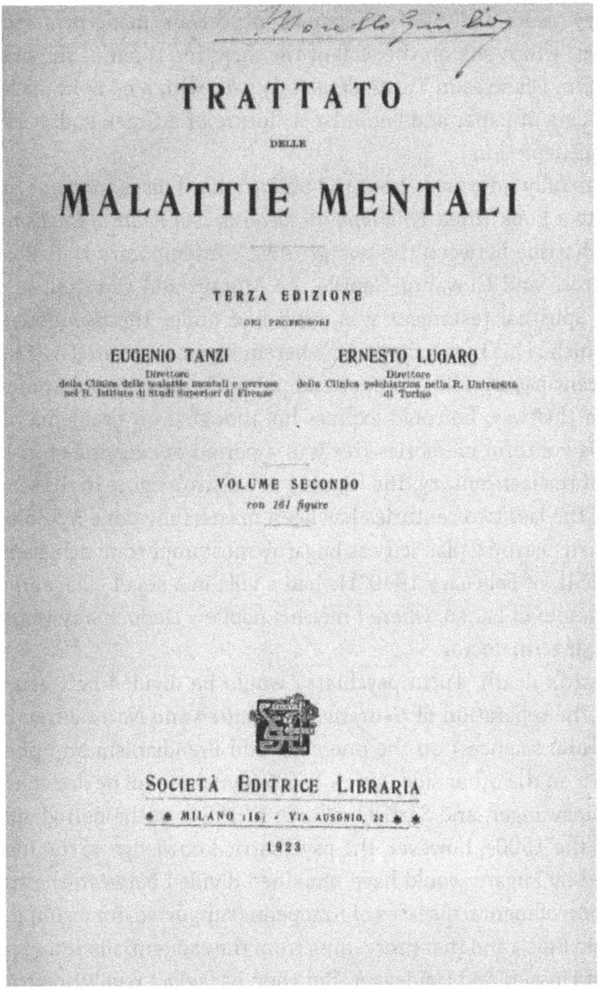

TRATTATO

DELLE

MALATTIE MENTALI

TERZA EDIZIONE

DEI PROFESSORI

EUGENIO TANZI
Direttore
della Clinica delle malattie mentali e nervose
nel R. Istituto di Studi Superiori di Firenze

ERNESTO LUGARO
Direttore
della Clinica psichiatrica nella R. Università
di Torino

VOLUME SECONDO
con 161 figure

SOCIETÀ EDITRICE LIBRARIA
MILANO (16) · VIA AUSONIO, 22

1923

Figure 14.2. Frontispiece of the *Trattato delle malattie mentali*, Società Editrice Libraria, Milano. Third edition, 1923.
Credits: Fondo Giulio Morello. Courtesy of Saba Motta from Carlo Besta Institute Foundation Library.

on an utterly organicistic concept of psychiatry, reducing the number of functional units in comparison with Kraepelin, but giving the maximum values to basic somatic pathognomonic symptoms. The authors underlined the existence of psychic cortical areas with neurophysiological and neuropathological arguments and were absolutely against Freud's ideas and psychoanalysis, accused of being closed in its hermeneutics. A merit of the work was undoubtedly its high literary value and the capacity to depict human characters and behaviors. For instance, how the figure of the "superior idiot" or even of the "depressed" man are described highly meritoriously even from the sheer literary point of view. A masterpiece of the *Treatise*, for example, was the description of Davide Lazzaretti, a paranoic who believed himself to be Jesus Christ and was shot by the carabineers in 1878 on Amiata Mount.

Lugaro was also a poet and a humanist. A portrait, made by a famous painter in those times, which sits on the wall of the direction room of the old Institute of Nervous System Diseases in Turin, depicts Lugaro with a book in his hands, near a table with sheets of paper and behind a sculpture of a Greek god: it is an accurate, and rhetorical, depiction.

Lugaro was fully informed about the philosophical discussions of his times, and he even wrote a book titled *Philosophical Idealism and Political Realism*, wherein he entered the diatribe between the two greatest contemporary Italian philosophers, Benedetto Croce and Giovanni Gentile. As Mutani and Chiò tell it, in 1952 his posthumous spiritual testament was published under the pseudonym of Leroué R. Gaston, which is his name anagram, wherein Lugaro appeared as a French doctor of the 16th century, as well as a poet and painter, who traveled around the courts of Europe. In this way, he could express his thoughts on problems of life, his infancy, and his youthful memories freely in a period of censorship in Italy, namely the thirties of the last century. The framing of Lugaro's figure in the world of Italian neurology of the last two centuries has been masterfully done by Bonavita (2011), who underlined neuronal plasticity as Lugaro's most important achievement. Lugaro died on the 15th of February 1940. He had a villa in a small village in the environs of Turin, Coassolo di Lanzo, where I met his nephew Dodo, many years later, when I was a young interin doctor.

After Lugaro's death, Turin psychiatry would be divided between the ideas of Dilthey with the separation of *Geisteswissenschaften* and *Naturwissenschaften* (spiritual and natural sciences) on the one side, and Freudianism and phenomenological psychiatry on the other side. A new psychodynamic will be drawn from Husserl, Heidegger, Binswanger, and Sartre by Torre in 1974. In the period spanning from the 1940s to the 1960s, however, the psychiatric knowledge at the Institute previously directed by Lugaro would have remained divided between the traditional organicistic vision of mental diseases of Kraepelin (supported, for example, by Lugaro's successor Dino Bolsi) and that proceeding from the existentialistic and phenomenologist views of Husserl and Heidegger. But then Basaglia's revolutionary ideas began to be disseminated (Babini et al., 2011).

REFERENCES

Babini V (2011) *Liberi tutti. Manicomi e psichiatri in Italia: una storia del Novecento*. Bologna: Il Mulino.

Berlucchi G (2002) The origin of the term plasticity in the neurosciences: Ernesto Lugaro and chemical synaptic transmission. *Journal of the History of the Neurosciences*, 11: 305–309.

Berlucchi G, & Buchtel HA (2009) Neuronal plasticity: Historical roots and evolution of meaning. *Experimental Brain Research*, 192: 307–319.

Boeri R, Peccarisi C, & Salmaggi, A (1994) Eugenio Tanzi (1856–1934) and the beginning of European neurology. *Journal of the History of the Neurosciences*, 3: 177–185.

Bonavita V (2011) The Italian neurological schools of the twentieth century. *Functional Neurology*, 26(2): 77–85.

Buchtel H A, & Berlucchi G (1977) Learning and memory and the nervous system. In R Duncan & M Weston-Smith (Eds.), *The Encyclopaedia of Ignorance*, vol. 2, pp. 283–297. Oxford: Pergamon.
Dieudonné S (2001) Serotonergic modulation in the cerebellar cortex: Cellular, synaptic and molecular bases. *Neuroscientist*, 7: 207–219.
Dilthey W (1991) *Introduction to Human Sciences*. Princeton, NJ: Princeton University Press.
Hebb D O (1949) *The Organization of Behavior: A Neuropsychological Theory*. New York: Wiley.
James W (1890) *Principles of Psychology*. London: MacMillan.
Jones E G (2000) Plasticity and neuroplasticity. *Journal of the History of the Neurosciences*, 9: 37–39.
Kandel E (2005) *In Search of Memory. The Emergence of a New Science of Mind*. New York: Norton & Company.
Lashley K S (1924) Studies of cerebral function on learning.VI The theory that synaptic resistance is reduced by the passage of the nerve impulse. *Psychological Research*, 31: 369–375.
Lugaro E (1894) Sulle connessioni tra gli elementi nervosi della corteccia cerebellare con considerazioni generali sul significato fisiologico dei rapporti tra gli elementi nervosi. *Rivista Sperimentale di Freniatria e Medicina Legale*, 20: 297–331.
Lugaro E (1898) Le resistenze nell'evoluzione della vita. *Rivista Moderna di Cultura*, 1: 29–60.
Lugaro E (1898) A proposito di un presunto rivestimento isolatore della cellula nervosa. Risposta al prof. C. Golgi. *Rivista di Patologia Nervosa e Mentale*, 3: 265–271.
Lugaro E (1898) Sulle modificazioni morfologiche funzionali dei dendriti delle cellule nervose. *Rivista di Patologia Nervosa e Mentale*, 3: 337–359.
Lugaro E (1899) I recenti progressi dell'anatomia del sistema nervoso in rapporto alla psicologia ed alla psichiatria. *Rivista di Patologia Nervosa e Mentale*, 4: 481–514, 537–547.
Lugaro E (1904) Sullo stato attuale della teoria del neurone. *Archivio Italiano di Anatomia ed Embriologia*, 3: 412–437.
Lugaro E (1906) *I problemi odierni della psichiatria*. Milano: Sandro.
Lugaro E (1907) Sulle funzioni della nevroglia. *Rivista di Patologia Nervosa e Mentale*, 12: 225–233.
Lugaro E (1909) *Modern Problems in Psychiatry*. D Orr & R G Rows (Trans.), Manchester: The University Press.
Mazzarello P (1999) *The Hidden Structure: A Scientific Biography of Camillo Golgi*. Oxford: Oxford University Press.
Meyer M (1912) The present status of the problem of the relation between mind and body. *The Journal of Philosophy, Psychology and Scientific Methods*, 9: 365–371.
Mutani R, & Chiò A (2010) La scuola neurologica di Ernesto Lugaro. *SIN Collana quaderni di Neurologia*, 1: 143.
Paillard J (1976) Reflexions sur l'usage du concept de plasticité en neurobiology. *The Journal of Psychology*, 1: 33–47.
Palay S L, & Chan-Palay V (1974) *Cerebellar Cortex: Cytology and Organization*. Berlin: Springer.
Schiefferdecker P (1906) *Neuronen und Neuronenbahnen*. Leipzig: Barth.
Sherrington C S (1897) The central nervous system. In M Foster (Ed.), *Textbook of Physiology* Vol 3. London: MacMillan.
Sherrington, C S (1925) Remarks on some aspects of reflex inhibition. *Proceedings of the Royal Society B: Biological Sciences*, 97: 519–545.
Tanzi E (1893) I fatti e le induzioni della'odierna istologia del sistema nervoso. *Riv Sper Fren Med Leg*, 19: 419–472.

Tanzi E, & Lugaro E (1923) *Trattato delle Malattie mentali*, 2 vols., 3rd Ed. Milan: Società Editrice Libraria.
Torre M (1974) *Esistenza e progetto. Fondamenti per una psicodinamica*. Torino: Edizioni Medico Scientifiche.
Visintini F (1940) Ernesto Lugaro. *Giornale della Reale Accademia di Medicina di Torino*, 18: 19–33.
Visintini F (1971) Ernesto Lugaro nel centenario della nascita. *Minerva Medica*, 62: 1–4.

CHAPTER 15

Ernesto Lugaro

Contributions to Modern Psychiatry

FILIPPO BOGETTO AND SILVIO BELLINO

Ernesto Lugaro (1870–1940), in line with his belief in brain-based psychiatry, authored the *Treatise on Mental Diseases* with Eugenio Tanzi (1856–1934). This textbook went through two editions, and significantly influenced modern psychiatry (1914–1916; 1924). Lugaro's career of psychiatrist took place in Florence, Sassari, Messina, and Modena. But his final position was as the Chair of Psychiatry in the Medical School of the University of Turin, which he occupied for 30 years, until he died in 1940. In Turin, early neuroscientific studies are linked with the charismatic and controversial figure of Cesare Lombroso, who taught forensic medicine, anthropology, psychiatry, and neurology. Ernesto Lugaro succeeded Lombroso in 1911.

Lugaro had remarkable merit: He was the first to champion the existence of neuronal plasticity, while supporting the neuron theory of brain functioning in contrast to the syncytial theory proposed by Camillo Golgi. In fact, the analytical index of the *Treatise of Mental Diseases* already contained the terms "psychic plasticity", "plasticity of neurons", and "plasticity of neurofibrils." Together with his contributions in neurology, Lugaro oriented his scientific interests toward mental disorders, and he proved to be a complete neuropsychiatrist. He adopted a particularly modern approach while dealing with psychiatric diseases: The current psychiatric nosography of the *Diagnostic and Statistical Manual of Mental Disorders—Fifth Edition* (*DSM-5*) has several points of contact with the classification proposed by Tanzi and Lugaro's *Treatise* more than a hundred years ago.

First of all, Lugaro observed that the causes of mental diseases involve the relationship between mind and body, between consciousness and organic cerebral processes. He argued that the mere psychological approach to mental disorders was not sufficient. Moreover, he suggested that psychiatry not only needed an intimate contact with medicine and biology but also with the social and moral sciences. Lugaro suggested that normal and pathological psychic phenomena must always be examined in relation to the underlying anatomical and physiological conditions. He believed that the states of consciousness are accompanied by objective organic processes taking place in the nerve centers and especially in the brain. These functional activities are not isolated but linked to all the other vital processes of the organism: "the organism is continually influenced, in its turn, by the forces of the external world, to which it can sometimes react on its own account without the intervention of the brain, while the brain may be influenced by some of the indirect effects" (Lugaro, 1906). This concept is somewhat similar to the modern bio-psycho-social approach to psychiatry: The integration of biological, psychological, and environmental factors can contribute to understanding mental disorders and to designing appropriate treatments. In the book *Modern Problems in Psychiatry*, Lugaro discussed this psycho-physical parallelism, namely the intimate relationship between the states of consciousness, which are subjective, and organic phenomena, which are objective. According to his view, a connection exists between states of consciousness and groups of special organic conditions, in both normal and pathological situations. In particular, because the structure of the peripheral nervous system and central nervous system organs varies, similarly the states of consciousness corresponding to the various nervous phenomena must also change. Lugaro stated that pathological phenomena of the mind are not only the result of the coordination of the internal and external factors acting on the organism along the usual paths, but they originate by the intervention of unusual and disturbing influences and to being carried out in altered organic tissues. Based on these concepts, he emphasized the need to study the psychic phenomena of patients by way of a rigorous anatomical and physiological examination of the brain and related organs (he uses the term "psychic organs") and to integrate psychiatry with general medicine.

Lugaro was also interested in the studies of psychotic symptoms such as hallucinations and delusions. He suggested that the healthy relationship between perceptions and representations can be inverted, to a certain extent, by pathological conditions. Normally, there is a continual passage of stimuli from the perceptive to the representative centers, where the stimuli leave their imprint of the images. But there is also a lesser known retrograde action, throughout specific neuronal fibers, which regulates the influx of the external impressions. In pathological conditions, the functional activity of these retrograde fibers or the representative centers increases, and the stimuli can pass backward and awaken images in the perceptive centers. This process, similar to those provoked by external objects, produces hallucinatory images. The biological genesis of the delusion is more complex to explain. The author maintained that delusions cannot originate from destructive lesions or localized excitation, but every delusion is connected with a total or partial disorder of the affections. From this point of view, the affective state is possibly the first to be altered, either through a congenital anomaly or by an acquired disturbance, and the delusion may only be a reflection of the affective disturbance on the course of ideas (Lugaro, 1906). Affectivity may impact on the association of ideas because it produces an influence favoring or inhibiting the associations, or chooses and arranges the images so that only those directly concerned with the matter at hand find their way into consciousness. Lugaro stated that the affective disturbance determines a change of general orientation of thoughts inducing the subject to select what exists in reality based on an idiosyncratic point of view. So, according to Lugaro, a strict link relates to affective dysregulation and psychotic phenomena. He proposed a model that is an anticipation of the modern approach, stressing the role of the interaction between affective and cognitive processes in the genesis of severe psychiatric disorders.

The nosological system proposed by Lugaro in the *Treatise of Mental Diseases* was characterized by some fundamental features that can be found in the current classification of *DSM-5*. Yet, although significant commonalities are present, several differences, due to progress in psychiatric research, are evident. On the one hand, in most disorders, duration of illness and exclusion criteria were not taken into account for the diagnosis in the Tanzi and Lugaro handbook. On the other hand, syndromic pictures were delineated by Tanzi and Lugaro with accurate, rich, and complete descriptions, providing a well-detailed portrait of psychiatric patients. Ethical interpretation of psychiatric illness, which we can summarize in the concept of moral madness dating back to Pinel (1809) and Esquirol (1819) in the Age of Enlightenment, is also a significant difference between the *Treatise* and *DSM-5*. It received particular attention from Tanzi and Lugaro, although it has been rejected in modern models of psychiatry and in the atheoretical approach of *DSM*.

Tanzi and Lugaro stressed the importance of the etiopathogenetic hypothesis to identify the organic-constitutional basis of mental diseases. Although contemporary psychiatry has made significant progress in identifying several etiopathogenetic factors, especially with the contribution of recent techniques of brain imaging, the main classification systems, namely DSM-5 and the International Classification of Diseases (ICD-10), lack a section about etiopathogenesis of mental disorders. Hypotheses on pathogenesis are much improved and are supported by a large amount of empirical data, but they are not sufficiently specific for every single diagnostic category.

In the following pages, we present some examples that allow us to compare the classification and description of the mental disorders as they have been displayed in the *Treatise of Mental Diseases* and in the *DSM-5*.

With regards to the disorders showing a cognitive impairment, the *DSM-5* indicates them as neurocognitive disorders and identifies several conditions based on the organic cause producing the impairment (Sachdev et al., 2014). The majority of these conditions were already listed in Tanzi and Lugaro's *Treatise* (except for the Lewy body disease). The two authors also emphasized distinguishing the types of dementia according to age groups. Still, in the context of organic cerebropathies and related disorders, the concept of delirium proposed by the *DSM-5* finds correspondence in the *Treatise* with the morbid picture of amentia, which was described by Tanzi and Lugaro as a clinical condition characterized by acute mental confusion with conscience obfuscation, hallucinations, and impairment of ideation processes, due to toxic, infective, or postinfective causes. Some differences already have been mentioned about the presence, among the *DSM-5* diagnostic criteria, of one criterion that identifies the short duration of the disorder and another one that excludes the presence of a preexisting neurocognitive disorder. These criteria of duration and exclusion were not considered in the *Treatise*.

Among organic disorders due to exogenous causes (use of psychotropic substances), a considerable overlap between the descriptions of the two manuals can be observed. In particular, both the *DSM-5* and the *Treatise* describe the phenomena of intoxication, tolerance, withdrawal, and dependence. In addition, the *DSM-5* highlights the most recent concept of craving. The list of substances covered by the *DSM-5* is undoubtedly more comprehensive than the list provided by Tanzi and Lugaro, and this is chiefly due to the diffusion of substances that were previously not known or absent, and also to the identification of psychopathological effects of substances that were accepted in the past as poorly harmful, such as tobacco and caffeine. The ethical criterion adopted by Tanzi and Lugaro in the interpretation of several psychopathological conditions is present in the description of cocainism in terms of moral decline and perversion of will. This yardstick finds no support in the modern psychiatric approach, but rather reflects traditional concepts of psychiatry in the 18th and 19th centuries (Jones, 2017).

In addition to this, Tanzi and Lugaro referred to schizophrenia as dementia praecox. Still, the authors stated that the term "schizophrenia" just introduced by Bleuler was preferable. In the *Treatise,* the description of this clinical condition is very accurate and mainly arranged around a psychopathological point of view in a tight correlation with the Bleulerian model of psychic dissociation. The *DSM-5* model does not show significant differences, but it is rather focused on the list and on the description of objectively detectable symptoms (Tandon et al., 2013). It does not explore the psychopathological interpretation, and it stresses some criteria that mark more recent nosological models: duration of illness, exclusion of similar conditions, and the fundamental criterion of functional impairment. The aim is to obtain a more standardized and objective diagnostic, but this result is obtained at the cost of providing a probably too schematic and synthetic framework.

Descriptions of delusional disorder or paranoia are very similar in the two manuals, except for the reference in *DSM-5* to functional impairment, which, in the delusional disorder, would be relatively mild; and the list of delusion types reported by Tanzi and Lugaro, which was more abundant and detailed, displaying the intention for accuracy and completeness that was typical of the treatises of the time.

In light of the relevance of etiopathogenesis of mental disorders, and in particular on the organic endogenous or exogenous causes, Tanzi and Lugaro devoted considerable attention to psychic diseases due to the effects of medical illness. They described several clinical conditions that were common and considerable at that time, such as neurosyphilis, pellagra, and rabies. The description of psychopathic states related to thyroid dysfunction and uremic psychosis is still interesting and useful nowadays, given that these diseases maintain a significant role in clinics.

A significant difference between the *Treatise* and the current nosological model concerns depressive disorders. It somehow reflects the long and intense debate about the organization of this psychopathological area that took place in the last decades. Discussing affective diseases, Tanzi and Lugaro referred to the syndrome of melancholia: "a general depression of the affective tone with limitation of thought to a narrow circle of sad reflections, pessimistic view of external realities and of the personality of the patient himself, delusions of sinfulness, of ruin, of unworthiness" (Lugaro, 1913, 225). This clinical picture corresponds to a specific type of *DSM-5* major depressive disorder: a major depressive disorder with melancholic features, which is the most severe and biologically determined depressive form (Tondo et al., 2020). In the *Treatise*, there was no reference to other forms of depression that the *DSM-5* identifies on the basis of the prolonged course, such as persistent depressive disorder (dysthymia), or of specific clinical conditions, such as premenstrual dysphoric disorder.

Tanzi and Lugaro described a typology of melancholic syndromes that was primarily based on the symptomatic features that were predominant in the clinical picture, distinguishing an apathetic, irritable, delusional, and hypochondriac form. Only the delusional form is found with the same description in the *DSM-5* classification. As for bipolar disorders, the relatively recent distinction between type I and type II bipolar disorder was not mentioned. Tanzi and Lugaro, apart from the obvious differences in terminology, identified manic-depressive insanity, characterized by the alternation of melancholic, hypomanic, and manic phases with no cyclicality and periodicity. This type of affective disorder is not easy to compare with the current definition of bipolar disorder (Kaltenboeck et al., 2016). The lack of periodicity should suggest some similarity with the cyclothymic disorder of the *DSM-5*. Still, the clinical picture described by Tanzi and Lugaro included more severe depressive and manic episodes and even amential phases. Yet affective psychosis, or circular madness, was presented in the *Treatise* as a disorder characterized by episodes of illness with variable duration and periodicity, two elements that distinguish the psychopathology and clinical course of bipolar disorder in contemporary conception.

When Tanzi and Lugaro dealt with obsessive-compulsive disorder, one of the more interesting aspects of their approach was the choice of a name for the disease: "obsessive psychosis." In so far as the psychiatric literature of the last decades, the term "obsessive psychosis" recalls the forms of obsessive-compulsive disorders with poor insight, namely the lack of awareness about the exaggerated or absurd content of obsessions and compulsions (Jacob, 2014). On the contrary, Tanzi and Lugaro used this term as an equivalent of obsessive-compulsive disorder. The use of the term "psychosis" is probably due to the purpose of stressing the clinical severity of this disease. Still, the authors were aware of the main psychopathological feature of patients with obsessions and compulsions. They clearly described this feature, stating that the subject suffering from this disease always showed an intrinsic, precise, and exact consciousness of their illness. As often seen in the *Treatise*, they listed obsessive contents in an accurate and detailed way and already mentioned in this list the rather modern concept of "impulsive obsession," defined as a mental representation of an action that the individual cannot ignore or suppress. This definition presents in surprisingly modern terms the egodystonic character of aggressive impulses in obsessive symptoms.

Within the section dedicated to the phobias, Tanzi and Lugaro took into account only specific phobias that they also indicated as affective obsessions, highlighting the significant psychopathological relationship between obsession and phobia that is mostly recognized today. Also, in this chapter of the *Treatise*, the list of various types of phobic stimuli was very detailed. The authors included agoraphobia, which was not identified in the list as a specific condition, but they did not cite social phobia or social anxiety.

With regard to hysteria, Tanzi and Lugaro adopted the classic psychopathological concept of a single neurotic disorder with a complexity of manifestations, involving traits of personality (hysteria, hysteric mentality), acute crises (hysteric crises), and somatic and dissociative symptoms. In the *DSM-5*, traits and symptoms of hysteria are presented in three separate chapters: personality disorders, dissociative disorders, and somatic symptoms and related disorders. Still, hysteria is no longer considered as a single, complex, clinical entity. The consequence of this choice is that a relationship between different and very heterogeneous clinical manifestations is not indicated and their reciprocal links are challenging to find with current criteria.

A relevant and innovative topic of the *Treatise* concerned the introduction of a trauma-related disorder: traumatic neurosis or traumatic hysteria. This significant novelty reflects the advanced approach to mental illness proposed by Tanzi and Lugaro. However, the pathogenesis of this disorder depicted by Tanzi and Lugaro was somewhat different from the *DSM-5* concept of post-traumatic stress disorder (PTSD; North et al., 2016). In fact, PTSD is induced by exposure to very severe traumatic events that threaten death or serious injury to the victim. On the contrary, Tanzi and Lugaro maintained that traumatic neurosis can be the consequence also of mild negative events and that the neurotic reaction was exaggerated and related to a particular subjective diathesis. So, the main characteristic of the disorder was the peculiar vulnerability of patients, who could not react adequately to the usual emotional stimuli that occurred in their lives.

Very significant differences separate Tanzi and Lugaro's *Treatise* from *DSM-5* in the section of sexual disorders, in relation to a completely different cultural environment. Some similarities regard only sexual perversions described by Tanzi and Lugaro and paraphilic disorders included in *DSM-5* classification. These disorders were defined very clearly by the two Italian authors, using terms that can be substantially accepted in the modern classification. They noted: "perversion occurs because a tendency clearly in contrast with reproductive function causes a rejection of normal sexual contact and a desire for abnormal ones" (Tanzi & Lugaro, 1923, 618).

The main difference between the two descriptions of sexual disorders is that in the *Treatise* homosexuality was called sexual inversion and was classified as a psychiatric disorder, in sharp contrast with current nosography. Other sexual disorders were not considered by Tanzi and Lugaro, but are included and described in *DSM-5* (Campbell et al., 2015). In particular, this is the case with sexual dysfunctions, including all the conditions in which sexual response or experience of sexual pleasure are compromised, and gender dysphoria, indicating an affective and cognitive incongruence between experienced and assigned gender. Both disorders are considered with attention in *DSM-5*, which provides a specific section for each of them.

In conclusion, sexual disorders represent one of the psychopathological areas that have been more significantly changed in about one century of psychiatric development. The comparison of the two classifications we presented until now clearly indicates that most of the other areas show remarkable and stimulating similarities. Of course, descriptions of psychiatric disorders in Tanzi and Lugaro and the *DSM-5* are not overlapping: A long period separates the two handbooks and a massive amount of data and new theories that have been produced in psychiatric research, in particular concerning biological and physiopathological correlates. So, the differences are considerable both in the general model and in the identification of specific disorders. The aim of our comparison is to highlight how Tanzi and Lugaro showed a surprising ability to analyze and to define the main clinical aspects of psychiatry based on the most advanced pieces of knowledge of their time. The expression of these efforts is a *Treatise* that can still contribute to the education of modern psychiatrists and trigger a debate on significant issues.

In contrast, Tanzi and Lugaro's *Treatise* and the conception of contemporary psychiatry are almost incomparable if we consider therapeutic instruments and treatment strategies. Both modern psychotropic medications and models of psychotherapy were entirely unknown to these authors. Their treatment recommendations for main psychiatric disorders are reported in Figure 15.1. Some therapeutic techniques are very unspecific or simply derived from traditional habits: For example, overeating and deprivation of rest in obsessive psychosis; wraps and work in

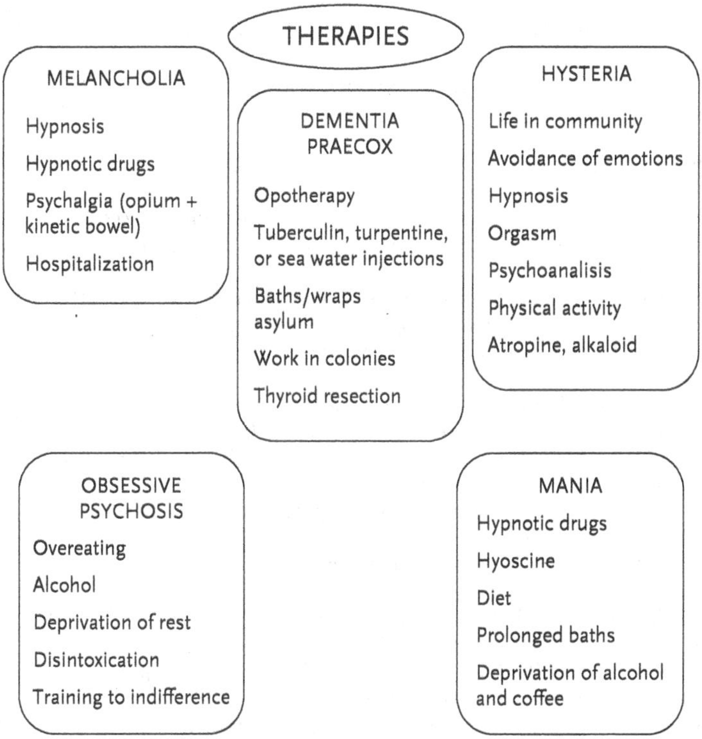

Figure 15.1. Treatment recommendations for main psychiatric disorders reported in Tanzi and Lugaro's *Treatise*.

colonies for schizophrenia; prolonged baths and deprivation of coffee and alcohol for mania; and life in the community for hysteria.

To identify criteria behind the choice of these kinds of interventions (apart from maintaining traditional habits), we can hypothesize that Tanzi and Lugaro proposed, or better re-proposed, a model of psychiatric disorders characterized by a strong ethical component. From this perspective, the treatment is also interpreted as a correction of moral deviations. It should be recognized, however, that Tanzi and Lugaro made an effort to include some initial rudimentary psychotropic drugs in their treatment recommendations, and suggested a role for psychoanalysis, which at that time was a very recent innovation, to treat hysteria.

ACKNOWLEDGMENT

We would like to thank Dr. Paola Bozzatello for her contribution to the drafting of this chapter.

REFERENCES

American Psychiatric Association (2013) *Diagnostic and Statistical Manual of Mental Disorders, Fifth Edition*. Washington, DC and Arlington, VA: American Psychiatric Association.

Bellino S, Patria L, Ziero S, & Bogetto F (2005) Clinical picture of obsessive-compulsive disorder with poor insight: A regression model. *Psychiatry Research*, 136 (2–3): 223–231.

Berlucchi G, & Buchtel H A (2009) Neuronal plasticity: Historical roots and evolution of meaning. *Experimental Brain Research*, 192 (3): 307–319.

Berlucchi G (2010) The origin of the term plasticity in the neurosciences: Ernesto Lugaro and chemical synaptic transmission. *Journal of the History of the Neurosciences*, 11 (3): 305–309.

Campbell M, Artz L, & Stein D J (2015) Sexual disorders in DSM-5 and ICD-11: A conceptual framework. *Current Opinion in Psychiatry*, 28 (6): 435–439.

Esquirol J-ED (1819) Monomanie. In *Dictionnaire des sciences médicales*, 34. Paris: Panckoucke.

Jacob M L, Larson M J, & Storch E A (2014) Insight in adults with obsessive-compulsive disorder. *Comprehensive Psychiatry*, 55 (4): 896–903.

Jones D W (2017) Moral insanity and psychological disorder: The hybrid roots of psychiatry. *History of Psychiatry*, 28 (3): 273–279.

Kaltenboeck A, Winkler D, & Kasper S (2016) Bipolar and related disorders in DSM-5 and ICD-10. *CNS Spectrums*, 21 (4): 318–323.

Lugaro E (1909, 1913) *Modern Problems in Psychiatry*. D Orr & R G Rows (Trans.). Manchester: The University Press.

North C S, Surís A M, Smith R P, & King R V (2016) The evolution of PTSD criteria across editions of DSM. *Annals of Clinical Psychiatry*, 28 (3): 197–208.

Papadimitriou G (2017) The "Biopsychosocial Model": 40 years of application in psychiatry. *Psychiatriki*, 28 (2): 107–110.

Pinel P (1809) *Traité médico-philosophique sur l'aliénation mentale*. 2. Ed. Entièrement refondue et très-augmentée. Paris: Brosson.

Sachdev P S, Blacker D, Blazer D G, Ganguli M, Jeste D V, Paulsen J S, & Petersen R C (2014) Classifying neurocognitive disorders: The DSM-5 approach. *Nature Reviews Neurology*, 10 (11): 634–642.
Tandon R, Gaebel W, Barch D M, Bustillo J, Gur R E, Heckers S, Malaspina D, Owen M J, Schultz S, Tsuang M, Van Os J, & Carpenter W (2013) Definition and description of schizophrenia in the DSM-5. *Schizophrenia Research*, 150 (1): 3–10.
Tanzi E, & Lugaro E (1923) *Trattato delle Malattie Mentali* (3rd Ed.). Milano: Società Editrice Libraria.
Tondo L, Vázquez G H, & Baldessarini R J (2020) Melancholic versus nonmelancholic major depression compared. *Journal of Affective Disorders*, 266 (1): 760–765.
Visintini F (1971) Ernesto Lugaro and the centenary of his birth. *Minerva Medica*, 62 (1): 1–4.

CHAPTER 16

Agostino Gemelli's Years in Turin

CARLO CRISTINI AND ALESSANDRO PORRO

In loving memory of Marcello Cesa-Bianchi (1926–2018)

INTRODUCTION

This chapter tells the story of a journey, more than the story of a character. It is a scientific journey starting and ending in Milan, but with a number of critical stages: Pavia, which is the city hosting an illustrious university; Rezzato, a small town 10 kilometers away from Brescia; several foreign locations (mostly in France, Belgium, and Germany); and, of course, Turin, which is, by far, one of the fundamental stages of this scientific journey.

This journey was undertaken by Father Agostino Gemelli (1878–1959; Figure 16.1, left), an accomplished and controversial scientist, physician, psychologist, philosopher, educator, friar, and priest. The use of the adjective "controversial" does not have a negative connotation here. Still, it indicates the extent to which the complexity of the figure and the work of Father Agostino Gemelli still provokes a lively historiographical debate (Pasqualini, 2016; Montanari, 2017). His positivist starting positions and neo-Thomist end position have not always been interpreted with due accuracy, especially by those who were active in the less sensitive part of the religious experience. This contributed to a form of prejudicial historiographical analysis, which often failed to grasp the complexity of the intellectual path of Gemelli, especially concerning his activities during the fascist regime in defense of scientific psychology in Italy. Even in works that are commendable for their quest for a balance (Marhaba, 1981; Cosmacini, 1985), this aspect of the historiographic complexity does not seem to be completely unraveled. More recently, other contributions attempted to evaluate the position of Gemelli in a more articulated manner (Foa, 2009). In our desire to focus our analysis on Turin and its university, we will stop with the end of the First World War. Afterward, Gemelli went on to develop his scientific, organizational, and educational activity in Milan, with the founding of the

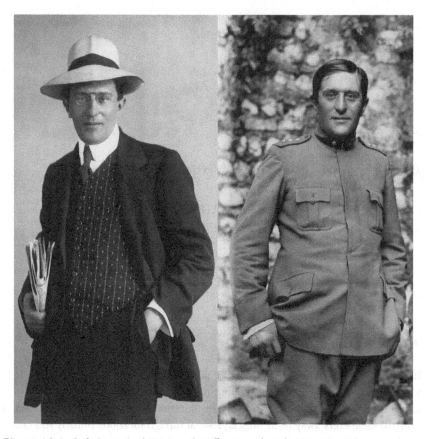

Figure 16.1. Left: Portrait of Agostino Gemelli as a student during a trip to Germany.
Credits: Archivio generale per la storia dell'Università Cattolica del Sacro Cuore, *Sezione fotografica*.
Right: Portrait of Gemelli as an official during the First World War.
Credits: Archivio generale per la storia dell'Università Cattolica del Sacro Cuore, *Sezione fotografica*.

Catholic University of the Sacred Heart. This did not mean a break of ties with the world of scientific psychology in Turin, but his perspective changed.

The first question to ask is the following one: What was the role of Gemelli in the development of scientific psychology (Ancona, 1960) and, more generally, in the development of neuroscience? Gemelli started and anticipated a significant proportion of the evolution of psychology in the 20th century (Cesa-Bianchi, 2000). However, this was due to several encounters, including the one with the world of psychology in Turin. On his path of psychological training, Gemelli met Federico (Friedrich) Kiesow (1858–1940) in Turin in the years leading up to the outbreak of World War I. In Turin, Kiesow founded an internationally important laboratory of Experimental Psychology.

The laboratory was based on the Physiology Laboratory set up by Angelo Mosso (1846–1910) at the local university (Lorusso et al., 2010). Mosso himself wanted Kiesow, a pupil of Wilhelm Wundt (1832–1920), in Turin, where he moved to from

Leipzig. From 1897 to 1901, Kiesow was a special assistant at the Laboratory of Physiology directed by Mosso, then a full-time assistant from 1901 to 1906. From 1901 to 1904 and in 1909–1910, he was an independent teacher in General Physiology. Kiesow also taught an official course of Experimental Psychology at the Faculty of Medicine of the University of Turin from 1902 to 1906. In 1906, he successfully competed for one of the three chairs of Experimental Psychology instituted in Italy, at the Faculty of Philosophy and Literature in Turin (Cesa-Bianchi et al., 2009). When Father Gemelli arrived in Turin, Mosso had been Director of the Laboratory and Institute of Physiology of the University of Turin, and had recently died. Gemelli's attendance at Kiesow's Experimental Psychology Laboratory was fundamental to the maturation of his skill as a psychologist. Also, Mosso played an influential role with his decidedly positivist positions, expressed, for example, during the inaugural speech of the academic year 1895–1896 made on November 4, 1895 (Mosso, 1896). In this significant speech, he outlined the crisis in positivism, as recalled in the introduction to this volume. Kiesow's positivist background is clear, not least from his adherence to cremationism (Tucci, 2003). We also must briefly retrace, however, the events preceding the "ergo biography" of Gemelli, given that they witness to a peculiar evolution from a human and a scientific perspective.

BIOGRAPHICAL NOTES

To better understand the figure of Father Gemelli, it may prove stimulating to read the biographical entry written by Nicola Raponi for the *Italian Biographical Dictionary* (Raponi, 2000). Gemelli was born in Milan, with the name of Edoardo, to a family who educated him without religious references, although he was baptized into the Catholic church. His father, Innocente, was anticlerical and ascribed to Freemasonry. His mother, named Caterina Bertani, was related to Agostino Bertani (1812–1886), a physician, patriot, and representative of radical ideas, famous for the elaboration of a scheme of Public Hygiene Code in 1885. As a result of such education, it seemed natural for the young Edoardo to approach the anticlerical and socialist circles of Milan and Pavia, thus acquiring positivist positions within the scientific field.

In Milan, he completed his secondary education at the *Collegio Longone* (1888–1896) and joined the University of Pavia (1896), where he studied Medicine and Surgery. It was not until 1898 that Gemelli succeeded in enrolling as a pupil in the *Collegio Ghislieri* in Pavia. This was one of the most illustrious colleges in Pavia, founded by Pope Pius V (Michele [known as Antonio] Ghislieri 1504–1572) in 1567. The particularity of the college education must be emphasized. Then, as today, the existence of a national network of colleges guaranteed an elevated level of quality of higher education, directed toward particularly gifted students, which complemented the training provided by schools and public universities. The students of *Collegio Longone* attended the courses of the *Liceo Parini*, the most prestigious high school in the city of Milan; the students of the *Collegio Ghislieri* attended the Pavia University courses, enjoying a *de facto* privileged status.

Adhering fully to the positivist ideas of that time, Gemelli engaged in the socialist ranks of Pavia, continued his university studies, and graduated under the guidance of the general pathologist Bartolomeo Camillo Golgi (1843–1926), future Nobel Laureate in Medicine or Physiology in 1906. In 1902, his year of graduation, Gemelli was expelled from the Collegio Ghislieri for his ideas.

GEMELLI, AN EXPONENT OF LATE 19TH-CENTURY NEUROSCIENCE

In 1902, Gemelli discussed a thesis on the anatomy and embryology of the pituitary gland, which was awarded the Polli Prize and published in part in the *Bollettino della Società Medico-Chirurgica di Pavia* ([Pavia Medical-Surgical Society Bulletin]; Gemelli, 1903). He had already published a work on the subject when he was still a student in 1900 (Gemelli, 1900). After graduation, he spent a period as a trainee at the *Ospedale Maggiore* of Milan (Pastori, 1960), which allowed him to continue his scientific research. In 1903, Gemelli's study on the pituitary gland failed to win the Cagnola Prize of the Lombard Institute, even though Golgi chaired the Judging Commission: Something significant in Gemelli's life had occurred in the meantime.

With regard to Mosso, Kiesow, and Golgi, reference should be made to the specific discussions included in other chapters of this volume. It was not by chance that the young Gemelli devoted himself to studying anatomy, histology, embryology, and histopathology of the central nervous system (Pastori, 1960). These were the main research interests of Golgi, ever since he developed the *reazione nera* (black reaction; Golgi, 1873), which opened up new avenues for studies in neuroanatomy and neuroscience, in the modern sense of the terms (Mazzarello, 2010). Edoardo Gemelli, not by chance very well-versed in Golgi's silver impregnation (Pastori, 1960), was more than just one of the young men in the Golgi circle, destined for a bright scientific career in medicine: He was probably Golgi's favorite pupil. Being initiated into a brilliant career was a common fate, however, for students admitted to the Laboratory and the Institute of General Pathology of Pavia. In essence, at least one year's training led to indelible scientific imprinting and a license of universally recognized methodological rigor.

After graduating in Medicine and Surgery, over a short period, and not suddenly as is often remembered in hagiography, the life of Edoardo Gemelli changed. In the spring of 1903, Gemelli approached Catholicism and soon became a Franciscan friar: We are in the stage of the journey that takes place at the convent in Rezzato, a Lombard village in the Province of Brescia, not far from the Lake Garda area, starting in November 1903. This choice caused a sensation, especially in the socialist circles that Gemelli had joined, having been destined for a career of political importance. In essence, there was talk of the *suicide of an intelligence* (Turati, 1903). Edoardo became Father Agostino, in memory of the conversion of Augustine of Hippo (354–430), but his interest in neuroanatomy, neurophysiology, and neuropathology did not end. For example, his studies on the pituitary gland continued during these years and were published by prestigious academic institutions, (Gemelli, 1905, 1906a, 1906b, 1906c, 1908a), triggering a scientific debate in international journals (Gemelli,

1906d; Sterzi, 1906; Gemelli, 1907). The value of Gemelli's pioneering reports on the pituitary gland has recently been recognized (Riva et al., 2011). In effect, it was a question of demonstrating the functions of a gland, namely, the pituitary, which was still shrouded in a sort of mystery and considered to be a rudimentary organ.

The opportunity that he was granted to conduct scientific research in the convent appears to have been of great interest (Pastori, 1960). This enabled him to continue his studies on the pituitary gland. Having ascertained that the pituitary gland was a functioning organ, but having excluded that it was essential for life, what was its function? Antitoxin, a regulator of skeletal growth, a sleep regulator? Other subjects he addressed are also worth remembering, such as the regeneration of the nerves, which was presented as a continuation of the histological and anatomical research deriving directly from his experiences in Pavia (Falconi, 2007). The experiences related to his medical training were central to Edoardo/Agostino's scientific development and should not be ignored (Sironi, 2009).

GEMELLI'S INTEREST IN PSYCHOLOGY

The origin of Gemelli's interest in psychology is a matter of absolute importance, and the complexity of the cultural landscape that allowed its development played a key role. It is not by chance that one of his students, Marcello Cesa-Bianchi (1926–2018), underlined how being a doctor and having been a pupil of Golgi formed the unavoidable reality leading to Gemelli's approach to psychology (Cesa-Bianchi, 1986, 2000), even if Gemelli himself defined his interest in this field as *tardo* (late) (Gemelli, 1952; Montanari, 2017). This definition is to be understood in a chronological and relative sense. It often has been mentioned that the impossibility of practicing as a doctor or surgeon, due to his status as a friar and the rules of canon law (Raponi, 2000), should be interpreted as the *primum movens* (or, at least, as a guiding factor) of Gemelli's decision to devote himself to psychology. This is partly true. Gemelli's decision was not entirely forced, however, and it allowed him to progress scientifically. The problem of how the disciplines and psychological connotations could, or should, fit into the more general context of the cultural maturation of the Catholic world, or even the more general one of the relationships between religion and science, is not examined here. We can, therefore, agree with the words of Cesa-Bianchi: "The research conducted by Gemelli tended towards a perspective of psychology as interdependent with the sciences that study the functioning of the organism, and in particular of the nervous system or endocrine system" (Cesa-Bianchi, 1986). It was not a matter of organicism, nor psychologism, but of integration, which we find as early as 1908, in a work dedicated to the role of the experiment in psychology (Gemelli, 1908b). Facing and recognizing the biological aspect was thus unavoidable (Gemelli, 1908c, 1908d, 1913; Cesa-Bianchi, 2000). It would have been equally inevitable to enhance it with a further evolution of integration at a higher level, which allowed movement from a limited to a broader world that includes it. It was in this sense that the passage from the histology of the nervous system to neurophysiology, and subsequently to psychology, was interpreted, just as the evolution in this last discipline from psychophysics to psychophysiology, and then to personality psychology (Cesa-Bianchi, 2000).

FROM REZZATO TO TURIN, VIA GERMANY

In light of this integration, we can interpret the attendance at qualified foreign institutions, which subsequently led Gemelli to encounter experimental psychology in Turin. Whereas, at a philosophical level, Gemelli's references were Leuven, his Catholic University, and Désiré Félicien François Joseph Mercier (1851–1926), who would become the Primate of Belgium. It was his continuous attendance at qualified scientific institutes and laboratories in Germany that determined the subsequent developments in Gemelli's research. We then must consider the break represented by the change in Italian political and military alliances during 1914, highlighted by Italy's entry into World War I alongside the Allies against the Central Empires in 1915. This did not prevent Gemelli from publicly acknowledging the value of German scientific institutions.

We can briefly retrace Gemelli's time spent abroad in the period leading up to the First World War. In the summer of 1910, he went from Paris to Leuven, where he frequented the psychology laboratory of the local Catholic University, and then to Munich. In the summer of 1911, he was in Bonn and Munich. His stay in Germany in the second part of the year led to more in-depth analysis of the subjects of physiology with Max Verworn (1863–1921), in Bonn; of biology, with Moritz Nussbaum (1850–1915), in Bonn, putting his histological skills to good use (Pastori, 1960); of clinical neurology with Ludwig Edinger (1855–1918), in Frankfurt am Main; and with Emil Kraepelin (1856–1926), in Munich. Later, he attended Oswald Külpe's lectures (1862–1915) in Munich, which brought him into contact with a psychological vision based on induced introspection (Ancona, 1960), very different from that of the school of Wilhelm Wundt (and of his pupils).

How could these experiences be exploited when Gemelli returned to Italy? The natural first step was to refer to the University of Turin and Kiesow. He was the representative in Italy of the Wundt school (Gemelli, 1952). The possible difference in development as compared to that of a pupil of Wundt who worked in Turin is often emphasized, and this is furthermore due to the evolution of Gemelli's positions in the field of psychology. There were no real alternatives, however, in terms of courses on Experimental Psychology, to that of the laboratories of the University of Turin. So Gemelli attended Kiesow's lectures and his Laboratory of Experimental Psychology. On the 13th of December 1913, he passed the teacher's examination in Experimental Psychology with flying colors, with the qualification officially awarded on the 20th of June 1914, and was posted with the Faculty of Philosophy and Literature (Yearbook, 1915). This meant he had to teach courses, but the war was about to break out.

Gemelli was able to hold his first course in the academic year 1915–1916 at the Faculty of Philosophy and Literature of the University of Turin. The lecturer in Experimental Psychology Agostino Gemelli already could be featured in the Turin University Yearbook with a long series of academic qualifications and awards. In addition to having a degree in Medicine and Surgery, he was an Adjunct Professor of

Histology at the University of Leuven, a Corresponding Member of the *Anatomisches Gesellschaft* of Jena, of the *Société de Biologie* of Paris, and of the *Accademia Pontificia dei Nuovi Lincei* in Rome. He was also a Director of *the Italian Society for Philosophical Studies* (Yearbook, 1916).

Gemelli was conscripted during the war, but he was posted as a Medical Captain of the *Supreme Command* and was not involved in operations or combat (Figure 16.1, right). Therefore, he was able to devote himself to applied psychophysiology (pilot selection; Figure 16.2). Still, he did not neglect the clinical aspects of what is today defined as a *post-traumatic stress disorder*, with even the institution of specialist hospital departments (Gemelli, 1917). We may recall that Golgi also supported the hypothetical constitution of specialist hospital departments, in relation, however, to neurology (and neurosurgery). Although no evidence of this exists in the Turin University yearbooks of the time, Gemelli is supposed to have held a free course in Experimental Psychology, also in the academic year 1918–1919. This is proven by a statement issued by the Rector of the University of Turin on the 20th of October 1925, included in the personnel file of Agostino Gemelli preserved in the Archives of the Catholic University of the Sacred Heart in Milan.

WHY TURIN?

In a diachronic dimension, we can wonder if and why the starting points for Gemelli's journey through psychology were Turin and Kiesow. Gemelli's period in Turin,

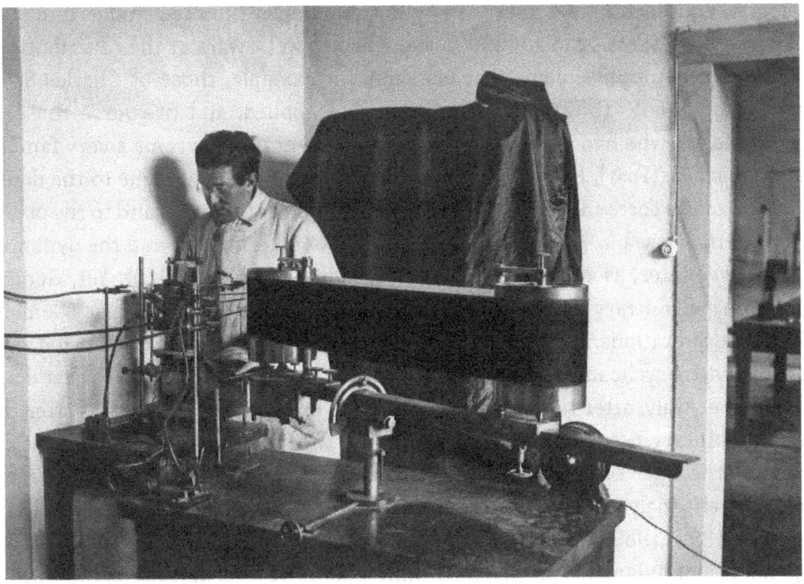

Figure 16.2. Agostino Gemelli in the "Laboratorio di psicofisiologia applicata" at the Supreme Command, at the front, 1915.
Credits: Archivio generale per la storia dell'Università Cattolica del Sacro Cuore, *Sezione fotografica*.

perhaps also due to the years of war, is usually covered by a few mentions, even by Father Agostino himself (Gemelli, 1952). There is typically an emphasis on the evolutionary dimension, starting with the connection with Wundt's ideas (also later evaluated by his pupil Kiesow), thus remaining within a context of human scientific knowledge (Ancona, 1960). The next step would be the encounter mentioned above with Külpe, perhaps to overcome a certain mechanical (or technical?) nature of the Leipzig School. The period ends in a thoroughly anthropological dimension, namely progressive personalistic unification. In general scientific terms, it was a matter of taking back the qualitative, subjective datum, which had been annihilated by mechanistic reductionism and homologation. The Turin experience was then interpreted as an opportunity for comparison and a platform on which to build other evolutionary stages, with an almost utilitarian vision: Gemelli's life and works would seem to support this hypothesis, which fits into the historiographical mainstream. The situation is, however, more complicated than it looks.

THE PARADIGM OF THE STUDY OF EMOTIONS AND FEELINGS

It is challenging to categorize Gemelli's research within the various psychological fields hierarchically. However, studies on emotions and feelings (Gemelli, 1952) can illustrate the experiences of Gemelli's period in Turin. Regarding this line of studies (Quadrio, 1960), the unavoidable nature of biological data (Gemelli, 1908b, 1908c, 1908d, 1913; Cesa-Bianchi, 2000) can be mentioned. This means that Gemelli never renounced his nature as biologist, histologist, anatomist, physiologist, pathologist, and doctor, as witnessed by the value he gave to case studies and clinical psychology (Cesa-Bianchi, 2000). Gemelli was well aware of the contributions of the main neurophysiologists of his time; for example, those of Charles Scott Sherrington (1857–1952), which he knew and applied, and of course those of Angelo Mosso, who had published in 1884 what went on to become a very famous work, *La paura* ([Fear]; Mosso, 1884; Porro, 2009). However, he came to the determination of the cortex as central to the expression of any emotion and to the observation of the close bio-psychological correlation in determinism and the dynamics of affective states, as recalled by Assunto Quadrio (Quadrio, 1960). Yet, Gemelli proved to be contrary to mechanistic (Zunini, 1960) or localizationist (Gemelli, 1909) interpretations. His work on emotions reminds us of his complicated relationship with psychoanalysis: Even in the most tragic period of Nazi-Fascist domination over Italy, after the armistice of the 8th of September 1943 and after the German military occupation of a large part of the country, Gemelli scientifically defended the value of psychoanalysis, which he did not approve for other reasons, and of psychoanalysts who had been hit by anti-Jewish racial laws, such as Cesare Musatti (1897–1989) (Cesa-Bianchi et al., 2009). What is very evident is the independence of judgment and the open-mindedness of Gemelli toward the various contributions of psychology, albeit in terms of prudence and caution: Within this context, eclecticism was placed at the service of a nonrigid and a priori position (Quadrio, 1960).

AFTER TURIN: BUILDING TO EXPLORE THE NEW

A common thread ties together the postwar student experience in Pavia, Turin, and Milan: the experimental dimension of psychology, which does not exclude the biological aspect (Cesa-Bianchi, 1986, 2000). More specifically, it consisted of the establishment of a laboratory that was in part yet to be invented: like Kiesow (Corallini Vittori, 2006), Gemelli found himself walking along unexplored roads. His first test of construction of an experimental psychology laboratory took place during the First World War, with the preparation of the Psychophysiology Laboratory of the Supreme Command of the Royal Army, as revealed by a report preserved in the Historical Archives of the Catholic University of the Sacred Heart (Report, 1924–1925). This activity was part of the experience gained at the time in the field of psychology in Turin.

In the postwar period, with the founding of the Catholic University of the Sacred Heart in Milan, the Gemelli Laboratory of Psychology and Biology represented an *unicum* within the Italian academic scene. For some disciplinary fields, such as the electro-acoustic analysis of language (Galazzi, 1985), Gemelli's pioneering research represented a disciplinary initiative of absolute value. The peculiarity of the instruments of the Gemelli laboratory is confirmed by the testimonies of his students (Cesa-Bianchi, 1986, 2009): electro-physiological and photographic devices, sometimes built *ad hoc* and marketed (Catalogue, 1952). We already have mentioned that Gemelli never abandoned the link with medicine and the biological sciences, also featured in the research of his students and associates (Cesa-Bianchi, 1986, 2000). We recall various works on perception and the first, pioneering investigations on the psychology of ageing (Cesa-Bianchi, 1951, 1952), subsequently expanded and developed in different contexts (Cristini & Cesa-Bianchi, 2009; Cesa-Bianchi et al., 2015; Cristini & Porro, 2015; Memo & Cristini, 2015; Cristini & Porro, 2017). The studies and research of Father Agostino Gemelli in the psychological field characterize his life as a man and a scientist, developed through these various experiences. In Milan, he founded his laboratory. In addition to this, a large part of his experimental work—as well as a school of distinguished students, among whom Professor Marcello Cesa-Bianchi most certainly stands out, from the second postwar period to the present day—represents the final stage of a journey of scientific and academic training. The years spent by Gemelli in Turin form an intermediate, and certainly not insignificant, stage of this journey.

REFERENCES

Ancona L (1960) Ricordo di Padre Gemelli. In *Padre Gemelli psicologo*, 7–17. Milano: Vita e Pensiero.

Annuario della R. Università di Torino 1914–1915 (1915) Torino: Stamperia Reale: XIII; 43.

Annuario della R. Università di Torino 1915–1916 (1916) Torino: Stamperia Reale: 75; 100; 250.

Catalogo di strumenti costruiti secondo modelli dell'istituto di Psicologia dell'Università Cattolica del Sacro Cuore. Milano: Capello & Boati.

Cesa-Bianchi M (1951) L'applicazione dei reattivi mentali nello studio dell'invecchiamento. *Archivio di Psicologia Neurologia e Psichiatria*, 12 (4-5): 390–393.
Cesa-Bianchi M (1952) Ricerche sull'attività psichica nell'età senile (con 2 tabelle e 11 grafici). *Contributi del Laboratorio di Psicologia* 16: 146–188.
Cesa-Bianchi M (1986) Padre Agostino Gemelli: psicologia sperimentale e dello sviluppo. *Contributi del Dipartimento di Psicologia* 1: 19–29.
Cesa-Bianchi M (2000) Gemelli e la psicologia. *Vita e Pensiero* 83 (2): 131–149.
Cesa-Bianchi M (2009) Ricordo di un allievo. In M Bocci (a cura di.), *Storia dell'Università Cattolica del Sacro Cuore. Volume VI. Agostino Gemelli e il suo tempo*, 223–226. Milano: Vita e Pensiero.
Cesa-Bianchi M Cristini C & Cesa-Bianchi G (2015) Emotività e creatività. In C Cristini, M Cesa-Bianchi, A Porro, & C Cipolli (a cura di), *Fragilità e affettività nell'anziano*, 207–235. Milano: FrancoAngeli.
Cesa-Bianchi M, Porro A, Cristini C (2009) *Sulle tracce della psicologia italiana. Storia e autobiografia*. Milano: FrancoAngeli.
Corallini Vittori A G (2006) *Nel labirinto della psicologia sperimentale. La strumentazione del '900. Catalogo (sui generis)*. Torino: Angolo Manzoni.
Cosmacini G (1985) *Gemelli. Il Machiavelli di Dio*. Milano: Rizzoli.
Cristini C, Cesa-Bianchi G (2009) Le emozioni invecchiano? In C Cristini & A Ghilardi (a cura di), *Sentire e pensare. Emozioni e apprendimento fra mente e cervello*, 45–67. Milano: Springer Verlag Italia.
Cristini C, & Porro A (2015) L'anziano e la psicogerontologia: percorsi storici nel e dal Giornale di Gerontologia. *Giornale di Gerontologia*, 63 (1): 16–31.
Cristini C, & Porro A (2017) Per un'ergobiografia di Marcello Cesa-Bianchi. *Ricerche di Psicologia*, 40 (4): 443–528.
Falconi B (2007) Un tema d'attualità nella Lombardia del 1906: la rigenerazione dei nervi. *Medicina nei secoli. Arte e scienza*, 19 (2): 361–371.
Foa A (2009) Gemelli e l'antisemitismo. In M Bocci (a cura di.), *Storia dell'Università Cattolica del Sacro Cuore*. Volume VI. Agostino Gemelli e il suo tempo, 211–220. Milano: Vita e Pensiero.
Galazzi E (1985) *Gli studi di fonetica di Agostino Gemelli*. Milano: Vita e Pensiero.
Gemelli E (1900) Contributo alla conoscenza della struttura della ghiandola pituitaria nei mammiferi. *Bollettino della Società Medico-Chirurgica di Pavia*, 15 (4): 231–240.
Gemelli E (1903) Nuove ricerche sull'anatomia e sull'embriologia dell'ipofisi. *Bollettino della Società Medico-Chirurgica di Pavia*, 18 (3): 177–222.
Gemelli A (1905) Nuovo contributo alla conoscenza della struttura dell'ipofisi dei mammiferi. Nota riassuntiva. *Rivista di Fisica, Matematica e Scienze Naturali*, 12: 136–145; 235–247; 338–346; 419–431.
Gemelli A (1906a) Contributo alla fisiologia dell'ipofisi. *Archivio di Fisiologia*, 3: 108–112.
Gemelli A (1906b) Su l'ipofisi delle marmotte durante il letargo e nella stagione estiva. Contributo alla fisiologia dell'ipofisi. Nota preventiva. *Rendiconti del R. Istituto Lombardo di Scienze e Lettere*, 39: 406–413.
Gemelli A (1906c) Contributo alla conoscenza dell'ipofisi, Osservazioni sulla sua fisiologia. In *Memorie della Pontificia Accademia Romana dei Nuovi Lincei* 24, 167–188.
Gemelli A (1906d) Ulteriori osservazioni sulla struttura dell'ipofisi: nota riassuntiva. *Anatomischen Anzeiger*, 28 (24): 614–628.
Gemelli A (1907) Replica alle osservazioni mosse dal Dott. G. Sterzi al lavoro: "Ulteriori osservazioni sulla struttura dell'ipofisi." *Anatomischen Anzeiger*, 30 (7–8): 202–204.
Gemelli A (1908a) Ulteriore contributo alla fisiologia dell'ipofisi cerebrale. *Memorie della Pontificia Accademia Romana dei Nuovi Lincei*, 26: 41–75.
Gemelli A (1908b) L'esperimento in psicologia. *Rivista di psicologia*, 4: 53–70; 149–170.
Gemelli A (1908c) Le fondament biologique de la psychologie. *Revue neo-scolastique de philosophie*, 15 (2): 250–277.
Gemelli A (1908d) *Psicologia e biologia. Note critiche sui loro rapporti*. Firenze: Libreria Editrice Fiorentina.

Gemelli A (1909) La teoria somatica delle emozioni. Osservazioni critiche e ricerche. *Rivista di Filosofia Neoscolastica*, 1 (1): 77–96; 1 (2): 241–268; 1 (3): 461–474; 1 (4): 570–590.
Gemelli A (1913) *Psicologia e biologia. Note critiche sui loro rapporti*. Firenze: Libreria Editrice Fiorentina.
Gemelli A (1917) *Il nostro soldato. Saggi di psicologia militare*. Milano: Vita e Pansiero.
Gemelli A (1952) Agostino Gemelli. In E G Boring, H S Langfeld, H Werner, R M Yerkes (Eds.), *A History of Psychology in Autobiography*. Vol. IV, 97–121. Worchester: Clark University Press.
Golgi C (1873) Sulla struttura della sostanza grigia del cervello. Ricerche [. . .] (Comunicazione preventiva). *Gazzetta Medica Italiana Lombardia*, 33: 244–246.
Lorusso L, Cristini C, Falconi B, Porro A, & Franchini A F (2010) Angelo Mosso's legacy and his laboratory: From physiology to psychophysiology. *Journal of the History of the Neurosciences*, 19: 48–49.
Marhaba S (1981) *Lineamenti della psicologia italiana 1870–1945*. Firenze: Giunti.
Mazzarello P (2010) *Golgi. A Biography of the Founder of Modern Neuroscience*. New York: Oxford University Press.
Memo M & Cristini C (2015) Emozioni e cervello: aspetti psicobiologici. In C Cristini, M Cesa-Bianchi, A Porro, & C Cipolli (a cura di), *Fragilità e affettività nell'anziano*, 165–189. Milano: FrancoAngeli.
Montanari I (2017) *Agostino Gemelli psicologo. Una ricostruzione storiografica*. Milano: EDUCatt.
Mosso A (1884) *La paura*. Milano: Treves.
Mosso A (1896) Materialismo e misticismo. In R. Università degli Studi di Torino. *Annuario accademico per l'anno 1895–1896*, 23–52. Torino: Stamperia Reale.
Pasqualini M (2016) Un enigma llamado Agostino Gemelli: catolicismo, fascismo y psicoánalisis en la Italia de entreguerras. *História, Ciências, Saúde-Manguinhos*, 23 (4): 1059–1075.
Pastori G (1960) Il lavoro istologico nell'ambito della educazione medico-biologica giovanile. In *Padre Gemelli psicologo*, 173–180. Milano: Vita e Pensiero.
Porro A (2009) Le emozioni per lo storico medico. In C Cristini, & A Ghilardi (a cura di), *Sentire e pensare. Emozioni e apprendimento fra mente e cervello*, 71–83. Milano: Springer Verlag Italia.
Quadrio A (1960) Le ricerche sull'emotività ed i sentimenti. In *Padre Gemelli psicologo*, 42–55. Milano: Vita e Pensiero.
Raponi N (2000) Gemelli, Agostino. In *Dizionario Biografico degli italiani*, 53, 26–36. Roma: Istituto della Enciclopedia Italiana.
Relazione sulla fondazione e sul funzionamento del Laboratorio di Psicofisiologia del Comando Supremo del Regio Esercito durante la guerra mondiale. (La presente relazione è di carattere riservato), s. i. e. (probabilmente 1924–1925).
Riva M, Cosmacini G, & Mortini P (2011) The history of the hypophysis: The pioneering studies of Edoardo Gemelli. *Neurosurgery*, 68 (6): 1483–1489; discussion 1490.
Sironi V A (2009) Il fascino per la medicina. In M Bocci (a cura di.), *Storia dell'Università Cattolica del Sacro Cuore*. Volume VI. Agostino Gemelli e il suo tempo, 19–27. Milano: Vita e Pensiero.
Sterzi G (1906) Osservazioni al lavoro del frate Agostino dott. Gemelli dal titolo: ulteriori osservazioni sulla struttura dell'ipofisi. *Anatomischen Anzeiger*, 29 (19–20): 543–544.
Tucci W (2003) Federico Kiesow (1858–1940). In G De Luna (Ed.), *Le radici della città. Donne e uomini della Torino Cremazionista*, 114–116. Torino: Fondazione Ariodante Fabretti.
Turati F (1903) Il suicidio di una intelligenza. *Il Tempo*, 27 Novembre 1903.

CHAPTER 17

Mario Ponzo and the Age of Visual Illusions

NICHOLAS J. WADE

Luigi Rolando, Cesare Lombroso, and Rita Levi-Montalcini were all concerned with vision, but they used it rather than investigating it. Rolando discerned the gross structure of the brain, Lombroso categorized criminals based on their appearance, and Levi-Montalcini peered down microscopes to detect cell growth. It is, however, to visual illusions that we turn, not to the uses of vision in the neurosciences, although there have been uses (see Wade, 1998b).

This chapter is concerned with visual illusions in general and geometrical optical illusions in particular. Mario Ponzo is a significant figure in the domain of the latter, and a configuration he examined (Figure 17.1) now bears his name. In 1912, Ponzo illustrated an illusion of extent with two circles of the same diameter; the upper one, which is closer to the converging lines, appears larger than the lower one. The size distortion even occurs with facial portraits. In 1928, Ponzo re-examined the illusion and presented a figure with two equal lines of dots rather than circles (Figure 17.1). Ponzo was recruited to the newly formed psychology group in Turin (within Mosso's Physiological Institute) by Kiesow. Kiesow had worked with Wundt in Leipzig and brought the "New Psychology" to Turin; this included the investigation of geometrical optical illusions. Such is Ponzo's association with this visual illusion that it has overshadowed many of his other contributions to the science of the senses.

One reason for the popularity of the Ponzo illusion, particularly with lines, is that it can be related to the possible perspectival features in the distorting elements. In essence, the converging lines could correspond to parallel lines (like railway tracks) receding into the distance (Gregory, 1966, 2009). If such interpretations are entertained, then the parts that are apparently more distant are apparently enlarged. The illusion has been the source of considerable experimental enquiry (Vicario, 2011), and its interpretation remains a topic of lively debate (Farné, 1975; Pressey, 2013). Ponzo (1912a) first published his observations in French, which was then the principal language for articles in the *Archives Italiennes de Biologie*, and they were repeated in Italian later that year in *Rivista di Psicologia* (Ponzo, 1912b). His

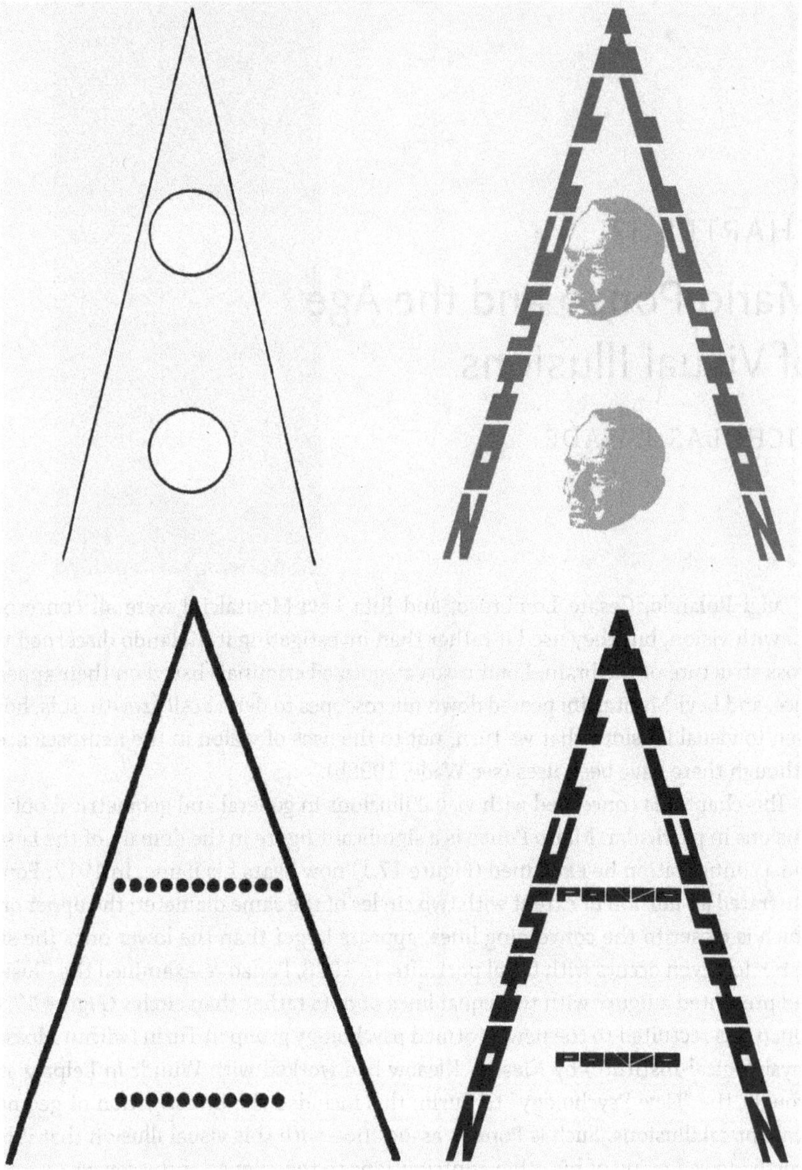

Figure 17.1. *Ponzo illusions* by Nicholas Wade. The figure on the upper left is taken from Ponzo (1912a), and that on the upper right contains two equally sized portraits of Mario Ponzo (1882–1960) but, like the circles, the upper one appears larger than the lower one. The figure on the lower left is derived from Ponzo (1928), and that on the lower right contains two equally sized letters of the originator's name.

second article on the illusion (Ponzo, 1928) was in German, and an Italian version was published later in the *Archivio Italiano di Psicologia* (Ponzo, 1929). Kiesow had founded this journal in 1919 as a vehicle for publishing the experimental research conducted at the Turin Institute of Psychology. Kiesow was appointed as an assistant in psychology in 1896 and became the Director of the Institute of Psychology in 1906 (Kiesow, 1930).

Illusions have provided a source of visual fascination since antiquity. For example, Ptolemy in the second century and Ibn al-Haytham (also known as Alhazen) in the eleventh were concerned with general features of perception as well as illusions (Sabra, 1989; Smith, 1996). Ptolemy drew a distinction between subjective and objective aspects of visual phenomena, and devoted considerable space to errors of perception. Indeed, he was one of the first writers to provide a detailed account of illusions. They are classified, and then considered under the headings of color, position, size, shape, and movement. Ibn al-Haytham adopted a similar analysis of the errors of direct vision, although he extended the range of phenomena for which they occur. He was more explicit in categorizing the three modes of vision in which illusions can occur. Illusions were to be understood in terms of the breakdown of the process of inference. Nonetheless, the categories Ibn al-Haytham gave for the errors of sight were fewer than the visible properties he listed. Errors of inference were confined to distance, position, illumination, size, opacity, transparency, duration, and condition of the eye.

Illusions can be considered as errors in perception. As such, they were remarked upon before the underlying neural and perceptual processes were either described or appreciated: It was possible to compare observations of the same objects over time and to note any discrepancies between them. Aristotle did entertain the possibility of illusions entering into a particular sense. The examples he mentioned were those of color or sound confusions, and errors in spatial localization of colors or sounds. The modern definition of illusions applies to differences between the perception of figures and their physical characteristics. Consensus concerning an external reality did not exist in antiquity, and so attention was directed to those instances in which changes in perception occurred. That is, when the same object appeared to have different properties under different conditions. According to this observational definition of illusions, all that is required is an assumption of object permanence; thereafter, changes in the appearance of the same object will be classified as illusions.

Geometrical optical illusions involving line drawings that induce small spatial distortions became a topic of experimental interest within visual science from the mid-19th century (see Wade, 2016, 2018). They were then, and remain, fascinating to look at, and many variations were described, often bearing the names of those who drew attention to them. Now, with the advent of computer graphics, their number has expanded enormously (see Shapiro & Todorovic, 2017).

An abiding example of a visual illusion is the variation in apparent sizes of celestial bodies at different locations in their transits through the sky. These have been exemplified in the moon illusion—its larger appearance near the horizon than high in the sky (Figure 17.2). Berkeley (1709) stated: "Now, between the Eye, and the Moon, when situated in the *Horizon*, there lies a far greater Quantity of Atmosphere, than there does when the Moon is in the *Meridian*. Whence it comes to pass, that the Appearance of Horizontal Moon is fainter, and therefore . . . it shou'd be thought bigger in that Situation, than in the *Meridian*, or any other elevation above the *Horizon*" (LXVIII). Berkeley was adopting an interpretation that had been voiced, but usually rejected, by others. That is, the moon appears of lower contrast

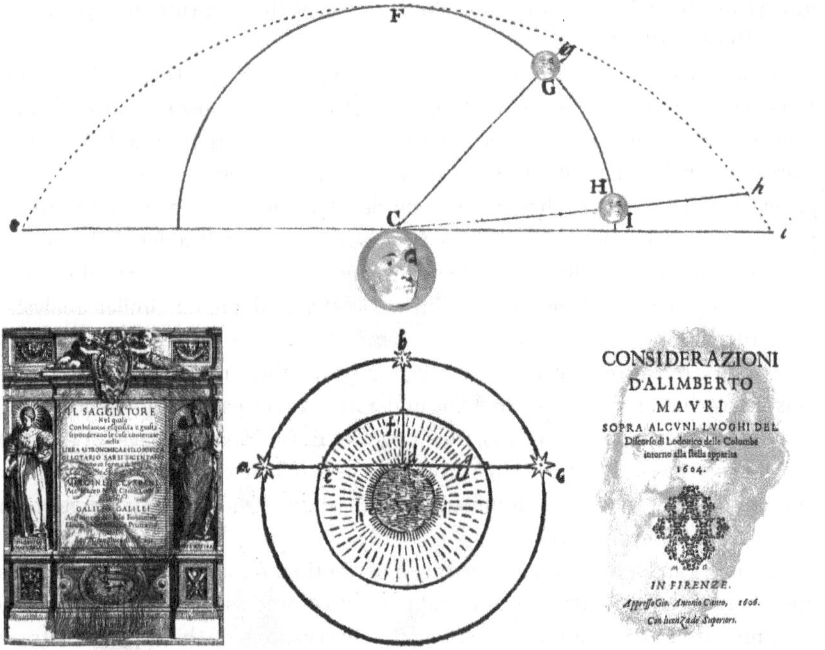

Figure 17.2. *Celestial illusionists* by Nicholas Wade. Upper, Berkeley described the moon illusion, and he is represented observing it in a figure derived from his contemporary Desaguliers (1739). Lower left, Galileo's portrait is embedded in the title pages of his books dealing in part with the senses and illusions. In the lower center is the diagram of the celestial illusion taken from the book shown on the lower right, the title page of which carries Galileo's portrait.

when near the horizon, and is seen as larger due to this blurred or confused appearance. The interpretation extends back to Aristotle, but the size/distance theory was then more widely accepted. The moon illusion is a size illusion, but it has also been interpreted as a distance illusion. It presented an enigma in the past, and it is one that still persists (Ross & Plug, 2002). Modern attempts at explaining it remain problematic (Hershenson, 1989). It provides a quintessential example of illusion because the observations have been consistent. Still, the interpretations have shown a progressive change: It was analyzed initially as a problem of physics, then physiology, and finally psychology.

Galileo (1623) spoke at length about illusions of the senses, including celestial illusions, and his interpretation represented a break with Aristotelian psychology. Galileo's general interest in the senses was of a psychological and philosophical character; it reflected the fallacies and limits of senses and how scientific knowledge of the world could be gathered from potentially deceptive sensory appearances. Galileo applied this approach to celestial illusions; he had visited this phenomenon previously, under the pseudonym of Alimberto Mauri (Galileo, 1606). Not only did he argue that the sun appeared larger near the horizon because it passed through more vapors, but he illustrated the situation, too (Figure 17.2). This represents a rare instance of Galileo applying an optical interpretation to a visual phenomenon (see

Piccolino & Wade, 2008, 2014; Wade, 2007). Paradoxically, despite his development of the telescope, Galileo did not contribute to the progress of optical science in his day, like that expounded by his contemporaries Kepler (1604) and Scheiner (1619). It was the moon illusion that stimulated Ponzo's (1912a) foray into visual illusions.

In a real sense, the systematic study of illusions has its origins in Italy. Pictures in perspective present us with one of the most common and compelling illusions we encounter. Marks on a flat surface appear to represent objects at different distances. Illusions played a significant role in the pictorial representations of objects, particularly when the Greek ideal of imitating nature was returned to in the Renaissance. Linear perspective was demonstrated by the architect and painter Filippo Brunelleschi and formalized by a contemporary architect and mathematician, Leon Battista Alberti. It was derived from the optics of Euclid, who analyzed vision in terms of a cone emanating from the eye (Figure 17.3). Perspective is the application of Euclid's visual cone to a glass plane intersecting it, and this device is now known as Alberti's window (Figure 17.3). Thus, the principles of reducing a three-dimensional scene to a two-dimensional pictorial image of it were formulated before the image-forming properties of the eye had been described. The optics of antiquity met the art of the Renaissance in the context of linear perspective. The technique of perspective painting was rapidly adopted by artists from that time onward, and many textbooks described its rules.

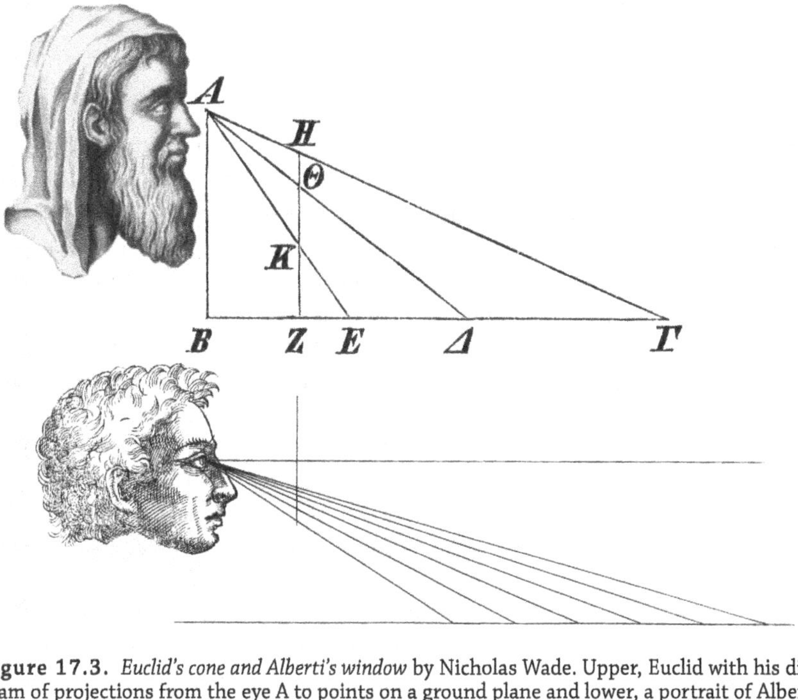

Figure 17.3. *Euclid's cone and Alberti's window* by Nicholas Wade. Upper, Euclid with his diagram of projections from the eye A to points on a ground plane and lower, a portrait of Alberti upon which is superimposed a drawing of rays from equally spaced tiles on the ground plane intersecting the vertical picture plane to meet the eye.

Linear perspective involves specifying a station point, picture plane, ground plane, and vanishing point, enabling depiction of a single image of a scene. Representations of solid objects on two-dimensional surfaces, following the rules of linear perspective, were assisted by using the *camera obscura*. Ibn al-Haytham described a rudimentary form of the instrument, and Leonardo da Vinci likened the eye to a camera. Despite these fertile suggestions, the *camera obscura* was used extensively by artists rather than scientists, because the optics and anatomy of the eye were only dimly discerned before the 17th century (see Wade, 1998a).

Leonardo saw not only the benefits that could derive from the application of the rules of linear perspective, but he also made the first systematic distortions of these rules (Figure 17.4). Soon after central perspective had been widely adopted in art, it was distorted in the form of accelerated and decelerated perspective architectures and anamorphic paintings. In anamorphic art, the appropriate viewpoint differs from normal or perpendicular to the picture plane, so that the pictorial content can only be seen when the picture is viewed awry or through some appropriate optical device such as a cylindrical mirror (Baltrusaitis, 1976). One of the most pervasive forms of manipulation, however, has been the many and varied attempts to fool the eye (trompe l'oeil) with flat paintings. Successful examples of trompe l'oeil are rare, and those that do succeed usually place constraints on the viewer. For instance, Andrea Pozzo's ceiling painting *Apotheosis of St Ignatius* in the church of St. Ignatius (Rome) has a disc on the marble floor which defines the correct viewing position; there is also a smaller trompe l'oeil dome in the church (Figure 17.4).

THE AGE OF ILLUSIONS

The 19th century was the golden age of visual illusions (Wade, 2014, 2016, 2018). The concern with confusions of color, contour, and motion can be traced to the ancients, but the pace quickened after 1800. Initially, the illusions of interest were those visible in the natural environment, such as the waterfall illusion, the apparent motion of the moon when clouds pass by, or the ambiguous direction of motion in windmill sails seen from afar. In the domain of color, practical problems of fabric dyeing resulted in formulating laws of color contrast. All was to change with the invention of photography and of instruments that presented paired pictures or sequences of slightly different ones. After that, pictures permeated perception transforming its study by transferring it from the natural environment to the laboratory. The nature of the transformation had two phases: In the early 19th century concern was with simulating in the laboratory what was visible in the environment—depth and motion. In the second half of the century, illusions became simpler and divorced from the external world.

Within visual science, the simple figures that induced spatial distortions were given the label, "geometrical optical illusions" by Oppel (1855) to restrict them to the relatively small, but reliable, distortions of visual space, mostly in the domains of size or orientation. Classifying them in this way is too restrictive, because some combine both dimensions and others involve different dimensions altogether. Vicario (2011)

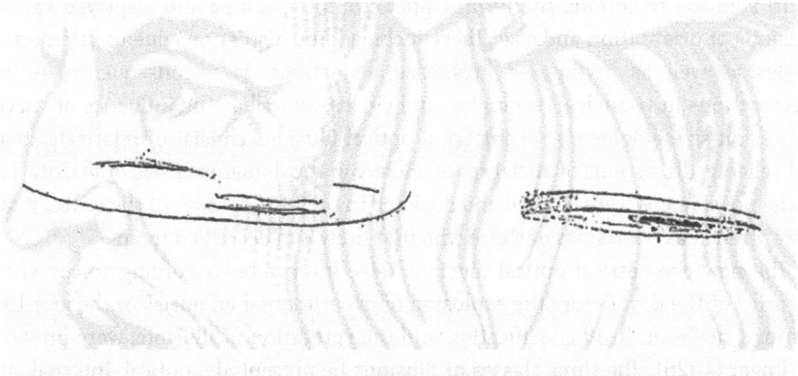

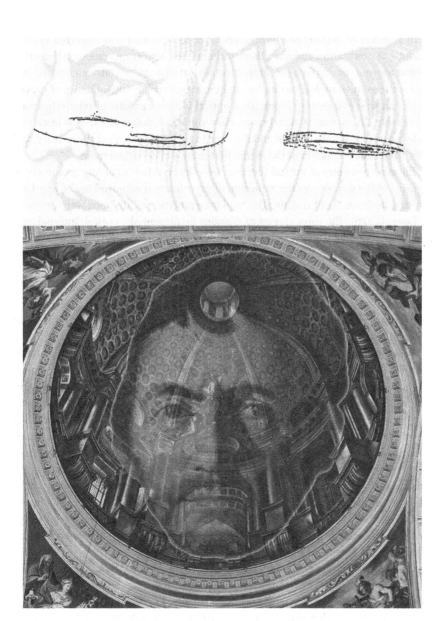

Figure 17.4. *Leonardo's eye and Pozzo's dome* by Nicholas Wade. Upper, Leonardo's portrait is combined with his anamorphic drawings of a child's face and eye. Pozzo's portrait can be seen in the trompe l'oeil dome in the church of St. Ignatius in Rome.

listed 26 different classifications! Perhaps the simplest is the one proposed by Boring (1942): extent, direction, and the rest. The common factors of the classifications are: direction (orientation), size, contrast, assimilation, and perspective. Some systems are concerned with the distorted dimensions (such as size and orientation), others involve possible underlying processes (such as assimilation and contrast, and eye movements), and yet others characterize the levels at which the illusions should be considered (e.g., physical, physiological, and psychological).

In addition to coining the term, Oppel (1855) described and displayed various illusions of orientation and size. These included line distortions due to intersecting angles as well as juxtaposed arcs, size distortions as a consequence of line intersections in triangles, rectangles, and circles, as well as the influence of curved figures on size judgments. Geometrical optical illusions consist of relatively small, but reliable, distortions of visual space, mostly in the domains of size or orientation. Many novel forms were devised and depicted in the final decades of the century, and they often bear the names of those who first drew and described them.

The new geometrical optical illusions were interpreted according to the visual theories of the day. Before the explosion of experimental enquiries in the late 19th century, however, lucid classification and interpretation of illusions were provided by Roget (1826). The three classes of illusions he presented—optical, internal, and mental—are similar to those that are applied in contemporary visual science of physical, physiological, and psychological (Gregory, 2009). Various approaches have been applied to interpret illusions essentially in the context of Roget's three categories. Illusions in the first class are generally interpreted in terms of geometrical optics. Interpretations of those in the second class have had some success concerning the burgeoning knowledge of neural processing. Most attention is now directed at those of the third class, for which there are competing theories.

Geometrical optical illusions are quintessentially phenomena of the late 19th century, when the likes of Bezold, Delbœuf, Helmholtz, Hering, Kundt, Lipps, Mach, Müller-Lyer, Oppel, Poggendorff, Wundt, and Zöllner described their eponymous phenomena (Figure 17.5). These illusions have a critical place in the history of psychology, because they were among the factors that led Wundt to establish his Psychological Institute at Leipzig in 1879—he could not envisage how illusions could be accounted for in physiological terms, and so they, along with consciousness, required a separate discipline. Wundt took as his yardstick the proximal stimulus (the retinal image)—and he could not accept that, say, two linear extents that produced equivalent retinal extents could yield perceptual inequality due to physiological processes. Thus, geometrical optical illusions are important in the context of establishing psychology as an independent discipline: there was considered to be no physiological correlate of perception.

The investigation of geometrical optical illusions started rather late in Italy, but its origin was in Turin. The stimulus was provided by Kiesow, who worked in Wundt's Institute in Leipzig and visited Mosso's laboratory to gain acquaintance with the new techniques developed in Turin: "As Turin was generally regarded as the foremost place for the study of graphic methods, I conceived the wish to go there during the vacation of our German universities, after the winter semester of 1893–94" (Kiesow, 1930, 177). On his return to Leipzig, Kiesow continued his research on touch and temperature sensitivity as well as introduced Mosso's sphygmomanometer to Wundt's laboratory.

Mosso and Kiesow were on good terms, and Kiesow (together with his fiancée Emily Lough) translated Mosso's *La Paura* into English. In 1896 Mosso invited Kiesow to become an assistant in psychology at the Physiological Institute at Turin, where he:

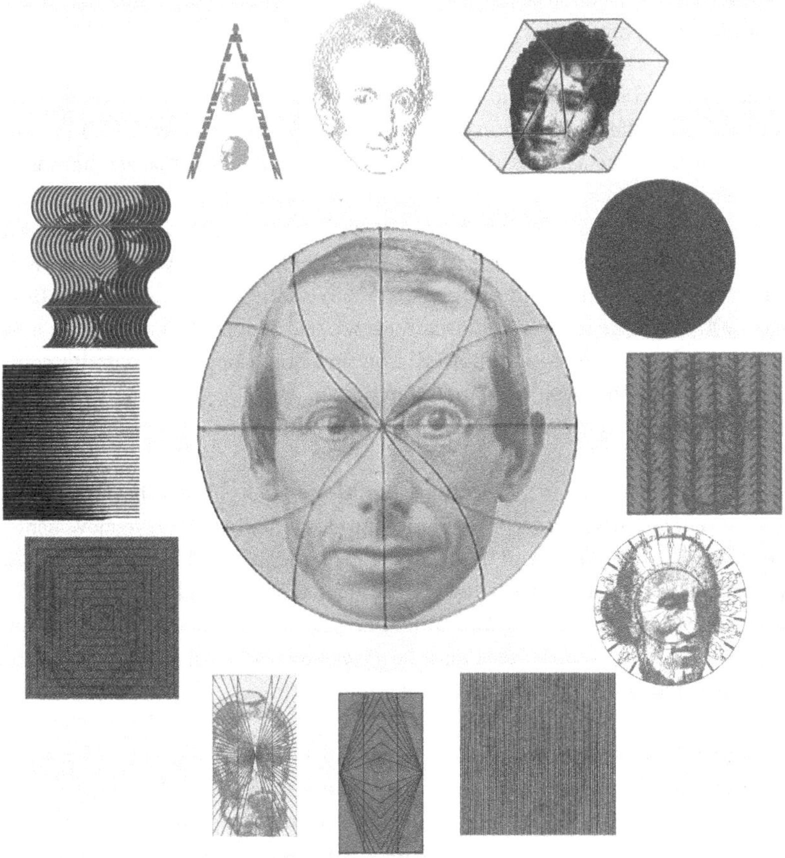

Figure 17.5. *Age of illusions* by Nicholas Wade. Pioneers of illusions embedded in the illusion figures with which they are associated. The central portrait is of Johann Joseph Oppel (1815–1894) in one of his illusion figures. The other portraits are (clockwise from the top in chronological sequence): Peter Mark Roget (1779–1869), Louis Albert Necker (1786–1861), Jan Evangelista Purkinje (1787–1869), Johann Christian Poggendorff (1796–1877), Joseph Plateau (1801–1883), Hermann Ludwig Ferdinand von Helmholtz (1821–1894), Wilhelm Maximilian Wundt (1832–1920), Karl Ewald Konstantin Hering (1834–1918), Johann Karl Friedrich Zöllner (1834–1882), Ernst Mach (1838–1916), Franz Carl Müller-Lyer (1857–1916), and Mario Ponzo (1882–1960).

began to gather a small group of young people about me, who aided me in my experimental work, and whom I advised as to the proper approach to psychological problems. To this circle belonged Luigi Agliardi, Mario Ponzo, Arturo Fontana, Raoul Hahn, Luigi Botti, and many others . . . Mario Ponzo was interested from the start in graphic methods, which he afterwards brought to a high degree of perfection in the course of his researches on the expression of volitional impulses in respiration-curves, as well as through other works performed at my Institute. Besides this, Mario Ponzo afterwards carried out many experiments concerning skin sensations, position sensations . . . Luigi Botti . . . devoted himself to a broad investigation of optical illusions. (Kiesow, 1930, 185)

Thus, it was not Ponzo who conducted research on visual illusions, but Botti (1906) who published his work on them long before Ponzo. Kiesow (1906) also wrote about illusions in the same issue of *Archiv für die gesamte Psychologie*; he was concerned with the perception of extent, as in the horizontal-vertical illusion, and a variety of Müller-Lyer figures. In this regard, Kiesow was influenced by a long paper on illusions from the pen of his mentor, Wundt (1898), which advocated the involvement of eye movements in illusions of extent. Wundt was also the first citation by Botti (1906) in the article that followed Kiesow's and addressed the influence of separation on judgments of extent. Both Kiesow and Botti supported Wundt's contention that the illusions were based on differences in eye movements over the illusory figures. In a review of the articles, Pierce (1907) commented:

> Is it not hazardous and to a large degree profitless to talk glibly of the influence of eye-movements in the absence of any exact knowledge of what these eye-movements actually are in any given case? In this day of registration possibilities, the cautious psychologist is not likely to find any satisfaction in the unverified assertion that the eyes are behaving thus and so. And until some graphic evidence can be furnished in support of such assertions, they must be viewed merely as hypotheses displaying cleverness but not carrying conviction." (118)

Remarkably, the graphical methods that had been introduced in America and Germany to investigate eye movements (see Wade & Tatler, 2005) had not penetrated the institute in which graphical methods had been championed. Kiesow was appointed to a professorship in 1906 and founded the Turin Institute of Psychology; he also returned briefly to the study of illusions.

Botti (1910) expanded his account of visual illusions and gave a historical review of research on them in the 19th century. As various commentators have noted (Arai & Arai, 2013; Farné, 1975; Vicario, 2011), even though Ponzo is known principally through his eponymous illusion, he was not the originator of it. Moreover, some of those precursors were cited by Botti (1910). Ponzo's illusion can be interpreted in terms of the cues for contrast or perspective from the converging lines. Several earlier illusions based on similar principles were produced in the late 19th century (e.g., Bezold, 1884), and original illustrations from many of them can be found in Wade (2014). A figure almost identical to that of Ponzo (1912a) was published in an American textbook on experimental psychology 14 years earlier (Sanford, 1898).

Even more precursors of the linear version of the illusion can be found, as is shown in Figure 17.6. Other examples exist of similar figures, but without the converging lines meeting (see Arai & Arai, 2013; Vicario, 2011). Both Thiéry (1895) and Sanford (1898) were explicit in describing the lines as physically equivalent but perceptually unequal. Moreover, Thiéry devised an apparatus for determining the perceived difference between the horizontal lines; these measurements are referred to by Sanford (1898).

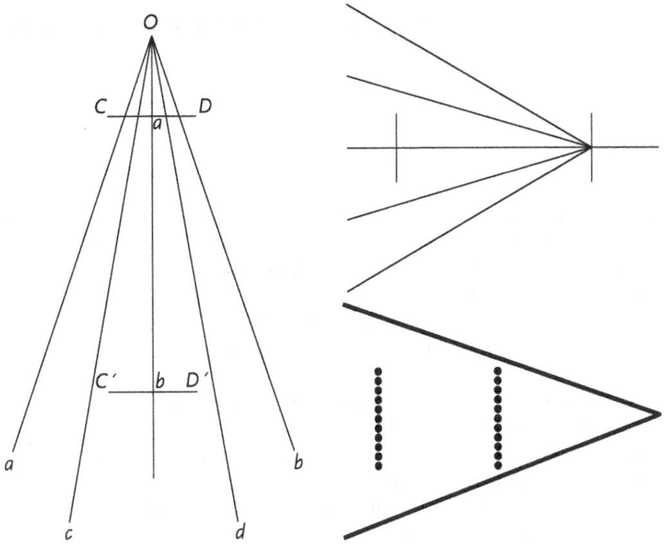

Figure 17.6. Left, a figure from Thiéry (1895) where the lines *CD* and *C′D′* are equal in length; upper right, Sanford's (1898) illustration in which the two vertical lines are equal in length; and lower right, Ponzo's (1928) figure with the two equal columns of dots. The figures are shown in their original orientations.

In the context of named visual illusions, such as the Ponzo illusion, it is not unusual for earlier versions to exist (see Vicario, 2008), but it is uncommon to find such a precise parallel. Ponzo's principal interest was in the skin senses rather than vision. One of his first publications was an experimental study of tactile localization (Ponzo, 1910), and he continued to investigate aspects of tactile perception. Nonetheless, his research was far broader than the senses, and he was an active representative of sensory perception in Turin and later an international ambassador for Italian psychology. In Ponzo's obituary in the *American Journal of Psychology*, Canestrelli (1960) did not even mention the Ponzo illusion. Instead, Ponzo's research on cutaneous sensitivity (initially with Kiesow) was emphasized as was his later work on psychomotor processes and on applied psychology. Still, it is with the illusion configuration, which Ponzo published in 1912, that he will be best remembered and, in many ways, it represented the end of the golden age of illusions.

CONCLUSIONS

Illusions have been grist to the visual scientists' mill for centuries, but there was an acceleration of interest in a subset of them in the second half of the 19th century. The investigation of geometrical optical illusions started rather late in Turin, stimulated by the arrival of Kiesow from Wundt's laboratory at Leipzig. Ponzo wrote two articles on illusions, but his name is now inextricably linked to a simple configuration of equal circles or lines contained with converging lines, which is known as the Ponzo illusion.

REFERENCES

Arai H, Arai S (2013) Tracing the history of Ponzo illusions. *Technical Reports of the Mathematical Vision Science Laboratory, Tokyo, Japan*. No.5 July 29:1–10.

Baltrušaitis J (1977) *Anamorphic Art*. (W J Strachan, Trans). Cambridge: Chadwyck-Healey.

Berkeley G (1709) *An Essay Towards a New Theory of Vision*. Dublin: Pepyat.

Bezold W von (1884) Eine perspectivische Täuschung. *Annalen der Physik und Chemie*, 23: 351–352.

Boring E G (1942) *Sensation and Perception in the History of Experimental Psychology*. New York: Appleton-Century.

Botti L (1906) Ein Beitrag zur Kenntnis der variabeln geometrisch-optischen Streckentäuschungen. *Archiv für die gesamte Psychologie*, 6: 306–315.

Botti L (1910) Recerche sperimentali sulle illusioni ottico-geometriche. *Memorie della Reale Accademia delle Scienze di Torino*, 60: 139–191.

Canestrelli L (1960) Mario Ponzo 1882–1960. *American Journal of Psychology*, 73: 645–647.

Desaguliers J T (1736) An explication of an experiment made in May 1735, as a farther confirmation of what was said in the paper given in January 30, 1734–5. To account for the appearance of the horizontal moon seeming larger than when higher. *Philosophical Transactions of the Royal Society*, 39: 392–394.

Farné M (1975) The Ponzo illusion: Some observations. In G B Flores d'Arcais (Ed.), *Studies in Perception. Festshrift for Fabio Metelli*, pp. 225–235. Milano: Martello-Giunti.

Galilei G (1606) *Considerazioni d'Alimberto Mauri sopra alcuni luoghi del discorso di Ludovico delle Colombe intorno alla stella apparita nel 1604. Considerazioni d'Alimberto Mauri sopra alcuni luoghi . . .* Firenze: Caneo.

Galilei G (1623) *Il Saggiatore, nel quale con bilancia esquisita e giusta*. Rome: Mascardi.

Gregory R L (1966) *Eye and Brain*. London: Wedenfeld and Nicolson.

Gregory R L (2009) *Seeing Through Illusions*. Oxford: Oxford University Press.

Hershenson M (1989) (Ed.) *The Moon Illusion*. Hillsdale, NJ: Lawrence Erlbaum Associates.

Kepler J (1604) *Ad Vitellionem paralipomena*. Frankfurt: Marinium and Aubrii.

Kiesow F (1906) Über einige geometrisch-optische Täuschungen. *Archiv für die gesamte Psychologie*, 6: 289–305.

Kiesow F (1924) Di una illusioni ottico-geometrica. *Archivio Italiano di Psicologia*, 3: 180–184.

Kiesow F (1930) F. Kiesow. In C Murchison (Ed.), *A History of Psychology in Autobiography. Volume 1*, pp. 163–190. Worcester, MA: Clark University Press.

Mosso A (1894) *Die Temperatur des Gehirns*. Leipzig: Veit.

Oppel J J (1855) Über geometrisch-optische Täuschungen. *Jahresbericht des physikalischen Vereins zu Frankfurt am Main*, 1854–1855: 37–47.

Piccolino M, & Wade N J (2008) Galileo Galilei's vision of the senses. *Trends in Neurosciences*, 31: 585–590.

Piccolino M, & Wade N J (2014) *Galileo's Visions: Piercing the Spheres of the Heavens by Eye and Mind*. Oxford: Oxford University Press.

Pierce A H (1907) Reviews of two papers on illusions, Ueber einige geometrisch-optische Täuschungen, and Ein Beitrag zur Kenntnis der variabeln geometrisch-optischen Streckentäuschungen. *Psychological Bulletin*, 4: 116–118.

Ponzo M (1910) Studio della localizzazione delle sensazioni tattili. *Memorie della Reale Accademia delle Scienze di Torino*, 60: 42–106.

Ponzo M (1912a) Rapports entre quelques illusions visuelle de contrast angulaire et l'appréciation de grandeur des astres à l'horizon. *Archives Italiennes de Biologie*, 58: 327–329.
Ponzo M (1912b) Rapporti fra alcune illusioni visive di contrasto angolare e l'apprezzamento di grandezza degli astri all'orizzontale. *Rivista di Psicologia*, 8: 304–306.
Ponzo M (1928) Urteilstäuschungen über Mengen. *Archiv für die gesamte Psychologie*, 65: 129–162.
Ponzo M (1929) Illusioni negli apprezzamenti di collettività. *Archivio Italiano di Psicologia*, 7: 1–37.
Pressey A W (2013) Clashing interpretations of Ponzo's illusion: Reconsideration of assimilation versus tilt-constancy theories. *Comprehensive Psychology*, 2 (14): 1–7.
Roget P M (1826) *An Introductory Lecture on Human and Comparative Physiology*. London: Longman, Rees, Orme, Brown, and Green.
Ross H E, & Plug C (2002) *The Mystery of the Moon Illusion*. Oxford: Oxford University Press.
Sabra A I (Ed. and Trans.) (1989) *The Optics of Ibn Al-Haytham. Books I–III. On Direct Vision*. London: The Warburg Institute.
Sanford E C (1898) *A Course in Experimental Psychology. Part 1: Sensation and Perception* (2nd Ed.). Boston: Heath.
Scheiner C (1619) *Oculus, hoc est fundamentum opticum*. Innsbruck: Agricola.
Shapiro A, & Todorovic D (Eds.) (2017) *Oxford Compendium of Visual Illusions*. Oxford: Oxford University Press.
Smith A M (1996) *Ptolemy's Theory of Visual Perception: An English Translation of the* Optics *with Introduction and Commentary*. Philadelphia: The American Philosophical Society.
Thiéry A (1895) Ueber geometrisch-optische Täuschungen. Fortsetzung. *Philosophische Studien*, 11: 603–620.
Vicario G B (2008) Optical-geometrical illusions: The nomenclature. *Gestalt Theory*, 30: 168–180.
Vicario G B (2011) *Illusioni Ottico-Geometriche. Una Rassegna di Problemi*. Venice: Istituto Veneto di Scienze, Lettere ed Arte.
Wade N J (1998a) *A Natural History of Vision*. Cambridge, MA: MIT Press.
Wade N (1998b) Illusions as neuro-signs. *Current Biology*, 8: R364–R365, R439, R509–R510, R593, R671, R743, R826.
Wade N J (2007) Galileo and the senses: Vision and the art of deception. *Galilæana*, 4: 259–288.
Wade N J (2014) Geometrical optical illusionists. *Perception*, 43: 846–868.
Wade N (2016) *Art and Illusionists*. Heidelberg: Springer.
Wade N J (2018, February) The age of illusions. *The Psychologist*, 54–59.
Wade N J, Tatler B W (2005) *The Moving Tablet of the Eye: The Origins of Modern Eye Movement Research*. Oxford: Oxford University Press.
Wundt W (1898) *Die geometrisch-optischen Täuschungen*. Leipzig: Teubner.

CHAPTER 18

Science and Literature at Giuseppe Levi's Home in Turin

MARCO PICCOLINO

GIUSEPPE LEVI, A MODERN CELL BIOLOGIST WITH A PARTICULAR INTEREST IN NEUROSCIENCES

As an introduction: the "Professore" and the others, science and literature in an haute—bourgeoisie home in Turin

Giuseppe Levi (1872–1965; Figure 18.1) was a prominent Italian scientist who carried out important research in various dimensions of cell biology and neurosciences. He was the leading figure in his area of studies in Italy in the first half of the 20th century, not only for the importance of his discoveries but also for his didactic texts. This was particularly the case for the treatises of histology and anatomy that he wrote or edited and which were reference manuals for generations of students in Italy and abroad. As a local consultant of the Rockefeller Foundation, which—starting from the 1920s—had launched a program for funding medical studies in Europe, Levi also played a significant role in the organization of medical and biological research in Italy.

With his immense scientific culture and his stunning personality, he was a memorable professor of anatomy and histology in Turin from 1919 until his retirement in 1948, and he succeeded in making his laboratory a lively cradle of scientific talents. Among his many students were several prominent scholars who have left milestone contributions in various fields of biological research. Outside Italy, Levi is probably best known for three of his pupils who were awarded the Nobel Prize: Renato Dulbecco, Rita Levi-Montalcini, and Salvador Luria.

In Italy, however, Levi is mainly known for another dimension, only loosely connected to his scientific and didactic achievements. Together with his wife Lidia Tanzi, he is one of the two main characters of *Lessico famigliare* ("Family lexicon") the book written by their daughter, Natalia Levi-Ginzburg, one of the greatest writers

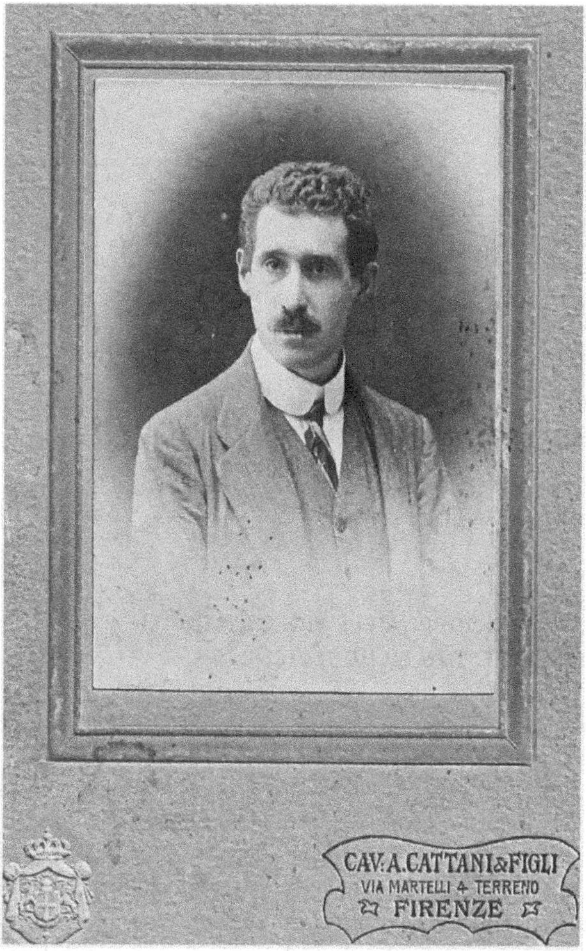

Figure 18.1. A portrait of Giuseppe Levi (1872–1964), probably dating back to the early years of his research in Florence. The photo was taken in a Florentine photographic studio (courtesy of the Levi-Ginzburg family ©).

of the Italian Novecento. In this book, Natalia provides a literary portrait of her family, with particular reference to the characteristic wording used by her parents and siblings, considered as an expression of the profound unity of its members. On one side, she represents her father, the *Professore*, as a paternal and severe authority, deeply absorbed in his studies and scientific interests and apparently alienated with respect to literature and art (see Piccolino, 2003, 2005). On the other side stands her mother, viewed as an intelligent and cultivated lady, deeply involved in the education of her children, with a delicate and graceful touch, powerfully attracted by literature (and particularly by Proust's *La Recherche*), by music, art, theater, cinema, but also by the relatively frivolous aspects of feminine life (fashions, silk clothes, luxury sweaters).

By portraying the Levi family in the pages of her book, Natalia succeeded in creating an extraordinary fresco of Italian intellectual *haute-bourgeoisie* during a complex and somewhat tragic period of modern European history. Her achievement accounts for the fact that—as already remarked—"Professor Levi" is best known as the father of the *Lessico famigliare* story, rather than as a great anatomist and biologist, or the teacher of a generation of great scientists.

The interests of Giuseppe Levi were very broad, and encompassed domains we could now label as cell biology, histology, microscopic anatomy, neurosciences, developmental biology, embryology, comparative anatomy, and more. He was an extremely prolific writer of numerous types of works, including research articles, review papers, treatises, discussion texts, and book reviews. He was capable of working and writing in the most demanding conditions, and, moreover, of taking advantage of any possible local opportunity for his research work.

In 1939, having been obliged to leave Italy because of the racial laws, he sets up a laboratory of investigation on nerve development in Liège, Belgium, and continues working and publishing important papers after Nazis invaded the city. Having returned to Italy in a fortuitous way, he works (at the age of 70) with his former student, Rita Levi-Montalcini, in the laboratory that Rita has been able to set up at her home. Forced eventually to leave the town and to wander in the countryside in search of uncertain refuge in the small villages of the region, he brings with him the abstracts of recent literature in order to prepare the third edition of his treatise of histology, and to write an important monograph on cell growth and senescence.

In this chapter, I will try to outline some aspects of Levi's scientific history, based on my first encounter with his figure when, many years ago—as a medical student—I was fascinated by the way he has succeeded in inserting in a potentially arid treatise of human anatomy a vibrant exposition of the modern achievements of cell biology. Many years afterward, I met Levi's writings again when my interests started turning from the experimental work on nerve physiology to the history of neuroscience.

In the next chapter, Giacomo Magrini will deal with the cultural and social history of the Turin in which Giuseppe Levi and of his family circle lived and with the complex and somewhat tragic events of the wartime period involving particularly his daughter Natalia and her husband Leone Ginzburg. Moreover, through the pages of *Lessico famigliare*, and of Natalia's other writings, he analyzes the complex intellectual relationship existing between the scientist and his daughter, also viewed as an expression of the dynamic conflict between two different gnoseological attitudes: that pertaining mainly, but not only, to the *Professore*, based on confidence on the value of the rationalistic approach to knowledge, and the less direct, but potentially more deep one, belonging to philosophy, literature, and religion.

In this chapter, I will not provide a systematic or chronological biography of Levi. I will follow, instead, a rather free, narrative discourse in which science, social and cultural history, and literature are intertwined. One of the points which I have grasped during the research that has led to this text, and that I hope to convey to the readers, concerns the historical and cultural richness of Italy in the period after the unification of the country, and the inventiveness and effort of innovation and of internationalism that characterized the generation of Risorgimento. One of Levi's great merits is to have kept and developed in his field of study the important legacy of the Risorgimento generation, and transferred, along the dark period of fascism, to his pupils, allowing them to flourish in their research in various directions, and undoubtedly at a very high level. Levi succeeded in being an important maestro for a generation of pupils, but he could be so because his endeavor had thrived in a rich cultural and social background that I will attempt to outline.

THE BEGINNINGS: THE MODERN IDEAS OF A YOUNG AND SHY PROFESSOR OF ANATOMY, AND A STUDENT IN SEARCH OF A VOCATION

Giuseppe Levi was born on October 14, 1872 in Trieste, the son of Emma Perugia and of Michele, a wealthy financier belonging to a lineage of bankers. Some of them, because of services rendered to the Austro-Hungarian Empire, had been honored with the title of Baron by the Habsburgs, then dominant in the region of Trieste. In 1886, after Michele's premature death, Emma, who belonged to the affluent Jewish bourgeoisie of Pisa (with tight Triestin connections), moved with her son to Florence, then a very lively cultural and scientific center, and a place of attraction for Triestins with strong roots in the Italian nationality and culture. A large part of Emma's wealth came from the family of her mother, Rachele De Parente (or *von* Parente, a family often mentioned in the *Lessico*). In 1889 Giuseppe enrolled himself in the medical section of the *Regio Istituto di Studi Superiori* (Royal Institute of Advanced Studies) where he had several important scientists of the time among his teachers, including the anatomist Giulio Chiarugi, the physiologist Luigi Luciani, the pathologist Alessandro Lustig, the chemist Hugo Schiff, and the clinician Pietro Grocco, some of whom held strong international connections.

The lively scientific and cultural atmosphere of the *Regio Istituto* was mainly due to the results of a process of renewal and de-provincialism initiated by the politicians and intellectuals of the Risorgimento. Among them, there was, in particular, Carlo Matteucci, the great physicist and physiologist born in Forlì, who had been for a short time Minister of Education in the Rattazzi Cabinet. Matteucci had invited to Florence Hugo Schiff and his brother, the physiologist Moritz (Maurizio) Schiff, who had been a student of Johannes Müller (and of other important scientists of the time). Moritz was the founder of the Florentine Institute of Physiology, located on the premises of Via Capponi, and, in the direction of this institute, he was succeeded by one of his assistants (and also a student of Carl Vogt), the Russian physiologist Aleksandr Herzen. There followed Luigi Luciani, a pupil of Carl Ludwig, particularly famous for his studies on the cerebellum, mostly conducted in Florence (and also for a famous handbook of physiology that was translated into several languages). Luciani taught Human Physiology to Levi, who passed the exam brilliantly with honors in 1892.

After Luciani, Giulio Fano (a pupil of Luciani, of Angelo Mosso, and of Ludwig) arrived in Florence, succeeding his master after he moved to Rome. Like his predecessors, Fano (who taught in Florence from 1894—during the years in which

Levi carried out his thesis work and then in the period of his subsequent research) was an influential scientist and a man of great culture and extensive international contacts. He professed a modern approach to physiology, based on nondogmatic materialism, open to the principles of Darwinian theory, and founded on a fruitful interaction of this science with physics and chemistry. Fano did not, however, push too far the reductionism typical of these sciences, and insisted against downgrading physiology to pure thermodynamic theories. He gave significant relief to the importance, for the mechanisms of life, of the structural organization and morphology.

Fano's ideas undoubtedly contributed to shaping the methodological approach to which Levi remained faithful throughout his scientific career, according to an attitude mainly characterized by a dynamic or functional conception of the morphological investigations. This was an attitude largely shared in the *Regio Istituto*, and it was, in particular, the *credo* of two eminent scientists who had a profound influence on Levi, the anatomist Giulio Chiarugi and the pathologist Alessandro Lustig.

It was in the Institute of General Pathology directed by Lustig that Levi carried out the research leading to his dissertation for graduation in Medicine in July 1895, with the maximum grade, cum laude, and with the dignity of publication (Figure 18.2). In the thesis—which was published in the same year as his graduation in the Florentine journal, *Lo Sperimentale*—Levi reported the results of a study, "Of the alterations produced in the kidney by Sodium Chloride" (*Delle Alterazioni prodotte*

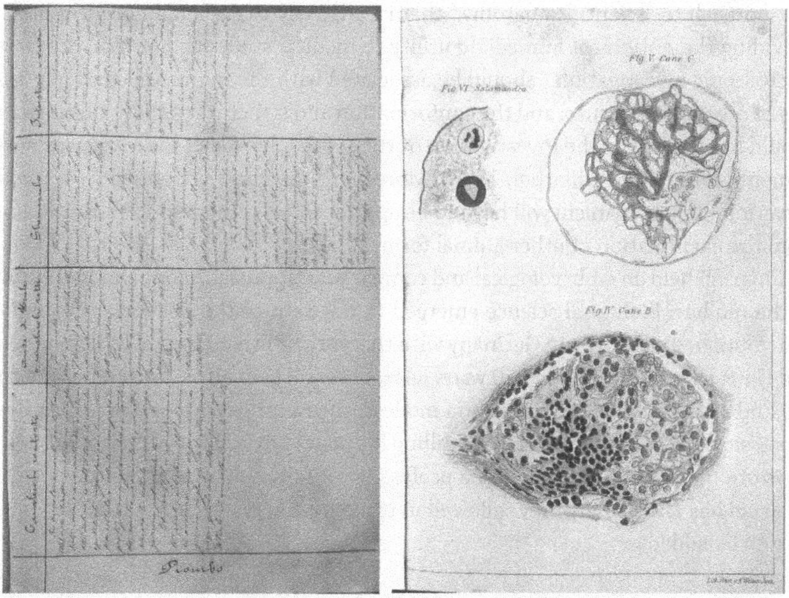

Figure 18.2. On the left, a page of Giuseppe Levi's manuscript thesis with the table summarizing the literature on the pathological effects of lead on the kidney. On the right, a table taken from the printed thesis, published in *Lo Sperimentale*, with images of the morphological alterations of the kidney structure in the dog and salamander (courtesy of the Biomedical Library of the University of Florence ©).

nel rene dal Cloruro di Sodio), performed on rabbits and dogs, as well as salamanders. The text of the thesis, which shows Levi's already mentioned dynamic approach to morphological investigation is remarkable also for the author's absolute mastery of the literature on the subject, in particular that in German (the language then widely dominant in the field of experimental pathology).

The thesis was the first printed work that Levi published alone. While working on the thesis, he collaborated with an important member of the Lustig laboratory, Gino Galeotti, with whom he established a friendship destined to last for a lifetime (also because of their shared passion for the mountains and for great journeys). With Galeotti, Levi had already published two works, one of which appeared in 1893, while Giuseppe was still a student, the other in 1895, the year of his graduation (Levi, 1893; Levi, 1895b). The two articles appeared in a German magazine (*Beiträge zur pathologischen Anatomie*). They deal with problems of tissue regeneration and are linked: The first concerns the regeneration of striated muscle fibers, the second the regeneration of nerve elements in newly formed muscle tissue. These works betray Levi's early orientation toward regenerative phenomena, a research path along which will emerge some of his most significant discoveries, both personal and of his students, especially in relation to the regeneration and development of nerve cells.

In addition, of great importance for Levi was the influence of Giulio Chiarugi, a young anatomist recently appointed at the *Regio Istituto*. In his inaugural lecture held in the anatomical theater on November 28, 1890 (and attended by Levi, then in the second year of his medical course) Chiarugi formulated some of the principles of his approach to "scientific anatomy," that is, anatomy that should not be limited to providing the notions of immediate utility to medical students. For him, the classic macroscopic investigation, "should be associated with the minute microscopic analysis of organs and tissues; and the conformation and structure of the adult organism should be clarified by the investigation of the process by which the history of development takes place" (Chiarugi, 1890). Moreover, "the results obtained from the observation of our organism will have to be appropriately compared to those obtained from the examination of other animal forms."

Chiarugi held an embryological and comparative approach, along the conceptions of the modern biological science emerged in the path of the Darwinian revolution and flourished especially in Germany with the work of Ernst Haeckel, Wilhelm Roux, and Hans Driesch. More than 50 years later, Levi still kept alive "the memory of that day and of that professor, young and modest, shy in his behaviour, but with a lively expression" (Levi 1946, p. 1918). Recalling his master in 1946, a year after his death, he wrote that this "prolusion was a profession of faith and a program to which the Chiarugi has always faithfully followed in teaching and research" (p. 1919).

And he added:

> In his concise, yet polished, style—this was one of his characteristics—he expressed the conviction that the description of the complete development of human forms must be integrated with the knowledge of those forms in progress during ontogeny, and with the similarities between the forms of man and those of animals. And, the embryological and anatomocomparative method is bound to give the raison d'être

of the mature human forms, of man's position in nature and of relationships existing between man and the lower forms. (Levi, 1946)

Although Chiarugi would have a profound influence on him, it is also true that neither at the time of the thesis work, nor in the years immediately afterward, did Levi orient himself toward the Institute of Human Anatomy in order to continue his research activity. Initially, he chose the Psychiatric Clinic, then located in the San Salvi Hospital, a choice that a posteriori seems difficult to understand given his declared dislike for clinical work. His decision could be due to the fact that in 1895 (the year of Levi's graduation) had been appointed director of the Florentine clinic Eugenio Tanzi, who was together with his pupil and deputy, Ernesto Lugaro, one of the leading figures of research on the microscopic anatomy of the nervous system. Tanzi and Lugaro were very famous, both for the importance of their research conducted and for the courage and lucidity with which they had supported the theory of the individuality of nerve cells ("neuronal doctrine"). This was particularly advocated by the Spanish anatomist Santiago Ramón Y Cajal, against the conceptions of "reticular" type then prevailing in Italy, which had been adopted by the famous histologist of Pavia, Camillo Golgi (Piccolino, 1988; Piccolino, Strettoi, & Laurenzi, 1989; Mazzarello, 1999).

In 1893, two years before his arrival in Florence, Tanzi published a famous critical review on *I fatti e le induzioni nell'odierna istologia del sistema nervoso* [On facts and inductions in today's histology of the nervous system]. In this text, in addition to exposing experimental data and theoretical considerations in favor of Cajal's neuronistic conceptions, he hypothesized possible mechanisms of functioning and plasticity of the connection between nerve cells that could represent the biological substrate of memory and of learning, of both the psychic and motor type. Tanzi assumed that the repeated activation of a nervous pathway, induced by psychic or motor exercise, could leave a more or less lasting change in the connection between communicating neurons (i.e., in the synapse, as it would have been called in 1897 by the English physiologist Charles Scott Sherrington). Tanzi supposed the existence, at this level, of "a resistance or, so to speak, as a kind of bad passage (*mal passo*) that the nervous wave will have to overcome, not without some difficulty," due to the anatomical separation between the two neurons in functional relationship (Tanzi 1893, 469; see Berlucchi & Buchtel, 2009). He suggested that this distance tended to shorten progressively with exercise and learning. These activities would increase "the conductivity of neurons, i.e. their functional capacity" (Tanzi, 1893, 469; see Berlucchi & Buchtel, 2009). Tanzi's pupil Lugaro will then return to these issues, hypothesizing that the transmission of interneuronal occurs through a "chemical modification" and being the first to introduce the term "plasticity" to indicate the synaptic changes due to exercise and learning (Berlucchi, 2002).

After leaving the San Salvi clinic in 1898, Levi decided to spend one year of research abroad and chose the laboratory of Oskar Hertwig in Munich. Hertwig was a German zoologist and biologist who had become particularly famous for having shown, with his experiments on sea urchins, that fertilization requires the fusion of the elements of male and female germinal cells. Levi probably derived the interest in the reproductive physiology from Hertwig, and this would lead him to study some aspects of the reproductive mechanisms, particularly in chiropters and amphibians. It is possible that the period with Hertwig favored Levi's decision to collaborate with Chiarugi on his return in 1899 to Florence. Chiarugi was then working on the reproductive mechanisms in invertebrates, and his orientation toward embryology and a dynamic form of anatomical research probably attracted the young Levi, finally determined for a research life and career.

Among the very important private events that occur in this period in Levi's life, there is the meeting with Lidia, the daughter of the Milanese lawyer Carlo Tanzi, brother of the director of the psychiatric hospital, and an active member of the socialist party. It is the beginning of a love story that will last for a lifetime. With her mother, Giuseppina Biraghi, Lidia had moved a few years earlier to Florence, where she had attended the high school courses at *Liceo Galileo*. The girl, who was younger than Giuseppe by six years (she was born in 1878), will also enroll in medicine (in 1898), but will attend the course only for two years. Despite brilliant grades in the exams, she moved to Natural Sciences in 1900, and then left the university because of her marriage with Giuseppe, and the birth, in 1901, of their first son, Gino. As I have already said, Lidia will be with Giuseppe (*Beppino*) the protagonist of *Family Lexicon*.

GIUSEPPE LEVI: THE IMPORTANCE OF FORM AND ORGANIZATION AGAINST DESTRUCTURED "CHEMISM"

Giulio Fano, the successor of Luciani in the Chair of Physiology, in his prolusion delivered in 1894, at the time of his inauguration in Florence, first underlined the importance of the study of the structure to clarify the functions of the nervous system. Fano then stressed the importance of morphological studies in connection with chemical investigations.
He said:

> From all this it is clear that with the study of the conditions and morphological changes that determine, accompany, follow a functional act, much more than with chemical research, we could perhaps one day explain the many and serious problems of Physiology. And perhaps also the most fundamental processes from which energy is accumulated and built up, of those that transform it and shape it, determining the most specific manifestations of a living being. And this, because the morphological facts, as we have said, express the elective actions accumulated slowly in the indefinite past. These actions, associating themselves with the current chemical acts, give results that are all the more unpredictable the more we ignore the intimate nature of the organization. (Fano, 1894, pp. 28–29)

It is no coincidence that these words of the physiologist Fano would resound, a quarter of a century later, in the lecture held by Levi in Turin at the time of his inauguration in the Chair of Anatomy, in 1919 (and published in 1920). Levi would spend the whole of his subsequent life of intense work, research, and teaching in Turin, and would live there until the day of his death (with more or less long interruptions linked, in addition to his scientific journeys, to the vicissitudes resulting from the proclamation, in 1938, of the racial laws, and from the tragedy of war). The inaugural lecture was dedicated mainly to the defense of the morphological and structural approach. This risked then being put aside by the most modern physiological conceptions (and also by the development of chemical theories of life mechanisms, particularly those based on the properties of colloidal systems. These views proposed the relative irrelevance of the morphological investigations for the understanding of functions, both at the level of organs and of cells. These conceptions had been reiterated—as Levi recalled—by Charles Richet in his inaugural address to the Congress of Physiology held in Vienna in 1910. Richet had referred then to the opinions of Claude Bernard. As George Canguilhem has stressed in modern times, Bernard had discovered the ability of the liver to synthesize sugar not through an anatomical study of the organ, but by following—with a biochemical and functional approach—the variations in the blood concentration of this substance in the various circulatory districts.

In particular, Richet contested the functional value of cytological and histology studies applied to nerve cells, then in full bloom, particularly after the great diffusion in this field of research of the staining method invented by the German pathologist Franz Nissl. This method allowed the detection, in the interior of the cell, of particular granules (the Nissl bodies as we now call them: formations that have a fundamental role in protein synthesis).

Richet wondered:

> Even though we can minutely describe the shape of a cell and the complicated network of the various granulations that make it up, we do not know anything about its function. From the existence in a nerve cell of 5 or 6 groups of differently colored substances could we deduce the amount of oxygen it consumes, the conditions of the reflex act and the laws of its irritability? (quoted in Levi 1920, p. 37)

In 1919, against the concepts of Richet, Levi reiterated the importance, in living beings, of structure and organization, with words that highlighted the intimate contradiction of a physiology and a "destructured" chemistry:

> The scepticism that has found its expression in the formula of Claude Bernard, that the knowledge of the form does not imply that of the function, does it really go so far to consider life independent of the specific form of organized matter? In this case the rules governing the latter resolve themselves in a "lusus naturae", and it would be implicitly assumed that life can manifest itself in amorphous matter without acquiring the specific constitution in living beings. But in reality no doubt can exist, that there is a definite relationship between structure and function. (Levi 1920, p. 42)

Levi recognized, on the one hand, the inadequacy of the solely structural investigation in "explaining the dynamic manifestations of life," and the inadequacy of a pure dynamism of the forms, detached from functional considerations (such as that which had been fashionable in the morphogenetic studies, on the wave of the Darwinian revolution). On the other hand, he highlights the limitations of a conception that saw life like the game of exclusively chemical forces; or even as the property of colloidal systems, whose model was then invoked by many (including some of his colleagues in Florence, as for instance the biochemist Filippo Bottazzi), as a possible reference for the explanation of the vital phenomena. "The notion that the colloidal environment is a necessary condition for the explanation of the life process—he said—did not advance us long in the knowledge of the latter."

He continued with words that now appear lucidly prophetic, if viewed from the perspective of the development of biological research that in the 20th century has—as we know—recognized one of the fundamental aspects of the functioning of biological systems as the results of the integration of physical–chemical processes closely related to cell structures and microstructures.

Levi said that:

> Life is not tied to a special substance, and it is not a special reaction, but it is a great system of processes and substances that cannot be dissociated; all these properties of the organized substance are in perfect harmony, appropriate to the function, from the most basic to the most complex. (p. 43)

He took up these concepts again in 1927, in the introductory section of what is undoubtedly his major work in the field of education, the already mentioned *Trattato di Istologia*, In the introduction to the work, Levi reaffirmed in a strongly assertive way the importance of organization in the understanding of the phenomena of life, and consequently the indispensable value of morphological research:

> The constitutive substance of living organisms has particular physical and chemical properties, but its most essentially specific character, which—more than any other—is related to vital manifestations, is given by structural properties, which are not reflected in the inanimate world. They are summarized in the word organization. There is no life without organization. And, this is quickly changed when a living person dies, and—after some time—cancelled. (Levi 1927, p. 1)

In 1927, by publishing his *histological treatise*, Levi was indeed giving birth to a text of cellular biology that was ahead of the times. It was intended to form the critical spirit of researchers in various fields of biological and medical sciences rather than to impart basic notions useful to medical students. From many points of view, he elaborated something that went even beyond the modern "physiological histology" advocated in those years by the French scholar Albert Policard. This was an approach that Levi himself would indicate as "histophysiology," when resuming his lessons in Turin in 1945, after his removal from teaching due to the racial laws and the vicissitudes of war.

In this new prolusion, which he titled, not surprisingly, *La struttura della sostanza vivente* [The structure of living substance], Levi takes up the long-cherished theme of the relationship between form and function, a theme that was then assuming new characteristics. This was due, on the one hand, to the development of biochemistry that was identifying organic macromolecules and was coming near to the identification of the chemical mechanisms of cellular functions and transmission of hereditary traits; and—on the other hand—to the introduction into the biological research of electron microscopy, a technique that began to reveal cellular structures with a resolution at the molecular level.

The successes of biochemistry were then reanimating the criticism against the importance of form and structure in the genesis of life phenomena, which Levi summarized by citing Bergson's words that "there is no organic form, because form is immobility, while—in the organic world—reality is movement." To the conceptions of the French philosopher, he opposed those of the German biologist Alfred Benninghoff, for whom "the flow of life is composed in innumerable stages of different speed; in this flow there are arrangements that are relatively constant over time" (Levi 1945, 82). And he concluded by reaffirming the profound value that—in his view—structure and form had for living organisms in:

> There is no living dynamics outside the form, the living process (*accadimento*) is ordered, and—in this order—it is at the service of the whole organism through the form; it constitutes the form and it maintains it (Levi 1945, 82).

THE ETHICAL DIMENSION OF SCIENCE IN GIUSEPPE LEVI

As mentioned, Levi addressed his didactic work more to provide the intellectual tools and critical spirit indispensable to those who were directed toward biological and medical research, than to inculcate the concepts immediately necessary for the medical profession.

This appears implicitly in many of his writings, but emerges particularly in the situations in which he can express himself on the directions of his teaching and research activity. Even then, as in his inaugural lecture in Palermo in January 1915, he strives to maintain a low profile as to the modernity of his scientific approach, and exalts for this reason—perhaps more than necessary—the importance of traditional anatomy. Concluding his lecture, held before the Rector, his new colleagues, and his students, he is mainly directed to the latter (whom he addresses as *giovani egregi*, probably in memory of Chiarugi's 1890 prolusion). He wonders—evidently in a rhetorical way—if it may have relevance to the predominantly didactic nature of the course of anatomy for medical students about to begin his extensive discussion of the problem of the growth of organisms that has been at the center of the lecture. This was based on a vast amount of data and reflections, above all of a functional nature, derived from the study of both animal and plant organisms, algae, and bacteria.

Afterward, he continues by saying: "If for educational needs we are then forced to impose limits on the various disciplines, these must not stop the researcher's initiatives" (Levi, 1915, 37), and finally concludes with words showing the profound ethical value that he attributes to research activity:

> Science imposes a severe and obscure activity on its devotees, and often requires the complete dedication of one's personality, without these dedications being compensated by evident success. Yet from the conscientious and disinterested work of the modest scholar, when he is animated by faith, we await the moral and intellectual elevation of our country. And this more for the educative function exercised by his work, than for the real conquests that he will be allowed to achieve. (p. 38)

The ethical dimension of the research work has a particular value for Levi. It protects the scientist from the flattery and vicissitudes of life. This value, which is a fundamental key to understanding his personality, will be recalled by Levi explicitly in the conclusion of the 1919 inaugural lecture in Turin. There, he encourages his students to pursue "the disinterested study, and not to care for the obvious success" because only on this condition can be genuinely realized "the cult of science." And then continues, taking up the words of a text of the Buddhist Canon, the *Dhammapada*: "As a massive cliff it is not shaken by the wind, so neither shall the sages wobble for praise" (Levi 1920, 125).

Giuseppe Levi, a Leonine Lust for Science and the Pursuit of the Ganglia of Whales

There is a passage in the *Family Lexicon* that seems of particular relevance to those who take into account the vastness of Levi's scientific interests. It is when Natalia narrates, almost certainly on the basis of maternal recollection, her father's early restlessness in the hotel room, when, traveling with his wife for some scientific congress, he woke up at dawn:

> He always woke up very early in the morning, and was, waking up, always hungry. Until he had had breakfast, he was in a ferocious mood; he whirled around the room, looking out, watching the first light of dawn. When they were finally five o'clock, he would hang on to the phone and order, screaming, for breakfast:—*Deux thés! Deux thés complets! avec de l'eau chaude!* (Ginzburg, 1963, pp. 117–118)

If we try to imagine this leonine vitality of the Professor channeled toward research activity, it will not be difficult to imagine how his scientific and didactic production, including experimental articles, review, and discussion texts, treatises, commemorations of masters and colleagues, really represents an extraordinary amount of pages rich in data, figures, reflections, hypotheses, and theories. Levi's immense scientific culture, combined with the desire to be complete and documented as far as possible, in what he asserted or discussed, led him, already from the first years of research, to make a comprehensive history of previous research on the problem that he faced experimentally. As a consequence, in his publications he used to cite a very considerable number of bibliographic references, which became really exuberant in the review texts. In his biography of the master, Levi's pupil, Rodolfo Amprino talks about the 650 bibliographic entries in the review article that

Levi wrote in 1925, for the prestigious German magazine *Ergebnisse der Anatomie Ergebnisse und Entwicklungsgeschichte*, about the morphogenetic factors of the size of cells and animal organisms. Nothing in comparison to the 1,270 references that the same Amprino counts in the review published in 1934, always in the same German magazine, about the in-vitro cultures of which Levi had been one of the pioneers in Europe. Personally, I have been able to count "only" 416 in Levi's monumental 1908 article on the cerebrospinal ganglia (*I gangli cerebrospinali, Studi di istologia comparata ed istogenesi*). A review article, made, to a large amount, of personal results obtained on numberless animal species, with 392 text pages, and 40 tables with 462 figures, almost entirely from Levi's own work!

This *natural vasto* (vast natural, to quote from the Don Giovanni's libretto), this "bulimia" of Levi as a writer of scientific texts, concerned many other aspects of his scholarly activity. In his article concerned with comparative cytological research on vertebrate nerve cells, published in 1897 (i.e., only two years after graduation, when the author was 25 years old), Levi compares the observations conducted in a remarkable variety of species: among the cells of mammals he examines are nerves of guinea pigs, dogs, oxen, bats, rabbits, mice, dormice, cats and even autoptic human preparations; among the reptiles, the snake and the turtle; among the anuran amphibians, the frog and the toad; among the urodeles, the crested newt, an Italian type of cave salamander, and the proteus; among the fish, the ray, the lamprey, the tench, and the catfish. If this variety of species can, at first sight, not seem impressive, we must consider that in almost all the species studied he examined a significant number of types of neurons (spinal ganglion cells, ventral and spinal cord dorsal horns, Purkinje and granule cells of the cerebellum, cells of the cerebral cortex and the basal ganglia, in the urodeles, the cells of the olfactory bulb). He also studied the cells of neuroglia, measuring in each element examined, both neurons and neuroglia, the dimensions of the nucleus and those of the cytoplasm.

In the 1925 review on the relationship between growth and size of animals, Levi reported the results of his experiments conducted in 44 chicken embryos, 36 embryos of other species of birds, 33 embryos of a small reptile, the *Gongylus ocellatus*, various bat embryos and the organs of fetuses and adults of various mammals. In each of these animals, he analyzed the volume changes in a variety of structures or organs during pre- and postnatal growth. An immense work, indeed, both in the research and experimentation phase and in the data processing and text writing stage!

In the long 1908 paper on the cerebrospinal ganglia, Levi reported the results of his investigation carried out in more than 50 species, some of which are exotic, and—moreover—he investigated the histogenesis of the ganglia in a large number of embryo or fetuses of birds and mammals.

To all the intense experimental work needed to perform these experiments, it should be added the extra work required to find some of the species used for the experiments. For Levi, however, this probably had, at least in part, a playful and delightful dimension. From various indications, it is to be presumed that, at least for the less common species, in this and other studies, he sometimes went to look for the experimental animals himself, during his walks on the mountains or elsewhere. He probably combined the apparently opposite pleasures of physical activity in the large spaces of natural environments with those—not less emotionally intense—of the long hours spent in the laboratory to observe the preparations under the microscope (or to cultivate cells, or to interfere with embryonic growth).

From the *Lexicon* we know of a very special search—though with an unsuccessful outcome—that had led him even toward the North Pole, at the time when he studied the correlation between the size of the large nerve cells of an animal and the size of its body. This would become one of his preferred fields of interest and would eventually lead him to formulate a law, generally referred to as "Levi's law" governing this relation. The episode took place in 1907, during one of Levi's trips to Norway, during the time in which he was looking for specimens suitable for his studies on the cerebrospinal ganglia, which he published in 1908. Some of the circumstances of this particular search for laboratory material resurface in the *Lexicon*, and particularly the reactions of Giuseppe's mother, Emma Perugia, and of his wife, Lidia Tanzi (Figure 18.3).

This is how Natalia puts the story, most surely from the recollection of Lidia:

- "Poor Thing—my father said [with reference to his mother, Emma]—When I came back from Spitzberg, where I had gone inside a whale's cranium to look for cerebrospinal ganglia, I brought back with me a bag full of my clothes covered in whale blood and she was too disgusted to touch them. I took them up into the attic and they stank beyond belief!"
- "I never did find those cerebrospinal ganglia,"—my father said.—My mom said: "He got all his good clothes dirty for no reason!"
- Maybe you didn't look hard enough, Beppino!"—my mother [i.e., Natalia's mother, Lidia] said—"Maybe you should have kept looking!" (Ginzburg N, 1963, p. 218; English translation by McPhee J in Ginzburg N, 2017).

There is another version of that search that attracted Levi in a particular way, because the particularly big size of the whales would allow for a particularly relevant test of his biological theories. This version, which contrasts with Natalia's, is referred to by Amprino in his biography and attributed to Levi himself. It resurfaces in other writings—very likely—based on Amprino's biography.

With reference to Levi, Amprino writes:

> In 1907, during one of his various trips to Norway, he spent several weeks at the Spitsbergen (Iceland) to collect sensory ganglia of whales; unluckily, the preservation of thee specimens was not sufficiently good for histology as he remarked in a footnote of his "I gangli cerebrospinali." (Amprino, 1967, p. 33)

Personally, I have gone through the many pages of this text and looked with particular attention at the footnotes, but I was unable to find there the source of Amprino's statement. So perhaps Natalia's version better corresponds to the real events (or maybe Amprino was writing based on his personal recollections from what he had heard from Levi himself).

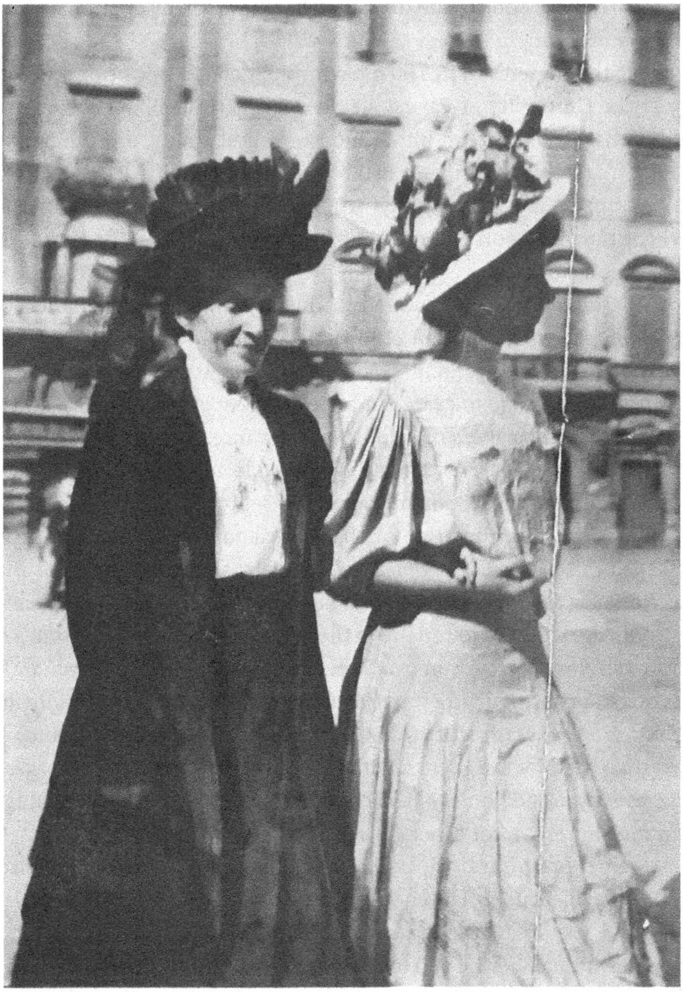

Figure 18.3. Lidia Tanzi, very young (on the right), in a rare photo from 1889–90, together with Anna Kuliscioff (on the left), a Russian *emigrée* who was a close connection of Levi's family. A very progressive and unconventional woman, Anna was, together with her partner Filippo Turati, among the founders of the Italian Socialist Party. A graduate in Medicine from the University of Naples, she carried out biomedical research in Pavia at the institute directed by Camillo Golgi. Anna considered Lidia to be her goddaughter (nicknamed "Lydiett"), to whom she transmitted part of her nonconformity (courtesy of the Levi-Ginzburg family ©).

A RAPID OUTLINE OF THE CAREER OF AN ANATOMIST POORLY INTERESTED IN ANATOMY

Levi's scientific interests correspond much more to those of a cellular biologist than to those of an anatomist. This despite the course of his academic career, which, since the years of his work in Chiarugi's institute in Florence, would develop exclusively in anatomy departments and culminate in 1919 with the Chair of Human Anatomy at the University of Turin.

No wonder therefore that, in 1907, having applied for a position as Professor of Anatomy at the University of Parma, he does not get the job. The examining committee finds that he shows "an uncommon technical ability, a profound biological culture and remarkable initiative, yet the part of his activity dedicated to research on gross Anatomy is much too scanty" (Amprino, 1965,12). Three years later, however, Levi got the professorship in a national competition and chose the University of Sassari as his destination.

Despite the difficulties encountered in this somewhat peripheral location, and notwithstanding the great burden of didactic activity to which he was obliged, together with his collaborators (and particularly Tullio Terni, who had followed him from Florence) he was able to carry out an intense experimental work schedule and publish many scientific papers of significant relevance, in both Italian and German journals (see Amprino, 1967). Among his notable investigations of this period, there was one on the development of photoreceptors in amphibians (toads and tritons), which was a continuation of that on salamanders conducted in Florence (and published in 1900 in *Lo Sperimentale*, the journal of the Florentine anatomical institute). The new research, published in 1914 in the German journal *Anatomischer Anzeiger*, confirmed his previous data on the origin of cone and rods from a common predecessor cell. It allowed, moreover, Levi to conclude that the strongly birefringent striations appearing in the "external article" (i.e., the outer segment) of the photoreceptors are discs of a cuticular type, and thus to exclude their mitochondrial nature (as suggested by the French authors Georges Leboucq and Georges Leplat). Levi also correctly argued for the mitochondrial nature of the ellipsoidal formation present in the photoreceptor inner segments.

During the period in Sardinia, Levi also published (in collaboration with Davide Carazzi, his old colleague in Florence and now in Sassari) a treatise of microscopic anatomy bound to gain a large regard among Italian microscopists for many years. Among the new researches he started in collaboration with Terni, there were those on the chondriome of various cell types, in particular of germinal elements, which led Levi to exclude the secretory or granular nature of this formation and to show that during cell reproduction it undergoes a different pattern of division compared to the cell nuclei (Levi, 1911a, 1911b, 1911c; Levi & Terni, 1912).

In November of 1914, Levi was appointed Professor of Anatomy in Palermo, undoubtedly a more important town than Sassari, but with no fewer difficulties for his research work.

Two years later, in Palermo, Natalia, the youngest of the children of Giuseppe and Lidia, was born. Despite the problems that the new birth created for the family, and even though, in the period 1916–1917, Giuseppe was mobilized as a medical officer in the World War I and sent into the war zone in the north of Italy, he eventually succeeded in setting up a laboratory for cell cultures that he would soon use for the study of various cell types and particularly of nerve cells. This was a really formidable achievement for Levi, considering the historical, social, and familial difficulties. It would endow him with an important technical tool for the investigation of the fundamental biological themes that he had started pursuing from his Florentine years and that he would carry on for the rest of his scientific life, even in conditions much more difficult than those encountered in Palermo. This occurred particularly during World War II and the period of persecutions following the emanation of the racial laws by the Fascist and Nazi regime.

CELLS CULTURES, A "WORLD FULL OF PROMISES," AND A "PROCEDURE OF EXPERIMENTAL CYTOLOGY"

There is a main nucleus in the multifaceted scientific interests of Levi. It has to do with some fundamental properties of life processes, those connected to growth and development, in their multiform aspects, including the relationship between cell size and organism growth, and those responsible for the senescence and death. The investigation along some of these research lines had a particular impetus after Levi succeeded in setting up the cell culture technique, which he applied first to muscle and mesenchymal cells, and soon afterward to nervous tissue studies. He became a strenuous supporter of this method, which—after the pioneer studies of Harrison and, after him, of Alexis Carrel—had received relatively little attention among cell biologists. The progress of Levi's research with the new technique was particularly vibrant in the Turin years, even in the difficult period of racial persecution and World War II, when he was obliged to leave Italy and to assume a false identity.

In a long paper written in 1918, during his stay in Palermo, in the period of World War I, Levi praised the importance of the method he had modified by using thin layers of clothed plasma as the main medium for the culture. He said that "despite the multifarious difficulties that in the present day hinder laboratory research, and despite the limitations in the international collaboration" due to the war, despite all that, "few times facts have gone beyond the hopes of scholars, as it has happened for the culture of tissues outside the organism, when the new method was known and its importance appreciated" (Levi 1919, 424).

It is a world "full of promises" that appears before his eyes through the microscope:

> The one who has spent long years of his life in the microscopic study of dead tissues, and can now follow the living cells of Metazoans for days and months in their most various manifestations, gets the sensation to have in front of him a new world full of promises, and it is perhaps by this way that we could arrive to discover the still mysterious domain of the morphological foundation of cellular functions. (Levi, 1919, 424)

What might seem a drawback of the technique, namely, the difference of the conditions of cells in culture with respect to their situation in the organism, becomes, in Levi's eyes, a valuable characteristic. As he puts it:

> The value of the method is not diminished by the fact that, in the culture, the character of the tissue undergoes substantial modifications. On the contrary, the

possibility of changing arbitrarily the properties of the medium in which the cells live, endows the method with the dignity of a procedure of experimental cytology. (p. 425)

Of particular importance for Levi was the use of the cell culture method with relation to the already discussed problem of the individuality of cells, in the context of the debates between the adherents to reticular theory and the supporters of the neuron doctrine, and of the criticism addressed by some scholars to the fundamentals of cell theory. In his first studies on cultured nerve cells, published in 1916, Levi had indeed observed the tendency of growing neurons to form reticular ensembles. The microscopic appearance suggested possible intercellular continuity, and this was one of the reasons why he was open to the prospect of reticular ensembles of nerve cells, and to other forms of continuity, possibly based on protoplasmic coalescence.

The cell culture method also showed, however, that the cells which seemed to have grown up as syncytia could regain their individuality, and—in the case of cells capable of multiplication like the myoblasts and mesenchymal cell—after separating from the syncytium could undergo mitosis and reproduction.

In a long memoir reporting the results of his first experiments on the culture of nerve cells, presented in 1916 at the *Accademia dei Lincei* (but published in 1917) he drew the following conclusion as to neuron individuality:

> Even when the processes of various neuroblasts do make anastomosis among each other in a reticular assembly, and apparently the anatomical individuality of the neurons has disappeared, we have reasons to believe that a part of the nervous protoplasm, made of the neurite and of its collaterals, which is under the dependence of the neuroblast, because of obscure biological reasons, maintains more intimate functional relationship with the neuroblast; as a consequence, it can become, at a given time, independent from the other neurones. (Levi 1917, p. 177)

Levi quoted the passage above, in an article published in 1918 and devoted to the problem of the individuality of various types of cells capable of forming syncytial networks in culture. He attributed the dependence that still seemed to exist between portions of protoplasm and the corresponding nuclei, despite the apparent syncytial arrangement of the ensemble, to a fundamental biological principle, the "law of the nucleo-plasmatic correlation" (Levi, 1918, 154).

Continuing his research on cell cultures, Levi arrived eventually at the conclusion that there is no real continuity between the cells that seem to form syncytia, even though, in most cases, cells establish "a so intimate union, that it is impossible to mark the limit between one cell and the other [. . .] even "by using the best objectives." He based his supposition on the great tendency that two nearby cells, apparently anastomosed, have to separate from each other and regain their individuality; and, moreover, on the observation that only in very exceptional cases there is a transfer of intracellular organelles (as, for instance, chondrioconts), between the elements of the reticulum.

He writes:

> The facts, derived from the prolonged observation of live cultures, thus demonstrate that in the great majority of cases the apparent continuity between the distinct elements, is nothing but an illusion, depending on the imperfection of our investigation methods. (Levi, 1923, p. 13)

The Paradox of "a Bad Lecturer" Who Was a Great Maestro

The considerations above show how Levi did not dogmatically stick to his theories and was capable of changing his opinion on the basis of substantial facts, when these were derived from prolonged observation. Despite his attraction to the great problems of biology, which necessarily implied the elaboration of theories and formulation of general principles, one of Levi's main legacies for the multitudes of his pupils and students (as well as for members of his family, such as his grandson, the historian Carlo Ginzburg; Ginzburg C, 2018), was the need to adhere to experimental facts, both in science and life. This did not imply, however, that he was in any way a realistic and pragmatic person.

As mentioned at the beginning of this chapter, Levi had been a formidable teacher. Among his pupils, there are great scholars, including the three Nobel prize winners, Renato Dulbecco, Rita Levi-Montalcini, and Salvador Luria, and other scientists of high international standards (e.g., Terni, Olivo, Amprino, and Angelo Bairati). As for his university lectures, however, even the most devoted of his pupils, Amprino, recognized that "Levi did not immediately appeal to the average medical student, since he was neither an elegant nor a fluent speaker" (Amprino, 1967, 32). On her side, Rita Levi-Montalcini remembered that the first lesson she attended in the anatomy amphitheater in Turin was "extremely boring" (*noiosissima*), adding that "Levi's complete lack of rhetorical skills was aggravated by the fact that he detested macroscopic anatomy" (Levi-Montalcini, 1987, 47).

How then could Levi be considered a great teacher? As for the medical students, Amprino responds that "so obvious were his tremendous knowledge, his deep respect and love for science, his force of conviction in the importance of a sound scientific basis in medical studies, that all his students felt that they were facing a great scholar and a unique personality" (Amprino, 1967, 32).

The feeling of "facing a great scholar and a unique personality" was particularly strong for the few select students who were admitted as interns in the Institute of Anatomy for research purposes, some of whom continued, afterward, a career in science. For them, Levi was important in various ways. He was an extraordinary example of complete dedication to science, had an immense scientific culture, an international dimension, and great intellectual and technical inventiveness. He was not only the first in Italy to set up cell cultures, but he was also the first to use cinematography in the microscopic study of living cells, and one of his students, Bairati, was among the first in Italy to apply electron microscopy to biological studies. Even during the difficult years of fascism, characterized by a great provincialism of Italian society and culture, with the tendency of the regime to control any aspect of life and institutions, Levi succeeded in keeping high research standards and strong international ties. He could thus pave the way for the international collaboration and for the study abroad of his collaborators. Some of his pupils could therefore go outside Italy, to the United States, England, France, and Germany (there, however, only until 1933, the year of the infamous racial laws). Moreover, Levi received in his laboratory in Turin, or collaborated with elsewhere, scholars of various countries, most notably the German Hertha Meyer (obliged to leave her native country in 1933 because of her Jewish ancestry), who would become one of the main experts of the cell culture technique. Among the foreigners working for relatively short periods in the laboratory of Levi, or collaborating with him elsewhere, there were the Spaniard Fernando de Castro (a student of Cajal), the Pole Zygmunt Szantroch, the Belgians Maurice Chèvremont and Simone Comhaire, the Japanese Shiro Esaki, the Pole Henry Grossfeld, and Wolfgang Jablonski (a Berliner of Jewish ancestry, who—after a series of vicissitudes—would eventually emigrate to Palestine in 1941 and would practice medicine in Jerusalem under the Hebrew name of אדם יובל, that is, Yuval Adam; see Piccolino, 2021).

Through his connections with the Rockefeller Foundation, Levi not only funded the work of his laboratory and his collaborators both Italian and foreign, but he also promoted the career and research of other talented Italian researchers (for instance, the Italian physiologist Giuseppe Moruzzi and his cousin Giovanni Moruzzi; see Gemelli, 2018 where, however, the two Moruzzi are supposed to be brothers).

The research of Levi and his group was always of a high standard and aimed at studying problems of great biological relevance. Levi's numerous texts in various languages contributed to the feeling of his students, not only that "they were facing a great scholar and a unique personality," but also—and importantly—that they were not at the remote periphery of the world of science. This was particularly important for those who decided to pursue biological research, even for those, among them Renato Dulbecco and Salvador Luria whose investigation themes would be far from those based on Levi's morphological approaches (Grignolio, 2018a, 2018b).

This was mainly because Levi's achievements and personality instilled in them the conviction that it was possible to carry out experimental research in Italy as well, a country that traditionally has never considered science as a valuable human and economic investment. As the science historian John Heilbron said in 1998, during the commemoration of the bicentennial of the death of Luigi Galvani, in science (as in other dimensions of culture and society) Italy needs particularly "great personages," and Levi was undoubtedly one of them.

Coming back to Levi's scientific career, after going through his numerous texts, one readily agrees with Amprino's statement, that, despite the importance of his research, and notwithstanding "his inventive and productive mind," Giuseppe Levi "did not perhaps open new ways" in his scientific endeavors. On the other hand, this was indeed the achievement of some of his pupils, and particularly of the aforementioned three Nobel Prize winners.

There is little doubt that, at the start of their careers, all of them benefited from Levi's teaching and from the institutional and cultural conditions that the maestro had been able to create in Turin, despite the difficult times of the Fascist and pre-war period. In the case of Rita Levi-Montalcini's research leading to the discovery of the Nerve Growth Factor, a scientific and historical continuity exists with the great research themes that have been at the heart of Levi's interest; particularly, neuroembryology and the problem of cell growth and death, with the use of the chick embryo and cell cultures as main laboratory techniques.

Indeed Levi and Levi-Montalcini collaborated on these themes during their forced emigrations to Belgium, at the times of racial laws, and especially during the war, when both left Belgium because of the Nazi invasion and re-entered Italy with great courage and some recklessness: first Levi-Montalcini at the end of 1939, and then, in 1941, Levi, through many difficulties and dangers. Here for a certain time, they could make experiments in the lab à la *Robinson Crusoe* that Rita was able to set up in her home in Turin (Levi & Levi-Montalcini, 1942, 1943). As will be detailed by Germana Pareti in the chapter 20 of this book, these particular studies were prompted by an article written by Viktor Hamburger, which Levi had given Rita. She had the occasion to read it—as herself put the story—in somewhat adventurous circumstances, in the summer of 1940, on a cattle train used for people transportation in the war period (Hamburger, 1934; see Levi- Montalcini, 1987). The results obtained by Levi and Rita would later attract the attention of Hamburger, a German-born scholar, who settled in the United States because of his Jewish ancestry. Of fundamental importance for Rita's future work in Hamburger's lab was her training in neurohistological techniques. But also her familiarity with experimental micro-manipulation of chick embryos, that were undoubtedly a legacy of Levi, as also was—on the cultural side—the instigation to pursue the study along great biological themes.

I have repeatedly remarked that, despite his deep interest in morphology, Levi was in no way a classical anatomist, and—as Rita acutely remarked—"he [even] detested macroscopic anatomy." He was instead—as I have said—a cell biologist, with excellent mastery and devotion for morphological studies at a cellular level, which would be of crucial importance in understanding the structural organization of life processes. Starting particularly from the mid-20th century, with the application of electron microscopy and molecular biology to the investigation of life mechanisms, it clearly has emerged that the basic processes of life are based on chemical and molecular reactions, which do not occur, however, in a liquid and unstructured phase of the cell. They require, instead, complex structures, or occur in specific compartments, like ribosomes, mitochondria, rough or smooth endoplasmic reticulum, Golgi apparatus, membrane pumps and carriers, complex receptor systems, peroxisomes, lysosomes, electron transport chains, and molecular motors. Surely Levi could not anticipate these discoveries. There is little doubt, however, that the progress of modern biology has greatly benefited from his insistence and the insistence of others who stuck to the importance of morphological studies at a cellular level in times of predominance of purely physiological and chemical approaches to life phenomena.

Much more than a researcher pursuing the "animated anatomy," according to the principles advocated by the 18th-century Swiss scholar Albrecht von Haller, Levi was an experimental biologist *à la façon* of Lazzaro Spallanzani. Their main interests were—as in Levi's case—the great themes of life, pursued in all possible directions. (Mazzarello, 2004; Piccolino, 2005; Dröscher, 2018).

The fact is that, despite his great cultural and scientific talents, Levi did not succeed in opening entirely new paths in science and making breakthrough contributions in his fields of study. This may be due, among other things, to the time and energy that he spent in his institutional duties, and particularly in the organization of his lab and the training of his research students. Because of his impulsive and intense character (which also emerges, at a personal level, in the *Family Lexicon*), and because of some of his deep scientific convictions, he could have created difficulties for some of his collaborators, despite the care he devoted to promoting their studies and careers.

In recalling with mixed feelings (together with Renato Dulbecco and another colleague, Ferdinando Morin, during her stay in the United States) the period spent in Turin with Levi, Rita Levi-Montalcini wrote:

> With Renato and Morin (or Fred as he is called here) we have tried to analyse the reasons underlying such a devotion that inspires respect even when one does not accept him. We have come to the conclusion that it was nice to have been his pupils, but it is even nicer today that we are no longer that. (Levi-Montalcini, 2000, p. 70; see Levi-Montalcini, 1965 on Morin, a student in Padua of Levi's pupil Tullio Terni, who worked in the Turin Institute in the period 1940–1946 and afterward emigrated to the United States to work as a neurophysiologist at Washington University of St. Louis.)

Despite her devotion to the maestro, Rita was particularly concerned when Levi visited her in St Louis and expressed his dissatisfaction with her ongoing experiments, and particularly with her interpretation of the results, which appeared to contradict some of Levi's fundamental theories on the growth of nerve cells. Good pupils know the value of having a good teacher, but know, even better, how important it is to go beyond his views and contradict some of the principles of the maestro (and of any received conception). Enjoying the benefits of the training received from a great, although impulsive and not easygoing teacher, Rita could be in shape to go beyond his views and arrive at one of the most significant discoveries of 20th-century biology.

On another dimension, there was another young woman who benefitted from the atmosphere created by the same authoritative, and somewhat cumbersome, personage. This was, as we shall see in the next chapter, his daughter Natalia.

One of the possible limits of the way she portrays her father in the *Lexicon*, "the Professor," is in the idea, which transpires from the book, that apparently science is devoid of the charms and the emotions of literature and art. When looking through the microscope at living nerve cells that emit their fibers and form delicate structures looking like artistic drawings, or at the singular aspects of the extremely large neurons of the sunfish that he had been the first to describe; or when considering the extraordinary adaptive mechanisms that allow bats or salamanders to reproduce in challenging biological situations, probably Giuseppe Levi felt the same pleasure and emotion experienced by his wife, Lidia, or his children, Paola or Mario, or his pupil Tullio Terni in reading Proust's *Recherche* or contemplating a painting.

This is at least what appears from the recollections of one of his last students, Antonio Barasa. With reference to the Zeiss-Winkel system for micro-cinematography that Levi had been able to install in Turin in 1953 in order to observe, for prolonged periods, the behavior of cultured cells, Barasa writes:

> The over eighty years old Professor Levi watched with this instrument (that was endowed with a powerful 100x immersion objective based on a Zernike-type phase-contrast optics) the behaviour of various types of cells and, above all, that of the arborisations of nervous cells cultured in vitro. Often the images aroused in the old Levi cries of joy and almost youthful manifestations of enthusiasm. (Barasa, 2018, p. 38)

Perhaps the best conclusion to this long chapter on Giuseppe Levi is this vision of the youthful enthusiasm of the old scholar looking through the microscope at his beloved cells in cultures. The wonders of nature were being made visible by the scientific endeavor that was at the very core of his long life, until his very last days.

ACKNOWLEDGMENTS

First I wish to express my deep gratitude to Antonio Barasa, who with great generosity has provided me with an extremely rich collection of materials concerning the life and work of Giuseppe Levi, his teacher. This includes a copy of many of his letters to several of his collaborators, numerous articles by Levi and on Levi, several pictures and other documents, some of which are originals by Levi's hand. Great gratitude also to Piera Levi-Montalcini for allowing me to consult many of the documents of her aunt Rita. This work would not have been possible without the collaboration and intelligent assistance of several librarians and archivists that I mention here more or less in alphabetical order because all have contributed with the same great dedication: Stefania Bagella of the University of Sassari, Livia Iannucci and Daniele Ronco of the University of Pisa, Daniela Lo Brutto of the University of Palermo, Fioranna Salvadori and Laura Vannucci of the University of Florence, Paola Novaria of the University of Turin, Luigi Balice of the "Stato Civile" Archive of Turin, Jennifer Walton of the Woods Hole Marine Laboratory Archive, Lee Hiltzik of the Rockefeller Foundation Archive, Chiara Giannotti of the Jewish Community Archive of Pisa and Livio Vasieri of the Jewish Community Archive of Trieste, Elisabetta Matticoli of the Library "Peppino Impastato" of Ladispoli. Thanks to Giacomo Magrini and Paola Raspadori for their helpful advice. Thanks to Dario Cantino and Enrica Strettoi who have discussed with me some aspects of Giuseppe Levi's science, to Giovanni Niccoli who has read and revised the text of the chapter. Thanks also to Giovanni Berlucchi, Elena D'Imporzano, Paolo Mazzarello who have critically read it. Thanks to Carlo Carta and Lorenzo Sbrenna for assistance with the computer software. I am deeply indebted to Luca Cono Drago for sending me material and information about the history of Palermo; to Marcia Attias for sending pictures of Hertha Meyer; to Carlo Ginzburg for sharing with me some recollections of his family and sending some pictures; and to Daria and Giovanna Visintini for materials and recollection concerning their father Fabio. A very great thank you to Nick Wade for generously and kindly revising the text and making less Italian my English. Thanks also to Patrick Hederman of the *The New York Review of Books* for kindly and rapidly granting permission to reproduce the two passages of the English edition of *Lessico famigliare*.

This chapter is a preliminary account of more ample research in progress on Giuseppe Levi and his scientific school (see Piccolino, 2021).

REFERENCES

Adelmann H B (1966) *Marcello Malpighi and the Evolution of Embryology* (2 vols.) Ithaca, NY: Cornell University Press.

Amprino R (1967) Giuseppe Levi (1872–1965). *Acta Anatomica*, 66 (1):1–44.

Barasa A (2015) Rodolfo Amprino e Giovanni Godina: due allievi della scuola torinese di Giuseppe Levi. *Medicina nei Secoli*, 30 (1) 31–74.

Cajal S R (1893) La rétine des Vertebrés. *La Cellule*, 9: 119–257.

Cajal S R (1901) Le réticule neurofibrillaire dans la rétine. *Trabajos del Laboratorio de Investigaciones Biológicas de la Universidad de Madrid*, 1 : 151–157.

Cajal S R (1909–1911) *Histologie du Système Nerveux de l'Homme et des Vertébrés* (French translation by L Azoulay). Paris: Maloine.

Cajal S R (1913–1914) *Estudios sobre la degeneración y regeneración del sistema nervioso*. Madrid: Moya.

Carazzi D, & Levi G (1916) *Tecnica microscopica: Guida pratica alle ricerche d'istologia ed embriologia animale, all'istologia patologica e alla parassitologia*. Milano: Società Editrice Libraria.

Chiarugi G (1890) I problemi dell'anatomia scientifica. *La Riforma Medica*, 6: 1742–1743, 1748–1749, 1754–1755.

Chiarugi G (1898) Produzione sperimentale di duplicità embrionali in uova di Salamandrina perspicillata. *Nota preliminare. Monitore zoologico italiano*, 9 (6): 131–136.

Chiarugi G (1899a) Sull'involucro delle uova di "Salamandrina perspicillata" *Lo Sperimentale*, 53 (1): 61–80.

Chiarugi G (1899b) *Receptaculum seminis* nella "*Salamandrina perspicillata.*" *Monitore zoologico italiano*, 10 (3): 60–61.

Chiarugi G (1929) *Trattato di embriologia: Con particolare riguardo alla storia dello sviluppo dei Mammiferi e dell'uomo*. Milano: Società Editrice Libraria.

Chiarugi G (1959–1965) *Istituzioni di anatomia dell'uomo* (5 vols.). Milano: Società Editrice Libraria.

Dröscher A (2018) Senescenza, rigenerazione e immortalità: Giuseppe Levi e il fenomeno vitale. *Medicina nei Secoli*, 30 (1): 105–125.

Fano G (1894) *La fisiologia in rapporto con la chimica e la morfologia*. Torino: Loescher.

Galeotti G, & Levi G (1895 b) Über die Neubildung der nervösen Elemente in dem wiedererzeugten Muskelgewebe. *Beiträge zur pathologischen Anatomie und zur allgemeinen Pathologie*, 17: 371–415.

Gemelli G (2018) LA Fondazione Rockefeller e le reti di eccellenza nella ricerca biomedica italiana: il ruolo di Giuseppe Levi. *Medicina nei Secoli*, 30 (1): 127–166.

Ginzburg C (2018) Giuseppe Levi, mio nonno. *Medicina nei Secoli*, 30 (1): 281–284.

Ginzburg N (1963) *Lessico famigliare*. Torino: Einaudi (English translation: *Family Lexicon* by McPhee J. New York: *New York Review of Books*, 2017).

Grignolio A, Guest Editor (2018a) "Medicina nei Secoli." Special issue dedicated to Giuseppe Levi, pp. 1–445.

Grignolio A (2018b) The path of three Nobel laureate students from their anatomical training in Turin to the American genetic-molecular model (1930–1950). *Medicina nei Secoli*, 30 (1): 167–209.

Hamburger V (1934) The effects of wing bud extirpation on the development of the central nervous system in chick embryos. *Journal of Experimental Zoology*, 68: 449–494.
Galeotti G, & Levi G (1893) Beitrag zur Kenntnis der Regeneration der quergestreiften Muskelfasern. *Beiträge zur pathologischen Anatomie und zur allgemeinen Pathologie*, 14: 272–287.
Levi G (1895) Delle Alterazioni prodotte nel rene dal Cloruro di Sodio. Manuscript Dissertation. *Biblioteca Biomedica, Università di Firenze* (printed in *Lo Sperimentale* 49: 426–485).
Levi G (1897) Ricerche citologiche comparate sulla cellula nervosa dei Vertebrati. *Rivista di patologia nervosa e mentale*: 2: 1–43.
Levi G (1900) Osservazioni sullo sviluppo dei coni e bastoncini della retina degli urodeli. *Lo Sperimentale*, 54: 521–539.
Levi G (1904) Nuovi fatti prò e contro la teoria del neurone. *Monitore zoologico italiano*, 15: 130–147.
Levi G (1907) Di alcuni problemi riguardanti la struttura del sistema nervoso. *Archivio di Fisiologia*, 4: 367–396.
Levi G (1908) I gangli cerebrospinali. Studi di istologia comparata e di istogenesi. *Archivio italiano di Anatomia e di Embriologia*, 7 :1–392.
Levi G (1911a) Sulla presunta partecipazione dei condriosomi alla differenziazione cellulare. *Archivio italiano di Anatomia e di Embriologia*, 10: 168–195.
Levi G (1911b) I condriosomi dei gonociti. *Monitore zoologico italiano*, 23: 116–121.
Levi G (1911c) I condriosomi nell'oocite degli Anfibi. *Monitore zoologico italiano*, 23: 149–163.
Levi G (1911) I condriosomi nelle cellule secernenti. *Anatomischer Anzeiger*, 42: 576–592.
Levi G (1914a) Ulteriori studi sullo sviluppo delle cellule visive negli anfibi. *Anatomischer Anzeiger*, 47: 192–199.
Levi G (1914 b) La modalità della fissazione dell'uovo dei Chirotteri alla parete uterina. *Monitore zoologico italiano*, 25: 101–107.
Levi G (1916a) Differenziazione «in vitro» di fibre da cellule mesenchimali e loro accrescimento per movimento ameboide. *Monitore zoologico italiano*, 27: 77–84.
Levi G (1916b) Migrazione di elementi specifici differenziati in colture di miocardio e di muscoli scheletrici. *Archivio di Scienze mediche*, 40: 14–21.
Levi G (1916c) Sull'origine delle reti nervose nelle colture di tessuti. *Rendiconti della Reale Accademia dei Lincei*, Serie 5, 25: 663–668.
Levi G (1917) Connessioni e struttura degli elementi nervosi sviluppati fuori nell'organismo. *Atti della Reale Accademia dei Lincei*, Serie 5, 12 (15): 142–182.
Levi G (1918) L'individualità delle cellule persiste in potenza nei sincizi. *Monitore zoologico italiano*, 29: 150–155.
Levi G (1919a) Nuovi studî su cellule coltivate "in vitro." Attività biologiche, intima struttura, caratteri morfologici specifici. *Archivio Italiano di Anatomia e Embriologia*, 16: 423–599.
Levi G (1919 b) Nuovi studi sull'accrescimento delle cellule nervose. Ricerche in *Orthagoriscus mola*. *Atti della Reale Accademia delle Scienze, Lettere e Arti di Palermo*, 11: 3–11.
Levi G (1920) Forma e funzione. *Archivio di antropologia criminale, psicologia e medicina legale*, 40: 37–57; 113–128.
Levi G (1923) Esiste una continuità protoplasmatica fra individualità cellulari distinte nelle colture in vitro? *Rendiconti della Reale Accademia dei Lincei*, Serie 5, 32: 11–13.
Levi G (1925a) Conservazione e perdita dell'indipendenza delle cellule dei tessuti. Elementi liberi, sincizi e plasmodi nelle colture «in vitro». *Archiv für experimentelle Zellforschung*, 1: 1–57.
Levi G (1925b) Wachstum und Körpergrösse. Die strukturelle Grundlage der Körpergrösse bei vollausgebildeten und in Wachstum begriffenen Tieren. *Ergebnisse der Anatomie und Entwicklungsgeschichte*, 26: 87–342.

Levi G (1927) *Trattato di istologia*. Torino: UTET.
Levi G (1934) Explantation, besonders die Struktur und die biologischen Eigenschaften der in vitro gezüchteten Zellen und Gewebe. *Ergebnisse der Anatomie und Entwicklungsgeschichte*, 31: 125–707.
Levi G (1945) La struttura della sostanza vivente. *Minerva Medica*, 36 (II, 34): 3–20.
Levi G (1946) Commemorazione del socio Giulio Chiarugi, Atti della Accademia nazionale dei Lincei. *Rendiconti della Classe di scienze fisiche, matematiche e naturali*, serie. 8, 1: 1218–1222.
Levi G, & Levi-Montalcini R (1942) Les conséquences de la destruction d'un territoire d'innervation périphérique sur le développement des centres nerveux correspondants dans l'embryon du poulet. *Archives de Biologie*, 53: 537–545.
Levi G, & Levi-Montalcini R (1943) Recherches quantitatives sur la marche du processus de différentiation des neurones dans les ganglions spinaux de l'embryon du poulet. *Archives de Biologie* 54: 189–206.
Levi G, & Meyer H (1942) Nouvelles recherches sur le tissu nerveux cultivé in vitro, Morphologie, croissance et relations réciproques des neurones. *Archives de Biologie*, 52 (2): 133–201.
Levi G, & Terni T (1911) Studi sulla grandezza delle cellule. II. Le variazioni dell'indice plasmatico-nucleare durante l'intercinesi. *Archivio italiano di Anatomia e di Embriologia*, 10: 545–554.
Levi-Montalcini R (1965) Ferdinando Morin (1912–1964). *Archives Italiennes de Biologie*, 10 (103) 335–337.
Levi-Montalcini R (1987) *Elogio dell'imperfezione*. Milano: Garzanti.
Levi-Montalcini R (2000) *Cantico di una vita*. Milano: Raffaello Cortina Editore.
Levi-Montalcini R, Piccolino M, & Wade N J (2010) Giuseppe Moruzzi: A tribute to a "formidable" scientist and a "formidable" man. *Brain Research Reviews*, 66 (1-2): 256–269.
Mazzarello P (1999) *The Hidden Structure: A Scientific Biography of Camillo Golgi*. H A Buchtel & A Badiani, Trans). Oxford: Oxford University Press.
Mazzarello P (2004) *Costantinopoli 1786, La congiura e la beffa, l'intrigo Spallanzani*. Torino: Bollati Boringhieri.
Piccolino M (1988) Cajal and the retina: A 100-year retrospective. *Trends in Neurosciences*, 11(12): 521–525.
Piccolino M, Strettoi S, & Laurenzi E (1989) Santiago Ramón Y Cajal, the retina and the neuron theory. *Documenta Ophthalmologica*, 71 (2): 123–141.
Piccolino M (2003) A "lost time" between science and literature: The " temps perdu" from Hermann von Helmholtz to Marcel Proust. *Audiological Medicine*, 1: 261–270.
Piccolino M (2005) *Lo zufolo e la cicala: Divagazioni galileiane tra la scienza e la sua storia*. Torino: Bollati Boringhieri.
Piccolino M (Ed.) (2021) *Rita Levi-Montalcini e il suo Maestro: una grande avventura nelle neuroscienze alla scuola di Giuseppe Levi*. Pisa: ETS.
Tanzi E (1893) I fatti e le induzioni dell'odierna istologia del sistema nervoso. *Rivista Sperimentale di Freniatria e Medicina Legale* 19, 419–472.

CHAPTER 19

Myth, Religion, Politics, and Literature in Giuseppe Levi's Turin

GIACOMO MAGRINI

TURIN

On the 17th of January 1920, in the pages of the weekly magazine "L'Ordine Nuovo" [The New Order], Antonio Gramsci, who was about to turn 29 years old, made a comparison between two great cities in northern Italy: Milan and Turin, as well as between their respective regions, Lombardy and Piedmont. Milan, with its glorious history of the *Risorgimento* and its highly active bourgeoisie, might have appeared to have all the elements to contend for primacy. Yet, "the Milanese bourgeoisie would never have been capable of creating a bourgeois state; it would never have been capable of freeing itself from the Austrian yoke. Barricades alone were not enough to achieve this, nor personal heroism, nor the Five Days; Milan alone was not enough—a liberal city, squeezed on all sides by the Austrian-sympathizing countryside" (Gramsci, 1994, 137). In contrast, "The decisive historical force, the historical force capable of creating an Italian State and firmly unifying the bourgeois class of all Italy, was Turin. The bourgeois population of Piedmont was not so rich or as daring as its Lombardy counterpart, but it was disciplined, it was solidly unified in a State, it had a stern military and administrative tradition and it had managed, through the intelligence of its politicians, to become part of the European balance of power. The Piedmontese State was a reliable apparatus of conquest, capable of carving out an Italian neo-formation; and it was able to provide the new State with a powerful military and administrative nucleus, and to give an organic form—*its own*—to the Italian people. Turin was the nerve-centre of this powerful Piedmontese system. Turin was the force that unified the population of Piedmont and it was the crucible of the Italian capitalist revolution. Today Turin is not the capitalist city par excellence, but it is the industrial city, the proletarian city par excellence. The working class of Turin is compact, well-disciplined and *distinct* as in few other cities in the world. Turin is like one great factory: its working population conforms to a single pattern and is powerfully unified by industrial production" (Gramsci, 1994, 137; italics by A.).

In 1919, in this city so vividly described by Gramsci, Giuseppe Levi arrived from Palermo and made his entrance. It could have turned out to be no more than a mere stage in his university career, but it became a fundamentally important and definitive place for him. But it was neither his city, nor that of his wife Lidia Tanzi. His city of origin was Trieste, and Milan that of his wife. When Levi moved to Turin, his family was already complete. Himself, his wife, and their five children: Gino, Paola, Mario, Alberto, and the three-year-old Natalia.

Giuseppe Levi met Lidia Tanzi in Florence: She lived there with her mother and studied at the Faculty of Medicine. The distinguished psychiatrist and neurologist Eugenio Tanzi, a paternal uncle, lived and practiced his profession in Florence, too. It was at San Salvi, the psychiatric clinic run by Tanzi, where the young Levi was doing his research work. This was the premise for the long and firm knot that would unite them for life. Cesare Garboli, a great literary critic and the closest friend of Natalia, notes that in *Lessico famigliare* [Family Lexicon], the book written by their youngest daughter Natalia (to which we will return later), there is, in reference to the relationship between father and mother, between husband and wife, a fertile and revealing contradiction: "We will observe [. . .] the rigorous absence of the scene that is mother of all things, the Freudian scene from which we all originate. This scene is not even touched upon, this scene is taboo, whilst at the same time being the very essence of the entire book, the most evident source of the noisy physical and moral well-being of Professor Levi and the gentle and ineffable zest for life of Signora Lidia." (Garboli, 2005, 90).

The Turin of the 1920s is commonly, and quite rightly, referred to as the city of Gobetti (Figure 19.1) and Gramsci. Two excellent minds (for both, the definition of "genius" would not be inappropriate). Strictly speaking, their presence ended just after the first half of the 1920s: Gobetti, age 25, died in Paris in 1926; in the same year Gramsci was arrested by the fascist police and began his long imprisonment, which ended with his death in 1937. Their influence, however, extended beyond that date: referring to Gobetti, the historian Angelo D'Orsi writes: "his companions, friends, disciples and masters survived, those who in some way would become his students; in short, Gobettism continued, indeed it was perhaps after his death, which left everyone astonished, that it really took off in earnest" (D'Orsi, 2000, 80). As for Gramsci, his influence only resumed with full vigor at the end of the 1940s, with the publication of *Quaderni del carcere* [Prison Notebooks], which is the most important among his works.

One of the features common to both Gobetti and Gramsci was their dissatisfaction with the theoretical paradigm and the practical findings of Positivism in all its forms. This attitude was shared by many of the more advanced contemporary cultures, not only in Europe; but likewise in Gobetti and Gramsci this found an original expression. And Russia, which both men were observing with extreme interest, it being untouched, or rather touched in a different and lateral way by Positivism, was, in a sense, the real and historical incarnation of such dissatisfaction.

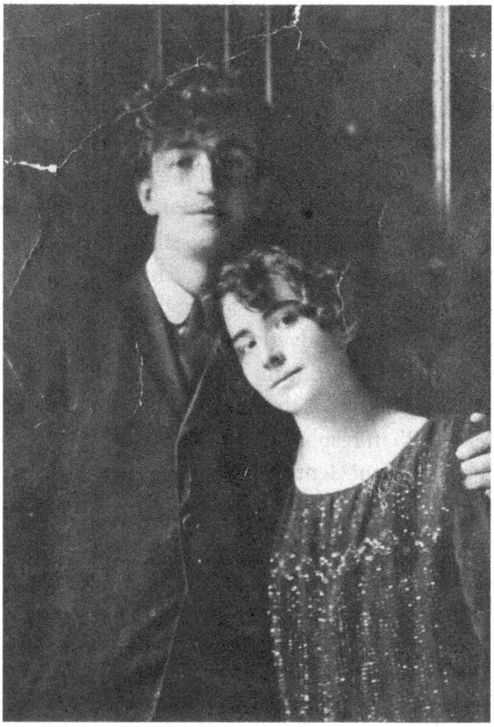

Figure 19.1. Piero Gobetti and Ada Prospero on their wedding day, 11th of January 1923. Credits: Archivio Fotografico del Centro Studi Piero Gobetti ©. Thanks to Alessio Bottai.

On the 23rd of December 1924, in the first issue of "Il Baretti," the last magazine to be founded by him, Gobetti published his editorial titled, *Illuminismo* [Enlightenment]. "In it"—states D'Orsi—"he somehow departs definitively from the Vocian movement and the intellectual experience of the pre-war years, moving towards a more mature awareness, not only of the aspirations, but also of the duties, and above all of the culpable weaknesses of men of culture." (D'Orsi, 2000, 72) The great political scientist and philosopher Norberto Bobbio senses a duplicity in the use of this word, Enlightenment. On the one hand, it is understood "as a historical category, that is to say, as the antithesis of romanticism" (D'Orsi, 2000, 72). On the other hand, it is "an ethical category, that is, signalling the autonomy of the man of letters from the prince" (D'Orsi, 2000, 72). We might also add that, with vigorous historical resurgence, Gobetti wanted to rid himself of Positivism, which nonetheless was on a certain continuum with the Enlightenment. The very city of Turin itself, in those years, could well be defined as a city of Enlightenment.

In the Italian culture, speaking of dissatisfaction and criticism toward Positivism means talking about Benedetto Croce. For Gobetti, Croce was a constant reference, naturally alongside others, among whom the economist Luigi Einaudi, of whom Gobetti was a student. Gramsci, in his *Prison Notebooks*, sets out a very meaningful, and indeed extraordinary, critique of Croce's historiographical and philosophical approach. The work of Croce, born in 1866, is expressed through a vast and consistently high-level production. It runs along two often converging parallel lines: one theoretical, the other of such meticulous historical investigation as to challenge even the most dogged positivist. Through the pages of *La Critica* [The Critique], the magazine founded in 1903 and largely written by him, the content of many subsequent volumes came out in installments: "the vehicle of journalism—Gianfranco Contini points out—immediately ensured a wide appeal in the endeavour of a general reviewing of the culture. This was a project in which, for the more strictly philosophical part, Croce had Gentile as both fellow and collaborator, until such time as their speculative divergences, with the advent of the fascist dictatorship, developed into irremediable political tension" (Contini, 1968, 425–426). Indeed, a coherent and militant expression of this discord is the *Manifesto of the anti-Fascist intellectuals* that Croce penned in May 1925 in response to, and in antithesis to, the *Manifesto of the Fascist intellectuals* by Giovanni Gentile. One of the subscribers to Croce's *Manifesto* was Giuseppe Levi.

LEONE GINZBURG

"New star rising," to repeat the ironic phrase with which Professor Levi tried to dampen the enthusiasm of his children, which was excessive in his eyes. On this occasion, however, it truly was a star rising. Leone Ginzburg, born in Odessa in 1909, working in Turin, intellectually ahead of his years, of exceptional talent and culture, who superbly mastered the Russian language and literature as well as the Italian language and literature. He also graduated in French literature, with a thesis on Maupassant. No one has been able to highlight the spiritual kinship of Gobetti and Ginzburg, with the imposing figure of Croce in the background, better than Bobbio in the following foundational page:

> The continuity of inspiration and Gobettian political thought in Ginzburg's work will be evident to those who read the few remaining political writings of his. Indeed, one of these writings is dedicated to an analysis of the *Paradosso dello spirito russo* [Paradox of the Russian spirit], which reveals, amongst other things, a common admiration for Trotsky (Ginzburg would translate much of the Trotsky's *Storia della rivoluzione russa* [History of the Russian revolution]. Ginzburg adopted the ethical conception of liberalism, as did Gobetti, a conception later delineated and canonised by Croce with the name «the religion of freedom». The juridical conception of liberalism, as a theory of the limits of the power of the state, had already been weakened, or at least set to one side, by the emergence of democratic ideologies according to which, once the power had been distributed to all, there would no longer be the need to limit it. The perennial, nourishing yeast of liberalism was manifested in the idea that the characteristic of modern ethics as opposed to ancient ethics, as has recently been aptly put, consisted in its being an agonistic ethics. That is to say an

ethics founded upon the principle that moral and civil progress can only exist where the maximum freedom of expansion of the individual, permitted by the obligations of peaceful coexistence, renders antagonism possible in all its forms, political, economic, social, religious, and cultural. If we fail to grasp this particular aspect of the liberal idea, advanced as a conception of the world and of history, we will not be able to understand the persistent loyalty to this tradition of men like Gobetti and Ginzburg, who broke all relations with the political liberalism of post-Risorgimental Italy. Nor will we be able to understand the influence of Croce on the anti-fascist groups of the younger generations, those who did not support political conservatism, in short, men whose politics were democratic rather than liberal. Faced with a fascism which had stifled the political struggle through violence, this ethical conception of liberalism became the most direct and outstanding antithesis of all forms of despotism, the most noble expression of resistance to tyranny. It can be said that it was not possible consequently, radically, to be antifascist without being liberal in this sense. (Bobbio, 2000, pp. LXII–LXIII)

A characteristic of Leone Ginzburg was his lack of interest toward religion. Indeed Bobbio, in the text from which several quotes have been taken, gives us the following biographical and autobiographical insight: "His morality had no supernatural foundations; though respectful of the faith of others, as a good liberal should be, he did not practice any religion himself, and I do not believe he had ever had a religious education. After all, the issue of religion was not one which people willingly addressed, be it for fear of discovering one's own feelings or concerns, be it because, emerging from adolescence, the reluctance to accept family values handed down by parents, paired with the desire to make a tabula rasa and to build one's own life, involved, first and foremost, religious beliefs" (Bobbio, 2000, p. LIII). This information is, at the same time, important and peripheral. On a more personal and specific note, an essay by Ginzburg on Čechov, which appeared in "La Critica" in 1931, can be revelatory. He reviews the publication, newly released in Mondadori's "Biblioteca Romantica" [Romantic Library], of some among Čechov's tales translated and presented by Leonardo Kocienski. And he demonstrates, as an excellent translator of Russian himself, with philological arguments, that the work of Kocienski is, by far, inferior to the work of Giovanni Faccioli published shortly before, and he adds: "as for the three novellas that were added to the more famous, main stories, perhaps they have the virtue of being unknown in Italy, however they are of little or no worth: indeed, *Lo studente* [The Student], and *Sul mare* [On the Sea] are among the ugliest and most declamatory pieces that Čechov has written" (Ginzburg L., 2000, 316). It should be noted here that the two stories mentioned are very different from each other, even from a chronological point of view: *On the Sea*, 1883, was among his first stories, whereas *The Student*, 1894, is an example of the full maturity of the writer. But what is most salient to us is that *The Student* is a small, that is, short, religious masterpiece. In making this judgment, we are comforted by the sensitivity and authority of the great scholar Vittorio Strada, who wrote: "In the work of Čechov, so strictly secular and therefore far removed from that of Dostoevsky and Tolstoy, and even more so from that of Gor'kij, which is animated by a dogmatic and political pseudo-religiousness, we find some of the most authentic and profound visions of religious life in such stories as *The Student* and *The Bishop*." (Strada 2005, 93). *Il vescovo* [The Bishop]—let us remind ourselves—is Čechov's penultimate short story, written in 1902 and the only tale produced that year. We would not have pointed out Ginzburg's distance from the question of religion were his position not shared by the vast majority of his intellectual contemporaries and beyond, albeit the religious dimension, that is to say reflecting upon religion, was essential and thus to elude it could have grave consequences. The contemporary works of Max Weber and Émile Durkheim are luminous and grandiose examples of this thinking. Almost in the same years, Gramsci, in his pre-prison writings, and then in his *Prison Notebooks*, paid constant and strong attention to the phenomenon of religion, both as an institution and as a sentiment. In the Piedmontese edition of "Avanti!" [Onward] on August 26, 1920, Gramsci stated that

> The Marxist Socialists aren't religious; they believe that religion is a transitory form of human culture, and that it will be superseded by a superior form of culture, a philosophic one. They believe that religion is a mythological conception of life and the world. It will be superseded by a conception based on historical materialism, i.e., the conception that recognizes and searches inside human society and individual consciousness for the causes and forces producing and creating history. But although they aren't religious, the Marxist Socialists aren't against religion. The Workers' State will not harass religion. The Workers' State will require of Christian Proletarians only the faithfulness that all States require from their citizens: it will require that if they insist on belonging to the opposition, this opposition be constitutional, not revolutionary. (Gramsci, 1987, 636)

In the momentous article *Il partito comunista* [The Communist Party], which was released in two parts in the weekly publication, *L'Ordine Nuovo*, on the 4th of and the 9th of October 1920, Gramsci noted: "At the present moment, the Communist Party is the only institution that may be seriously compared with the religious communities of primitive Christianity. To the extent that the Party already exists on an international scale, one can hazard a comparison and establish a scale of criteria for judging between the militants for the City of God and the militants for the City of Man. The communist is certainly not inferior to the Christian in the days of the catacombs." (Gramsci, 1987, 653–654). Then: "Rosa Luxemburg and Karl Leibknecht are greater than the greatest of Christian Saints" (Gramsci, 1987, 654). What mattered most of all was having established that relationship and having made that comparison.

In the 1930s, Ginzburg became a close member of the Levi household: He was good friends with Mario and in love with Natalia, whom he married in 1938 (Figure 19.2) and with whom he had three children. Not that it were necessary, but his presence strengthened and polarized even further the already obvious antifascism of the entire family. The tragic death of Leone Ginzburg, not yet 35 years old, in the Roman prison of Regina Coeli, tortured by his Nazi-fascist jailers, left an indelible scar on his wife's heart. She did not return to her maiden name, nor did she adopt that of

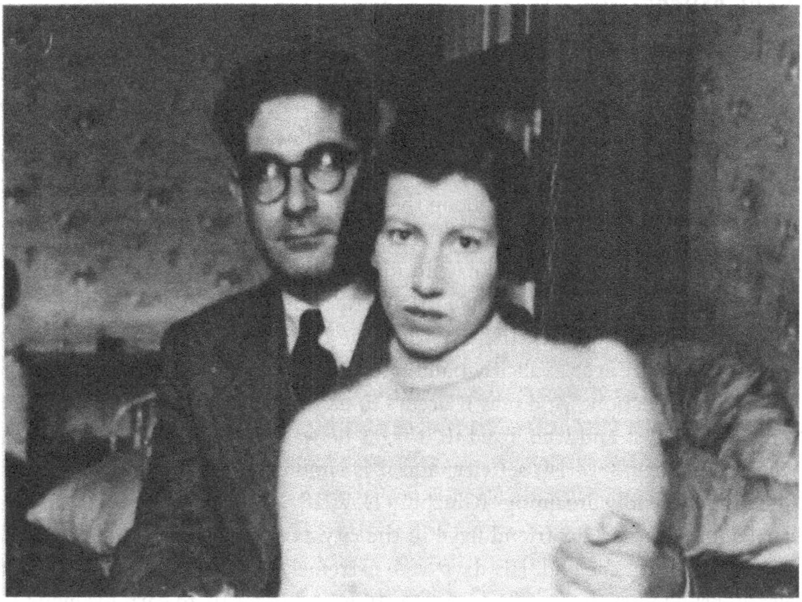

Figure 19.2. Leone and Natalia Ginzburg on their wedding day, 1938. By courtesy of the Ginzburg family ©. Thanks to Carlo Ginzburg.

her second husband in 1950, but continued to call herself Natalia Ginzburg. Leone is present in many of her literary works, either directly or in a veiled guise. But, even more important than his memory, or this transformation–transfiguration, is the dialogue. And she knew precisely how to establish this, particularly on the theme of religion. Toward the end of the essay, *Sul credere e non credere in Dio* [On believing and not believing in God], published in the collection *Mai devi domandarmi* [Never must you ask me] in 1970, Natalia infers the nonpeaceful, problematic existence of God with a stringent and unique, almost bizarre logic: "That believing in God makes life happier is false; and that it makes men better is false once again. Therefore, believing or not believing would seem irrelevant. But if believing or not believing is irrelevant, it means that everything about God is then of immense, inexplicable and essential importance: it means that God is more important than our believing or not believing in him" (Ginzburg N, 1987, 175).

The uniqueness of this logic lies in its being decidedly nonsubjective. And, in fact, immediately before that she had written: "If God exists, he can be found in the instants and in the places where one abandons the leaden weight of one's being, and looks up from the dark and poisonous seething of his gloomy conscience; looks at himself as if he were someone else; looks at his neighbour as his neighbour; and see God as God." (Ginzburg N, 1987, 175) Wherein, obviously, the key phrase, the most profound and novel element is: "looks at himself as if he were someone else." Thus, Ginzburg was working on an integration, or rather, an internal correction of Leone's omission. To achieve this is one of the greatest tasks in literature.

Activities of the newly established Einaudi publisher, founded in 1933 by Giulio, Luigi's son, revolved for the most part around Ginzburg and his friend Cesare Pavese (Figure 19.3). A stronghold of antifascism, Einaudi was defined the *Laterza* of the North, in reference to the southern publishing company linked to Croce. Pavese, born in 1908 in Santo Stefano Belbo in the Langhe region, was a notable writer and an excellent translator of Anglo-American English. He committed suicide in Turin, just before his forty-second birthday. In *Ritratto di un amico* [Portrait of a Friend], in the collection *Le piccole virtù* [The Little Virtues] in 1962, Natalia Ginzburg spoke both of Pavese and of Turin, the city where he had lived and died, as if in a joint epicedium, without ever explicitly naming either of them. The following describes their mutual reflection: "And now it occurs to us that our city resembles the friend whom we have lost and who loved it; it is, as he was, industrious, stamped with a frown of stubborn, feverish activity; and it is simultaneously listless and inclined to spend its time idly dreaming" (Ginzburg N, 2018, 23). And she spoke of Pavese's eternal adolescence: "Our friend lived in the city as an adolescent, and he lived in the same way until the end. His days were extremely long and full of time, like an adolescent's; he knew how to find time to study and to write, to earn his living and to wander idly through the streets he loved; whereas we, who staggered from laziness to frantic activity and back again, wasted our time trying to decide whether we were lazy or industrious" (Ginzburg N, 2018, 24). "In his last years his face was lined and furrowed, laid waste by mental torment; but his build and figure retained

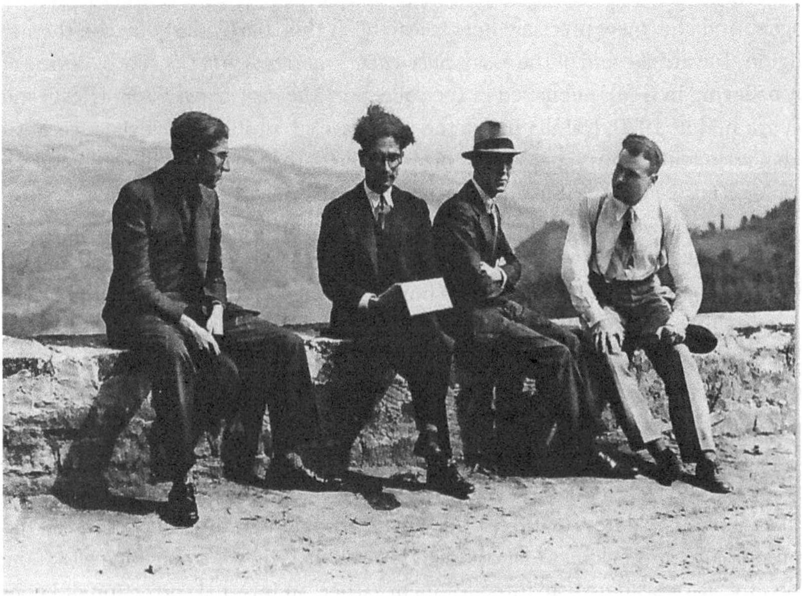

Figure 19.3. Cesare Pavese, Leone Ginzburg, Franco Antonicelli, and Carlo Frassinelli at San Grato di Sordevolo, Biella, approximately 1940.
Credits: Centro Studi Cesare Pavese ©.

their adolescent gracefulness to the end" (Ginzburg N, 2018, 29). Moving on from the viewpoint of memory and commemoration to a purely critical perspective, in an essay by Contini titled, *Un esperimento di poesia non aristocratica* [An Experiment of Non-Aristocratic Poetry], dated June 30th 1944, we find insightful observations on the first two works by Pavese, the book of poetry *Lavorare stanca* [Hard Labor], from 1936, and the novel *Paesi tuoi* [The Harvesters], from 1941. Referring to *The Harvesters* and to *Conversazione in Sicilia* [Conversations in Sicily] by his colleague and contemporary Elio Vittorini, released in the same year, Contini writes: "In both cases, the linguistic style used is full of coquetry, violence, formulas and *poncif* (clichés): in these works by Pavese full of syntactic and slang contortions, all is amiss from the very outset, that is to say, false in all its elements; however, a plenary and positive result overall" (Contini, 1972, 170). Falsehood, therefore, generates the truth: an apparently paradoxical logic, yet alluding to that of Aristotle, no less: "from true premises—writes the philosopher Enrico Berti—false conclusions cannot be drawn, that is to say only a true conclusion can be drawn, on the other hand a true conclusion may be drawn from false premises—and Aristotle determines in which cases this happens—equally, a false conclusion may be drawn—and again Aristotle determines in which cases—[...] Thus, while the falsehood of the conclusion necessarily presupposes the falsehood of the premises, the truth of the conclusion cannot infer that of the premises." (Berti, 2004, 102–103). As regards *Hard Labor*, Contini informs us: "In the geography of the publishing world, Pavese is supportive of the Piedmontese Gobettians, all united around the Frassinelli and Einaudi publisher's (as an indication of his orientation, two of the poems are dedicated to Augusto Monti and Leone Ginzburg, the old master and one of the group leaders, now tragically suppressed)" (Contini, 1972, 171). And he later writes: "For Pavese it is a matter of writing the poetic diary of a character very similar to those of *The Harvesters*, a townsman migrating towards the suburbs, intent on being a part of the very first movements, indistinguishable (and this is fundamental) from his environment of very humble souls, primitive souls; an "objective" poetic diary for which the farmer, locally born and bred, the rebellious boy, the mechanic, the drunkard, the convict, the vagabond, the slut, the estranged father (and to complete the list: the deceased) all emerge subtly, into existence and into consciousness" (Contini, 1972, 171).

NATALIA GINZBURG

Leone Ginzburg followed the first stories, the narratives, of the 20-year-old Natalia very keenly and attentively; Pavese urged her, almost challenged her, to produce a work of greater depth and breadth. He also sent a postcard to her, she who, with her sons, had followed her husband to confinement in Abruzzo, in which he said: "stop making children and write a book that is better than mine." The fruit of this plea-challenge was Ginzburg's first novel, *La strada che va in città* [The Road to the City], released in 1942, a year after *Paesi tuoi* [The Harvesters]. The works of Ginzburg are best known for their overriding theme of the family. She is renowned for her celebration of the family, for the way in which she describes it, analyzes it, and dissects it. Three of her works contain the word family in the title: *Lessico famigliare* [Family Lexicon] from 1963, *La famiglia Manzoni* ([The Manzoni Family] from 1983, two major works; *Famiglia* [Family] from 1977, a long novel. Generally speaking, the complete works of Ginzburg, from the point of view of this conception of the family, are considered to be similar to the trajectory of an arc, a parabola, which after the ascending phase culminating in the *Lexicon* irreversibly declines under the weight of reality: the family deteriorates, crumbles, and falls apart. Literature, in effect, particularly when realistic (as Ginzburg's is), reflects reality and its changes throughout both time and history. But if it is the mirror of reality, it is not merely a passive and desultory mirror; furthermore, realism does not necessarily mean being driven by reality. Thus, we can say that this widespread and common consideration is substantially wrong. And, moreover, we can say this not on the basis of mere theoretical deduction. There is also another word, another theme, of utmost importance: road. It is prominent in the title of her first novel, yet never reappears in the later titles, although it does find refuge in the epigraphs, almost all of them, as well as featuring in the twists and turns of the texts. The road is the exact counterpoint, the very counterweight to the family, the only youth (or adolescent, like Pavese) able to measure up to such a giant. And, as we can see, this is done right from the very outset. The road here is to be understood, not so much as a thrilling pagan adventure, but rather as a wearying and murmuring biblical exodus. It is impossible to fully document, in these pages, the scope and power of the road. We will limit ourselves to just two examples, one tiny, the other so huge that it is difficult to conceive of any greater example. The first is a curious improper linguistic usage. In normal Italian, when we say "crossing a road," we mean "going from one side to the other," crossing its width. Ginzburg, however, also uses the expression to mean "to travel its entire length," to follow it, to walk along it forever:

"I was thinking about my old life, about the city where I went every day, about the road that led into the city and that I had crossed in all seasons, for so many years" (*La strada che va in città* [The Road to the City] in Ginzburg N, 1986, 41); "Then they walked, talking endlessly, through streets that seemed strange and new to him one moment, and welcoming and easy to walk along the next. In fact, they were the same streets he walked along [in Italian text: *che egli attraversava*] every day, and normally he found them boring, hostile and inhospitable." (*Famiglia* [Family] in Ginzburg N, 1987, 2021, 48).

It could be that in this usage by Ginzburg, an element of her Piedmontese or Turinese substratum is re-emerging. We do not know which of the two it may be, but this does not matter. It does not matter because what is important here is the way that she, most certainly intentionally, makes use of it (note that the second quote is from a text of her later, rather than her more naive, earlier years). The second example is the whole of *The Manzoni Family*, where these two poles face each other on an absolutely equal footing. On the one side, the complex family relationships, some suffocating, others less so. On the other side, the roads with the various walks and journeys that take place along them, each involving a greater or lesser degree of uncertainty and danger. This is the beauty of Ginzburg's longest work. But—you may ask—was it really necessary for an equal and opposite force to the family to have been developed? The answer is affirmative: Yes, it was absolutely necessary, because the family is the source par excellence, to the highest degree, of "mythical powers," to use the apt expression by Walter Benjamin, who built his extraordinary work upon a critical analysis of this phenomenon. Literature has since its very origins, at least in the West, been the calling into question and the struggle with, rather than against, mythical powers to which we are, or at least we are constantly at risk of being subjected (a truth that the apologetic and senseless mythologism of our times tries to hide or to distort). Were this not the case, neither literature nor science would ever have come into being. Ginzburg created a literary masterpiece. And it would not seem excessive or out of place to say that she also created a scientific masterpiece. Despite having been raised in a predominantly high-level scientific family environment, she came to realize that their science was not enough, not nearly enough, to make them immune to, or even critical toward, the mythical powers to which they were enslaved and within which they were immersed. Thus, she decided to open their eyes via her own means. To open the eyes of other families as well as her own. In a single word, Family with a capital F.

"At the dinner table in my father's home when I was a girl if I, or one of my siblings, knocked a glass over on the tablecloth or dropped a knife, my father's voice would thunder, 'Watch your manners!' If we used our bread to mop up pasta sauce, he yelled, 'Don't lick your plates. Don't dribble! Don't slobber!' (Ginzburg N, 2017, 5).

This is how *Family Lexicon* opens, but we should not limit ourselves to merely rejoicing and enjoying this memorable introduction, immediate and theatrical, a snippet of that very lexicon after which the book is named. Something much bigger is at stake here. "En archei": referring to the two opening words, the incipit of both the Old Testament and the Fourth Gospel, fits well with what the philosopher Giorgio Agamben argues in *Creation and Anarchy*, with the following proposal of an alternative translation to that normally adhered to: "a word that is at the beginning, before anything else, can only be a command. I believe that perhaps the most correct translation of the famous incipit should be, not 'in the beginning was the Word,' rather 'in the command—that is, in the form of a command—was the Word.' Had this translation prevailed, many things would be clearer, not only in theology, but also and above all in politics" (Agamben, 2017, 92–93). It is hardly necessary to point out that the incipit of *Family Lexicon* is both a beginning and a command, actually more of a command than a beginning. But let us follow some key points of the very insightful Agambenean argumentation. It speaks of the "fundamental division of linguistic utterances that Aristotle establishes in a passage from *Perì hermeneias*, whereby, the exclusion of part of them from philosophical consideration has proven to be at the origins of the lack of attention that Western logic has paid to the command. "Not every discourse," writes Aristotle (*De int.*, 17 a 1-7), "is apophantic, only that discourse in which it is possible to say a truth or a falsehood (*aletheuein e pseudesthai*) is so. This does not happen in all discourses: for example, prayer is a discourse (*logos*), but it is neither true nor false. We will not therefore deal with these other discourses, because their investigation falls under the competence of rhetoric and poetics: apophantic discourse alone will constitute the subject of this study" (Agamben, 2017, 97). Agamben, after showing that Aristotle had told a few half-truths, did not keep his promise, however, because even in *Poetics* he continues to marginalize nonapophantic discourse, continuing with: "Consider this great caesura that, according to Aristotle, divides the field of language, and, at the same time excludes a part of the professional competence of philosophers. There is a discourse, a *logos*, which Aristotle calls 'apophantic' because it is able to manifest (this is the meaning of the verb *apophaino*) whether something exists or not, and is therefore necessarily either true or false. Then, there are other discourses, other *logoi*—such as prayer, command, threat, narration, questions and answers (we could also add exclamation, greeting, advice, curse, blasphemy etc.)—which are not apophantic, do not manifest the being or otherwise of something and are, therefore, indifferent to truth and falsehood. Aristotle's decision to exclude nonapophantic discourse from philosophy influenced the history of Western logic. Logic, namely the reflection on language, for centuries focused only on the analysis of apophantic propositions, those that can be considered true or false, and left aside, as if it were impracticable territory, that enormous portion of the language of which we make use every day, that nonapophantic discourse, which can be considered neither true nor false and, as such, when not being simply ignored, was abandoned to the competence of the rhetoricians, moralists, and theologians." (Agamben, 2017, 98–99). An "enormous portion," indeed, the other half of our linguistic and discursive universe, which is referred to as performative, and which is performative. Without making use of this category (introduced by John Langshaw Austin in the study, *How to do things with words,* 1962, just a year before *Family Lexicon*), Giacomo Magrini, in his monograph on *Lexicon*, described the work of Natalia Ginzburg as being applied to the "vast field of interrogation and exclamation, of doubt, of desire, of nostalgia, of prayer, of regret, of deprecation, of imprecation, of lament, of invective, of criticism, of command, of prohibition, of judgement, of blame and of praise" (Magrini, 802). From this point of view, we might share the opinion of Garboli, when he says that, in "a unique and original book filtered by countless models"(Garboli 2005, 95), he finds "just one error, the single page on the writers of the post-war period and the excessive portraits of Balbo and Pavese towards the conclusion, inspired by a non-fiction writing style alien to the tone of the book" (Garboli 2005, 96). "Non-fiction," in this case, means "apophantic": and, in fact, those pages are the most apophantic, or the least performative, of the entire work. Why are memoirs often unspeakably boring and irritating? Because they are based on a mystifying operation, which consists in hiding and transforming a joyous and anti-hierarchical performative plurality into a monolithic apophantic solemnity. *Family Lexicon* is the exact opposite. Let us once again use Agamben's words: "Corresponding to this linguistic partition is the partition of the real into two distinct but related spheres: the first ontology defines and governs the sphere of philosophy and science, while the second that of law, religion and magic.

"Law, religion and magic—which originally were not always easy to distinguish—constitute a sphere in which the language is always in the imperative form. In fact, I believe that a good definition of religion would be one which characterises it as the attempt to construct an entire universe upon the foundation of a command. And it is not only God who expresses himself in the imperative, in the form of the commandment, but, curiously, men also turn to God in the same way. In the classical world, as well as in Judaism and in Christianity, prayers are always formulated in the imperative form: 'Give us this day our daily bread'" (Agamben, 2017, 103–104).

"If we consider the increasing success of the performative, not only among linguists, but also among philosophers, jurists and theorists of literature and the arts, it would be reasonable to put forward the hypothesis that the centrality of this concept actually corresponds to the fact that, in contemporary societies, the ontology of the command is progressively supplanting the ontology of the assertion.

"This means that in a sort of, what psychoanalysts refer to as 'return of the repressed,' religion, magic and law—and, with these, the whole sphere of nonapophantic discourse which had been rejected in the shadows—in reality, secretly govern the functioning of our laic and secular societies" (Agamben, 2017, 105–106).

Consider, in *Lexicon*, the account that Ginzburg gives of a political meeting, one of the few, perhaps the only one where Giuseppe Levi gave a speech:

"They brought him into a theater, got him on stage, and my father began his rally with these words: 'Science is the pursuit of truth.' He spoke exclusively about science for nearly twenty minutes as people silently looked on, stupefied. At a certain point, he said that scientific research was far more advanced in America than in Russia. The people, even more confused, remained silent. He then unexpectedly happened to mention Mussolini and the fact that he usually referred to him as the "Jackass from Predappio." The audience erupted into resounding applause and my father looked around him, now stupefied himself. This was my father's political rally" (Ginzburg N, 2017, 193).

We must not imagine that Ginzburg wanted to belittle the cumbersome father figure, or that she intended to make fun of Professor Levi; but, in this passing from an initial, almost pathetic apophantic subtlety to the subsequent, amusing, performative insult, she plunges even him, him first and foremost, into the performative that pervades and envelops our lives. This questioning of mythical powers, which we have looked at, and the very accurate exploration of the performative that we are now seeing, with its discrete but grandiose effects of the "return of the repressed," are both intimately and profoundly correlated.

ACKNOWLEDGMENTS

I acknowledge with gratitude my debt to Marco Piccolino. A great thanks to "the person of my life." The translations of the essays I quoted are mine, unless otherwise specified. As for Natalia Ginzburg, I quote from the English editions of her work, when available. However, I couldn't view the English or American translations of *Mai devi domandarmi* and *La strada che va in città*.

REFERENCES

Agamben A G (2017) *Creazione e anarchia* [Creation and Anarchy]. *L'opera nell'età della religione capitalista*. Vicenza: Neri Pozza Editore.

Berti E (2004) *Nuovi studi aristotelici. Epistemologia, logica e dialettica*, Brescia: Morcelliana.

Bobbio N (2000) Introduzione. In D Zucaro (Ed.), *Leone Ginzburg, Scritti*, pp. XLVII–LXVI. Torino: Einaudi.
Contini G (1968) Benedetto Croce. In *Letteratura dell'Italia unita 1861–1968*, pp. 423–482. Firenze: Sansoni, pp. 423–482.
Contini G (1972) Un esperimento di poesia non aristocratica. In *Altri esercizi (1942–1971)*, pp. 169–172. Torino: Einaudi.
D'Orsi A (2000) *La cultura a Torino tra le due guerre*. Torino: Einaudi.
Garboli C (2005) Lessico famigliare. In *Storie di seduzione*, pp. 86–96. Torino: Einaudi.
Ginzburg N (under the pseudonym of Alessandra Tornimparte) (1942) *La strada che va in città*. Torino: Einaudi (English version: (2012) F Frenaye (Trans.), *The Road to the City* . New York: Arcade Publishing; originally published in London: Hogarth Publisher, 1952).
Ginzburg L (2000) Čechov. In D Zucaro (Ed.), *Scritti*, pp. 312–321. Torino: Einaudi.
Ginzburg N (1962) *Le piccole virtù*. Torino: Einaudi (English version: (2018) D Davis (Trans.), *The Little Virtues*. Foreword by B Boggs. New York: Arcade Publishing; originally published in Manchester: Carcanet Publisher, 1986).
Ginzburg N (1963) *Lessico famigliare*. Torino: Einaudi (English version: (2017) J McPhee (Trans.), *Family Lexicon*. New York: New York Review of Books.).
Ginzburg N (1970) *Mai devi domandarmi*. Milano: Garzanti (English version: (1973) I Quigly (Trans.), *Never Must You Ask Me*. Introduction by I Quigly. London: Joseph Publisher.).
Ginzburg N. (1986–1987) *Opere*. Collected and chronologically ordered by the Author. Two vols. Milano: Mondadori.
Gobetti P (1960–1969–1974) *Opere complete, I Scritti politici*, P Spriano (Ed.); II, *Scritti storici, letterari e filosofici*, P Spriano (Ed.); III *Scritti di critica teatrale*, G Guazzotti & C Gobetti (Eds.). Torino: Einaudi.
Gramsci A (1987) *L'Ordine Nuovo 1919–1920*. V Gerratana & A Santucci (Eds.). Torino: Einaudi.
Gramsci A (1994) *Pre-prison Writings*. R Bellamy (Ed.) V Cox (Trans.). Cambridge: Cambridge University Press.
Gramsci A (1975) *Quaderni del carcere*, edited by Valentino Gerratana, Torino: Einaudi, 4 vols. (English version: (2011) *Prison Notebooks* J A Buttigieg with Antonio Callari (Trans.) New York: Columbia University Press.
Magrini G (1996) "Lessico famigliare di Natalia Ginzburg." In *Letteratura italiana. Le Opere*, IV, 2. *Il Novecento. La ricerca letteraria*, pp. 771–810. Torino: Einaudi.
Strada V (2005) La Russia di Čechov come "Anima del mondo." In Vv. Au. *L'anima del mondo e il mondo di Čechov*, pp. 89–99. Genova: il Melangolo.

CHAPTER 20

A Real Imperfection? Rita and the Long Story of the Nerve Growth Factor

GERMANA PARETI

WARNING TO READERS

Any historian who wishes to illustrate the intellectual biography of Rita Levi-Montalcini (Figure 20.1) has to be aware of at least three challenges. These must be put on the table immediately: not as a *captatio benevolentiae*, but for the sake of truth and clarity.

First of all, the historian will have to know how to properly handle the many articles written about Rita Levi-Montalcini, both after the award of the Nobel Prize and after her death, in a *neutral* way. These works often led to conflicting judgments about her personality. In Italy, as it has been observed, she was (and continues to be) seen as a heroine, "a national treasure" (Abbott, 2009, p. 567) while in countries of Anglo-American culture the undeniable merit of her discovery does not exclude moral judgment.

Secondly, Rita Levi-Montalcini herself published the autobiography, titled *In Praise of Imperfection* (1988) as well as other autobiographical works (Levi-Montalcini, 1992, 2000, 2002). Although, on the one hand, they seem to facilitate the historian's work, on the other hand, they lead the historian to repeat prior-known information. She was a prolific and passionate writer, having published 21 popular books (Levi-Montalcini, 1993, 1996, 1998, 1999, 2001). She was an equally passionate reader of classics, including *Wuthering Heights* by Emily Brönte, and the works of Primo Levi, Italo Calvino, Virginia Woolf, and Franz Kafka. However, even her autobiography received conflicting reviews, ranging from praise to criticism (Hollyday, 1989; Purves, 1988). Nevertheless, *In Praise of Imperfection* is still a fundamental contribution, in which—it should be emphasized—the pages dedicated to her youth occupy half of the book.

Thirdly, the discovery of Nerve Growth Factor (NGF), which is the end product of this complex story (Hamburger, 1993), is a result on which scientists have never

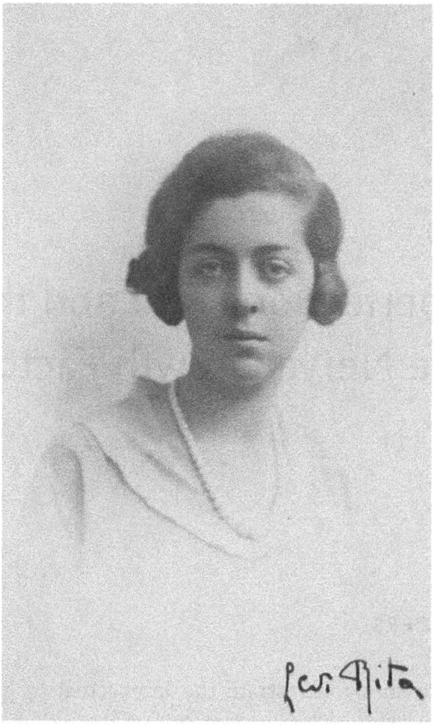

Figure 20.1. Portrait and signature of Rita Levi-Montalcini. This picture was originally attached to the request for enrollment at the Faculty of Medicine and Surgery of the University of Turin in 1930. Credits and source: Archivio storico. Fascicoli degli studenti e tesi di laurea; Archivio storico dell'Università di Torino, 2013. Thanks to the Historical Archive of the University of Turin and Paola Novaria.

stopped working (Bradshaw et al., 2017). Even today, more than 50 years after its discovery, the NGF is the subject of extensive literature, which describes its considerable potential effects on the therapeutic field. Rita Levi-Montalcini published more than 200 scientific articles, which contributed to progress in neuroscience. The discovery of NGF was interpreted as "a saga of determination to overcome hurdles that were personal and social as well as scientific" (Watts, 2013). The obstacles were due to religious discrimination, sexism, totalitarian regimes, and war (Chao & Calissano, 2013). Still, she was, as Primo Levi wrote, "a tiny lady with an indomitable will and a countenance of a princess."

To substantiate this assumption, this work will be articulated around three major thematic areas: her youth, the American adventure, and her return(s) to Italy.

THE YOUNG RITA: TWO REBELLIOUS SPIRITS?

In the pages describing her family environment, Rita (as Levi-Montalcini is generally referred to in the United States) mentioned the Victorian atmosphere. In doing so, she mainly referred to the attitude of her father, Adamo, who considered a woman's role in society to be a good wife and mother. All decisions were made by Adamo, who had a "traditional" conception of the role of the woman, which would see her relegated to the domestic sphere. "When I was a child, I was a very unhappy child because my family was totalitarian, I mean a Victorian kind, my father," Rita recalled in a "Conversation" with Moses Chao at the European Brain Research Institute in 2010. Adamo Levi shared with his children the importance of "free thought" and raised them to consider culture a priority. But despite this open attitude, once his daughters had completed lower secondary school, he enrolled them in an all-female high school (the "Scuola superiore femminile Margherita di Savoia" in Turin), which blocked direct access to the university (Sandrone, 2013).

At that time, boys' high school included humanistic and scientific subjects—the latter of which were simply "not conceivable" in the girls' school. In this respect, biographers agree in emphasizing the young Rita's rebellious attitude. She succeeded in convincing her father to allow her to attend private lessons to, eventually, enroll in the university. Nevertheless, we should not overlook the equally combative attitude of her twin, Paola, who expressed her interest in mathematics and the exact sciences, despite having a notable propensity toward the arts. Although she eagerly accepted her father's decision, Paola would subsequently embark on an artistic career, enrolling in the "Libera Scuola" of Painting, founded in Turin by the painter Felice Casorati, one of the principal exponents of Magic Realism. At this point, Paola also demonstrated a precocious, creative autonomy. Both twins had strong, determined characters.

FAMILY STORY

"It is true that Aunt Rita was a public character, but she also had a family," remarked Piera, Rita Levi-Montalcini's niece, while commenting on the Nobel Prize awarded to the scientist on the 10th of December 1986. "Our family was a Piedmontese Jewish one, the Levis were Turinese and the Montalcinis from Monferrato." The surname Montalcini seems to suggest Tuscan origin, likely indicating the village of Montalcino, in the province of Siena, where Rita's ancestors might have lived before installing themselves in Piemonte. The matronymic Montalcini was first added to the last name "Levi" by Gino, the oldest child, and then by the twins, to distinguish them from other professionals with the same, rather common, surname.

Even though Rita's parents came from Sephardic families, they "went neither to church nor the synagogue" (Levi-Montalcini, 1988, p. 19). "We commemorated traditional Jewish celebrations [like the Passover ritual], but we were secular," Piera remembers:

> among the objects of my aunt I have found books of prayer, even though she certainly didn't use them to pray. I believe that she inherited a lot from the Jewish culture, to which, despite being decidedly irreligious, she had a great sense of affiliation: asking questions in order to find answers is at the base of the Jewish search

and culture. *There is time for everything*, it is written in *Ecclesiastes*. And for her it was all a matter of organization. She knew how to spend and to distribute her time. She got up very early to read, before having breakfast and then working. This was her daily routine until the very day she died. ("La Stampa", September 8th, 2016)

In this regard, Rita's family looked like that of Primo Levi. Primo Levi came from a fundamentally secular family, like many families in the early 1900s in Italy. Regarding the Jewish character, the integration of Italian Judaism was unique. But, perhaps, the equilibrium of Turinese-Piedmontese Judaism was even more particular: It integrated quickly without abdicating its own identity. The same was true of the Levi-Montalcini family, which resided in Turin in a building on Corso Umberto I, called "the sacred hearth."

Rita and Paola were born on the 22nd of April 1909, the youngest daughters of Adamo Levi (called *Father* in her autobiography) and Adele Montalcini (*Mother*). The couple had gotten married in 1901, and was blessed with the birth of Luigi (Gino) in 1902 and with that of Anna, called Nina, in 1904. Adamo had a big handlebar moustache "*à la Umberto*" (Levi-Montalcini, 1988, p. 13), and he was nicknamed by the family *Damino the terrible* for his energetic and irascible character. He was an electro-mechanical engineer and a mathematician. Adelina, also known as Lina, was described to be as beautiful as a Pre-Raphaelite figure and was an artist during her youth.

Paola and Rita were heterozygous twins; they did not look alike and were complementary. Looking at childhood photos, Paola was shorter and "chubbier" compared to Rita, who was tall and slim. Paola's features resembled those of her father. Rita was, instead, the living portrait of their maternal grandmother: gray-green eyes with a melancholy gaze, a slight asymmetry of the face, and a delicate and slender conformation of the bone structure.

Paola, an extrovert by nature, adored their father, and she was profoundly affected by his death in 1932. She also shared a passion for art with Gino, who was a sculptor and architect. Rita, who was rather shy, felt a deep affection for her mother, but not for her father, with whom she had a problematic relationship. Nevertheless, the loss of her father caused an intense pain in Rita. Over 50 years later, she felt somehow obliged to dedicate her autobiography, "To Paola and to memory of our father, whom she adored while he lived and whom I loved and worshiped after his death."

Rita and Anna were passionate readers of the Swedish author Selma Lagerlöf, who was the first female writer to win the Nobel Prize (in 1909). But Anna abandoned her dream of becoming a writer to devote herself to the role of wife and mother. This path was not followed by the twins, who had no maternal instincts and, without regret, commented: "No children, just other satisfactions" (Vetrano, 2018). If Paola immediately understood her destiny was painting, having shown propensity for art, Rita took more time to realize hers. After completing her studies, Rita spent three years in complete uncertainty about her future. She was attracted to philosophy, but the high school she attended did not allow her to enter university. She was convinced she did not have any particular talent and the biological sciences were not included in her high school's curriculum. She reached a turning point when the family's beloved governess, Giovanna Bruatto, died of cancer. Propelled by the affection she had felt for this woman, Rita decided to enroll in medicine:

> It was on that day that my decision took form, and I felt that I would be able to convince my father to give me his authorization and I would have studied medicine. (Levi-Montalcini, 1988, p. 37)

Rita was encouraged by her mother to discuss her decision with her father and try to make him understand that she could not accept the role of wife and mother.

A NEW WORLD

In just eight months, and with the help of two tutors, Rita caught up in Greek, Latin, and mathematics. She obtained a high school diploma, and she enrolled at the Faculty of Medicine and Surgery of the University of Turin on the 31st of October 1930. A new scenario opened up: For the first time, Rita entered the amphitheater of the Institute of Anatomy in Corso Massimo d'Azeglio, where Professor Giuseppe Levi (no relation to Rita) had sovereign authority. Holder of the chair of Human Anatomy at the University of Turin, and a "dominant personality in the medical school," Levi was a leading figure in the biology of that period (Bentivoglio, 2006; Grignolio, 2018; Piazza, 2018; Ribatti, 2018). He also was celebrated for his bold antifascist stance. Particularly gripping are the pages of *In Praise of Imperfection* describing the legendary irascible temper of the professor (nicknamed *Levipom* due to his red hair), who was pushed over the edge whenever he saw personal belongings left on the tables in the library ("the library is not a bar!").

In the second year of Medicine, Anatomy lessons were also attended by two other students and future Nobel laureates: Renato Dulbecco and Salvador Luria, who both took internships at the Institute of Anatomy. They met either in the laboratory or in the library, even though their profound knowledge of Rita would only have been possible in the postwar period. Together with her cousin Eugenia Sacerdote, enrolled in Medicine at the same time, Rita enthusiastically attended Levi's lessons. However, she initially showed some difficulties in handling the histological technique: Rodolfo Amprino, Levi's "most gifted student" and his favorite pupil, used to frown and shake his head every time he was inspecting the slides Rita had prepared. But things were about to change.

Levi gave to his interns the task of assessing whether mice from the same brood shared the same number of cells in the sensory ganglia or not. Rita and Eugenia considered this task "tedious," and were not sure about the accuracy of their counts. Another task was about the formation of cerebral convolutions in human fetuses. But in the early 1930s it was difficult to obtain this material, and Rita was worried that Levi could consider her "a pain in the neck" (as he tended to describe those students found on his "blacklist"). Fortunately, Levi allowed Rita to change her topic, and the new research was on how nerve cells grow in vitro.

Studies on the differentiation of cells in in-vitro cultures were done by Ross Granville Harrison in the first decade of the century by using the lymph drop technique (in which he placed a tiny portion of amphibian medullary tube); after this, Rita relied on the numerous contributions by Levi and his coworker Hertha Meyer. The new topic constituted Rita's doctoral research, and she graduated with top marks in 1936 with a thesis titled *Research on the in-vitro formation of collagen and reticular fibrils from explants of various organs.* "For the first time, I became passionate about research, and the enthusiasm with which we gave ourselves to his new project did not go unrewarded" (Levi-Montalcini, 1988, p. 60). She could observe, for the first time, that the formation of reticular fibers, as revealed by argentic staining, was not exclusively a property of the connective tissue, but of the muscular and epithelial tissues as well. This experience would prove useful many years later in discovering the nature of the nerve growth factor.

SINISTER PRESAGES

The year 1936 was one of personal satisfaction, but also of tragic events for Rita and her family: the anti-Semitic campaign began in the spring of that year. In 1938, after the promulgation of the racial laws, she was prevented from continuing her research at the Institute of Anatomy. On the 16th of October 1938, Rita was suspended from academic work and from the Clinic for Nervous and Mental Diseases where she was a "voluntary assistant" (Figure 20.2). Rita, together with the neurophysiologist Fabio Visintini, had started a research project on the differentiation of the nervous centers and circuits in chicken embryos, wherein she used a modified silver impregnation technique inspired by Santiago Ramón y Cajal. Due to the racial laws, the results of this research could not be published in any Italian periodical. They appeared in a Swiss journal and received praise for their experimental rigor (Visintini & Levi-Montalcini, 1939). In 1939, Rita obtained the "Specialist Diploma" in Neuropathology and Psychiatry, because Article 5 of the *Provisions for the defense of the race in Fascist Schools* allowed already enrolled Jewish students to complete their studies without financial help (Strata, 2018).

Rita could not work at any Italian university or institute. In March, she accepted the invitation of Dr. Lion Laruelle, the director of a neurological institute in Brussels. This invitation was particularly appealing, because Professor Levi—invited by Professor Jean Firket—was already in Liège, and he had established a tissue-culture center there. With both of them in Belgium, they would be able to continue their collaboration. In December, due to the imminent German invasion, Rita decided to return to Italy to practice medicine, albeit in a clandestine way. A particularly decisive event in Rita's future was her encounter with Amprino, who urged her not to "lose heart in the face of the first difficulties," recalling the example of Cajal, who did fundamental research on the nervous system of vertebrates working in a modest laboratory in Valencia. Rita became convinced that chick embryos were the ideal material to carry out Cajal's research program, and she gained the family's approval to set up what became famous as "a private laboratory *à la* Robinson Crusoe [. . .] a minuscule

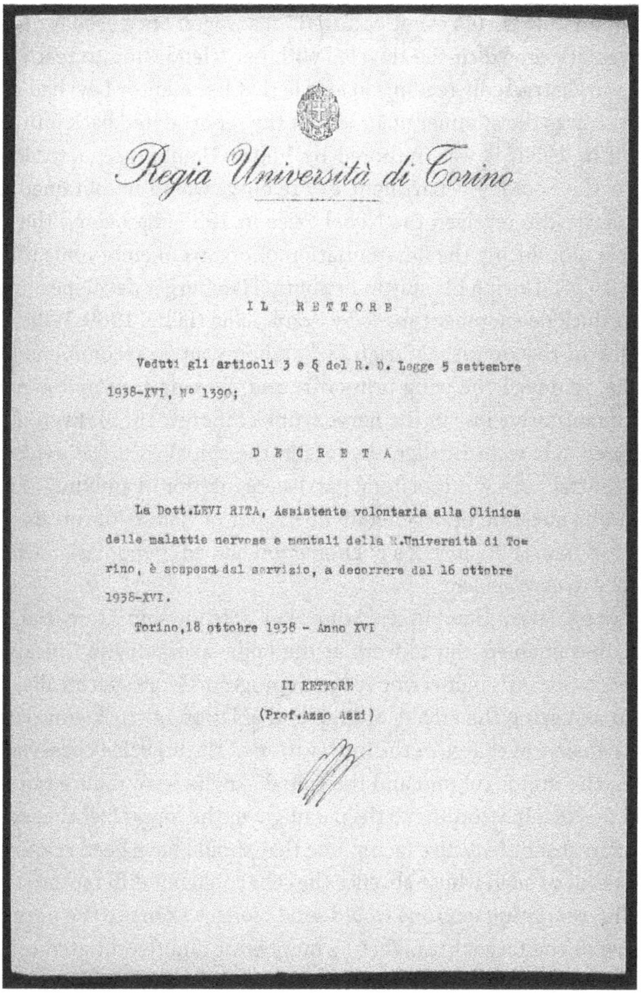

Regia Università di Torino

IL RETTORE

Veduti gli articoli 3 e 8 del R. D. Legge 5 settembre 1938-XVI, N° 1390;

D E C R E T A

La Dott.LEVI RITA, Assistente volontaria alla Clinica delle malattie nervose e mentali della R.Università di Torino, è sospesa dal servizio, a decorrere dal 16 ottobre 1938-XVI.

Torino,18 ottobre 1938 - Anno XVI

IL RETTORE
(Prof.Azzo Azzi)

Figure 20.2. Letter notifying the suspension from the Clinic for Nervous and Mental Diseases where Rita Levi-Montalcini was a voluntary assistant, 16th of October 1938. Credits and source: Archivio storico. Fascicoli degli studenti e tesi di laurea; Archivio storico dell'Università di Torino, 2013. Thanks to the Historical Archive of the University of Turin and Paola Novaria.

laboratory not unlike a convent cell" (Levi-Montalcini, 1988, p. 92). A small thermostat served as incubator, and other instruments, such as a stereomicroscope, a binocular Zeiss microscope, and other makeshift devices, constituted her laboratory equipment. When asked if she had a fellowship, Rita replied that she worked in her bedroom, and she just had her microscope.

Her aim was to analyze the influence of noninnervated tissues in peripheral territories, such as limbs, on the differentiation and development of motor and sensory cells, in the spinal cord and in the dorsal root ganglia respectively, in the early stages of embryonic life. Rita was dissatisfied with the results obtained on amphibian tadpoles. But an unexpected event occurred. In a wagon once used for the transportation of livestock on which she traveled with her friend Gino to reach a mountain village, she was distractedly reading an article that her mentor Levi had sent her two years earlier. It was the summer of 1938, but the report dated back four years.

Published in 1934, it was authored by Viktor Hamburger, a student of Hans Spemann, at the zoology department in Freiburg, where he obtained his PhD in 1925. Spemann, who received the Nobel Prize in 1935, discovered the *organizer*, a factor capable of inducing the differentiation of organs in embryonic life (Spemann & Mangold, 1924). During his stay in Freiburg, Hamburger developed an interest in the work on chick development made by Frank Lillie (Lillie, 1909; Willier, 1957). At the beginning of the century, Marian Lydia Shorey, upon recommendation by her mentor Lillie, removed the wing primordia and, looking into motor neurons, she observed a quantitative loss in the nerve trunks (Shorey, 1909). Even if the ganglia in the operated side were smaller, the loss in the spinal cord was evident, and the cells of the ventral horn (anterolateral part) were inferior in amount. She concluded that it was not a question of degenerate fibers, but of "failure of certain neuroblasts to develop" (Shorey, 1909, p. 51): a phenomenon named "hypoplasia," which was due to a deficiency in *development*.

Twenty years later, Hamburger, who won a fellowship from the Rockefeller Foundation that enabled him to work at the Lillie laboratory in Chicago, aimed at expanding Miss Shorey's pioneering research program. More specifically, Hamburger was keen on analyzing the effects of limb bud ablation in chick embryos on spinal cord motor neurons in charge of the innervation of the limb. He observed that, after the ablation, the motor column and the spinal ganglia were reduced in volume. He interpreted this result according to the paradigm of the "organizer theory," that is, as the effect of an absent *inductive* factor, one that should have been released from the innervated tissues and in whose absence the cells could not differentiate. He thought that early differentiating neurons would send pioneer axons to the periphery to explore the size of the target area. Then, a number of undifferentiated cells would be recruited by retrograded signals to the demand of the periphery in a quantitative way: "each peripheral field controls the quantitative development of its nerve center [. . .] The stimuli going from the peripheral fields to their nerve centers are probably transmitted centripetally by the nerve fibers" (Hamburger, 1934, p. 491).

Deprived of their fields of innervation, motor nerve cells in the segment of the spinal cord innervating the limb failed to undergo growth and differentiation. This finding suggested to the author that, under normal conditions, the pioneer nerve fibers, after reaching their target limb tissues, send signals to their nerve centers, which at this stage consist mainly of still undifferentiated nerve cells. Upon receiving the "signal", they would be induced to undergo differentiation (Levi-Montalcini, 1997, p. 1).

Rita was impressed by Hamburger's "limpid style and the rigor of his analysis—in sharp contrast with those of previous authors who had described the same phenomenon in amphibian larvae" (Levi-Montalcini, 1988, p. 98). Rita and Levi repeated Hamburger's experiments when Levi returned from Belgium. They investigated the effect of the limb bud removal in three-day-old chick embryos. Twenty hours after the extirpation, they sacrificed embryos every six hours, to fix them with the silver staining technique (following De Castro's modification of Cajal's silver impregnation), and they observed the sections through the optical microscope. Unlike Hamburger, who worked on motor neurons of the spinal cord, Rita and Levi focused their attention on the sensory cells of the dorsal root ganglia ("dans lesquels il est plus aisé, pour des raisons bien connues à chaque histologiste d'entreprendre des recherches quantitatives") (Levi-Montalcini & Levi, 1942, p. 539). They focused on lumbar ganglion 25 for the cell counts. They observed an enormous reduction in number and size of the differentiated elements on the operated side, but only the neurons whose neurites reached on one side the skin and muscles, and on the other side the medulla, were affected by the elimination of the peripheral innervation territory. Therefore, limb ablation resulted in regressive changes culminating in a massive degeneration of motor and sensory neurons deprived of their peripheral field of innervation. This regression depended on the impossibility of establishing connections with the peripheral structures (muscles and skin), "on the failure of the sensory cells to establish synaptic contact with their end organs." For the differentiation, there was no need for an early contact with the wing or limb primordia, and this ruled out their role as inductive factors. Unlike Hamburger's interpretation, it was not about the *absence* of an inductive factor, but of a *trophic factor* normally released by the innervated tissues. In recalling the history of this discovery, Hamburger commented that Rita and Levi did not mention his "recruitment hypothesis," but referred unambiguously to an "arrest of development":

> This means that the removal of the target did not interfere with proliferation and early differentiation of spinal ganglion cells, but that it had an adverse effect on their survival. (Hamburger, 1992, p. 1119)

These results could not be published in any Italian periodical, because the racial laws prohibited the publication of articles by non-Aryan authors. The results appeared first in a Belgian journal (Levi-Montalcini & Levi, 1942, 1943) and then in a more extensive Italian publication of a Vatican periodical with an abstract in Latin (Levi-Montalcini & Levi, 1944).

WAR AND PEACE

But this discovery was destined to be "quiescent" for a while. In 1942, due to the bombings on the cities of Northern Italy, and in particular on Turin, Rita's family decided to move to the hills surrounding Asti. Levi lived in another place, but he returned daily to continue his experiments despite the prohibitive conditions. On the 10th of September, German tanks were in Piedmont. After returning to Switzerland, Rita and her family stopped in Florence, where Levi arrived that spring. In Florence, Rita and Paola dedicated themselves to the only activity that was not forbidden to them: filling out false ID cards and distributing them to the friends who needed them.

On the 11th of August 1944, at 6:10 AM, the National Liberation Committee of Tuscany (CTLN) ordered the attack. At 6:45 AM the bell of Palazzo Vecchio (known as "Martinella") gave the signal of insurrection. During the battle, all the antifascist forces fought among the houses and in the streets: the scenario of the popular mass, between the expulsion of the Germans and the arrival of the Allied Forces, was the subject of one of Paola's paintings, "The Walking City." In September 1944, Rita served as a medical doctor at the Allies' health service. It was her only experience as a doctor, and she contributed to dealing with the epidemics that plagued the refugee population. In May 1945, Rita could return to the liberated North and to Turin. Levi was able to offer her an assistant position. But how could Rita's future depend on that one past experiment, albeit executed with rigor and with great success? Between her intention to enroll in Biology and her renewed friendship with Dulbecco, who came back to Turin as well, an unexpected event changed her life forever.

Viktor Hamburger had read their article in the Belgian *Archive de Biologie* and was convinced of the importance of their results, despite the fact that they did not confirm his interpretation. While in Chicago, in 1933, Hamburger received a letter from Spemann, notifying him that the Rector of the University of Freiburg, the philosopher Martin Heidegger, had signed his dismissal because of his Jewish origins. Hamburger accepted an offer by Washington University in St. Louis, where he became Chairman of the Department of Zoology. In the summer of 1946, Viktor, as he was called in the international scientific community, wrote to Levi and asked him if Rita could spend a semester in St. Louis. "He was very impressed by my results, so he wanted to know how. We were so much different. He was a student of Spemann, was thinking that periphery acted through induction. I did say no, it is not induction. We had entirely different views," said Rita more than half a century later (Chao, 2010, p. 8).

Hamburger strongly emphasized the importance of that paradigm shift in their interpretations:

> To an experimental embryologist of the Spemann school, the idea that we might be dealing with the *death* of neurons would have been hardly conceivable. Embryonic induction, on the other hand, was a familiar theme, and I had formulated the recruitment hypothesis after the fashion of assimilative induction which plays a role in the activity of the organizer. But the neurologist of the Levi school was not encumbered by the mindset of experimental embryology. Dr. Levi-Montalcini had no difficult imagining a loss of neurons during development. Her background in neurology had another advantage: she mastered the silver impregnation technique of Cajal–De Castro which enabled her to distinguish between undifferentiated cells and neurons with axons. This played an important role in the later investigations. (Hamburger, 1992, p. 1119)

Meanwhile, Luria, who worked at Indiana University in Bloomington, had offered Dulbecco a fellowship. On the 19th of September 1947, sailing from Genoa on the Polish ship *Sobieski*, Rita and Dulbecco embarked for the United States together. The initial idea was that she would stay for a single semester; instead, she spent

26 years in the United States, with a three-month leave every year to be spent in Italy (Strata, 2018).

Turin ceased to be the primary location of Rita's story, and a new life began. Rita familiarized herself with the informal atmosphere that characterized the Rebstock Building, which was home to the zoology department and that was so different from the austere environment of the Institute of Anatomy in Turin. Despite her having doubts about the validity of her experimental approach, Rita got along well with Hamburger. Therefore, on alternate Sundays, she went to Bloomington to discuss it with Luria, who, albeit without enthusiasm, urged her to continue neurobiological research. Rita was at the cusp of an experimental change. She was on the right track, but she did not know whether to continue. She was about to leave the nervous system to work with Luria and Dulbecco. Finally, she decided to focus on the problem for which Hamburger had initially invited her to St. Louis: the effects of the amputation on the development of the nervous centers in charge of the innervation of excised limbs.

In the autumn of 1947, Rita examined some silver-salt impregnated chick embryo sections: the nerve cells began to differentiate. Her attention was drawn to the spinal cord, which revealed "a surprising variety of scenarios," a spectacle not unlike that of a battlefield, even in the same segment in embryos at the same stage of development. According to the functions carried out by nerve cells, the nervous system adopted different strategies: it eliminated unnecessary cells; cell populations migrated according to their functions; cell populations with the same functions were destined to innervate different peripheral tissues and organs. It was a matter of studying these two ontogenetic processes—migratory and degenerative—at the early stage of development of the nervous system. Surprised by the enthusiasm of his new Italian researcher, Viktor gave her the green light to continue on that line of research, which led to an article published the following year (Hamburger & Levi-Montalcini, 1949). It was a work that required a lot of effort in the precise reconstruction of the observed processes, but the "lifelong alliance" between the nervous system and Rita was definitive.

TUMORS AND VENOM

Luck played an important role in this alliance. Specifically, a letter exchange with a former pupil of Hamburger, Elmer Bueker, from Georgetown University. Bueker had continued to investigate the effects of the peripheral tissues on the differentiation of the nerve cells innervating them (Bueker, 1948). This constituted a variation on the investigations undertaken in Viktor's laboratory. In fact, instead of grafting additional limbs, Bueker grafted tiny pieces of cancerous tissues, characterized by high proliferative activity, such as chicken Rous sarcoma and mouse tumors. Following implantation of a small portion of a tumor known as mouse sarcoma 180 (henceforth S. 180) into the body-wall of three-day-old chick embryos, the nerve fibers originating from the ganglia in the surroundings ramified in the neoplastic tissue in embryos fixed at the eighth day of incubation. Also, they were larger than the contralateral fibers innervating the limb. The tumor was strongly invaded by sensory fibers, whereas the motor nerves did not enter it. The selective nature of tumor innervation could be deduced from the hyperplasia in the spinal ganglia and the coincident hypoplasia in the motor column of the tumor innervating segments. In January 1950, Viktor and Rita repeated Bueker's experiments. She grafted fragments of tumors onto three-day-old chick embryos. "Up to 6 days, the tumor is not invaded by nerve fibres [. . .] From the 7th day on, nerve fibers begin to invade the tumor in large quantities, and by 11 days, the tumors are richly supplied with nerves" (Levi-Montalcini & Hamburger, 1951, pp. 331–332).

The yellow tumor mass was penetrated by bundles of nerve fibers stemming from the sympathetic ganglia (hyperplasia and hypertrophy with a maximum of 600%), and in a smaller percentage (250%) from the sensory ganglia. Effects of S. 180 were different from those of grafted limb buds or other tissues. Also, another mouse tumor known as S. 37 was invaded by a network of nerve fibers: "Sarcomas 180 and 37 [. . .] were supplied with a denser net of nerve bundles than any normal tissue at any stage of development. The sarcoma tissue provides an extremely favourable medium for the outgrowth of nerve fibres" (Levi-Montalcini & Hamburger, 1951, p. 346). Veins were also penetrated, which suggested the humoral nature of that substance with a neurotropic effect, a "chemotactic directing force" that caused the growth of the nerve fibers in a particular direction. The nerve fibers entered the tumor without any contact with neoplastic cells, because it was a "diffusible agent," a soluble factor released by the neoplastic cells, which gained ganglia cells through embryonal blood circulation and stimulated growth and differentiation of developing nerve cells. Therefore, the new evidence opposed Hamburger's previous hypothesis of an *inductive* factor acting as pioneer and organizer necessary to cell differentiation. Furthermore, the results of this study reiterated the importance of a "dynamic approach [for] an adequate understanding of the entire process of nerve differentiation, and that observations made on one stage only may be misleading" (Levi-Montalcini & Hamburger, 1951, p. 346).

Unexpectedly, Levi, who was visiting the States, happened to be at the Institute of St. Louis while Rita was examining preparations under the microscope. Observing her sections, he completely disagreed with Rita's interpretation: those were not nerves, but connective fibers. Dulbecco's reaction was the opposite, given that he defined the event described by Rita as "sensational." However, this mysterious "nerve-growth promoting agent" had yet to be identified. It was clear that biochemical techniques were needed. This was a challenge. Rita remembered the in-vitro culture technique learned in Turin under the guidance of Levi's colleague, Hertha Meyer, who now was in Rio de Janeiro at the Institute of Biophysics directed by Carlos Chagas. In 1952, with a grant from the Rockefeller Foundation, Rita flew to Rio, not before having implanted cells of S. 180 and S. 37 into two mice, which she would have hidden for the flight in the pocket of her overcoat.

The first experiments conducted in Rio were unsuccessful. This was due to the fact that fragments of neoplastic tissues did not stimulate the development of the nerve fibers, probably because of some toxic factor that masked tumor activity. Another option was to use previously transplanted tumors that had taken in chick embryos, and this proved to be a successful choice. The in-vitro and in-vivo results showed "striking similarities." Examining the hanging drop tissue cultures, from the ganglia in proximity of the previously transplanted tumor "an extraordinarily dense halo-shaped outgrowth of nerve fibres" stemmed (Levi-Montalcini, 1988, p. 156). Other mouse sarcoma did not stimulate nerve growth and control experiments with heart tissue from chick embryos were negative. At some point, however, the same effect, although less pronounced, could be observed in the presence of normal mouse tissue. Rita wondered if the difference was merely quantitative, not knowing at that time that growth factors could be released also by normal tissues.

"It was a spring day in 1951, when [. . .] it dawned on me that the [transplanted mouse] tumor acted by releasing a growth factor of unknown nature." (Levi-Montalcini, 1997, p. 78)

In a 1954 article published with Meyer and Hamburger, two problems came to their attention: the chemical nature of the agent and its mode of action. In both experiments (in vivo and in vitro) "the agent acts at distance, and the tumor does not require contact with the ganglion or with the nerve fiber to exert its influence. [. . .] At the present, it seems that the agent [. . .] is restricted to some sarcomas" (Levi-Montalcini, Meyer & Hamburger, 1954, p. 54). Though radially straight in all directions, the higher density of nerve fibers was on the side facing the tumor, and this effect could be interpreted in terms of *neurotropic guidance* as described by Paul Weiss in 1934.

Upon returning to St. Louis, Hamburger informed Rita she could count on the collaboration of a young biochemist, Stanley Cohen. Stan turned out to be a very successful new addition to the team.

"Neither Dr. Hamburger nor Dr. Levi-Montalcini were biochemists, so they went to several of Washington University's departments looking for a biochemist 'mad' enough to study this problem. I was interested in embryology and knew biochemistry, so I thought, 'Il have a go at it'." (Cohen, 2008, p. 33794)

From 1953 till 1959, Rita and Stan formed a close and collaborative team. They were complementary: Stan knew biochemistry and Rita knew neuroembryology. "You and I are good, but together we are wonderful." To obtain a good amount of neoplastic tissue for Cohen to analyze, Rita had to extract it from dozens of embryos. Her hands continued to dissect under the microscope even when she was talking with colleagues (McGrayne, 1993, p. 215). In a paper published in 1954, Stan, Rita, and Viktor announced that their purest preparation of the 3% of the dry weight of the tumor contained "66 per cent protein, 26 per cent ribosenucleic acid and less than 0.3 per cent desoxyribosenucleic acid." They indicated as a priority the "elucidation of the nature of the active material" (Cohen, Levi-Montalcini, & Hamburger, 1954, p. 1017, p. 1018). Therefore, the substance they had to identify was certainly a compound of proteins and nucleic acids. But what was the active ingredient? The enzyme biochemist Arthur Kornberg, who was based at the microbiology department, suggested to Stan to treat the factor with snake venom. This contained enzymes that break down nucleic acids, thus leaving the protein unaltered. The results of the test of the snake venom were surprising:

"The next day I saw the most incredible culture I had ever seen. The ganglion in culture had produced a massive number of nerve fibers in a single day." (Cohen, 2008, p. 33794).

It produced a "stupendous halo radiating from the ganglia," a much bigger halo (three thousand times richer) than that produced by the mouse tumor. "Treatment of the sarcoma factor with snake venom enhanced its activity, and subsequent tests showed that snake venom contains a very potent growth-promoting agent. [. . .] approximately 3.000–6000 times as active as crude tumor homogenates [. . .] in promoting nerve fibers outgrowth in spinal ganglia in vitro." (Cohen & Levi-Montalcini, 1956, p. 571) The venom itself probably contained a substance with the same property stimulating the growth of the nervous fibers and its behavior was "similar to that shown by the 'protein factor' isolated from sarcoma 180" (Cohen & Levi-Montalcini, 1956, p. 571). The inhibitory effect of the antiserum suggested that the active factor was associated "with one of the protein components of the venom," and the effects of the most purified venom preparation had specific activity in promoting the growth of the nerve fibers in the spinal ganglia "1.000 times as high as the purest tumor fraction." But it was improbable that two chemically identical proteins were found in such unrelated substances.

In control experiments, using venom and not the tumor, the same effect was observed. Stan had brilliant intuition: because the venom came from snake salivary glands, he investigated mammalian salivary glands. He discovered that the submaxillary salivary glands of male mice produce high levels of a homologous substance—a readily available and cheap source of the factor. He was able to purify it.

"What could be the connection between nerve growth, tumors, and snake venom?" Nothing obvious—but I thought 'where does snake venom come from, a modified salivary gland?' So, at random, I tested extracts of the salivary gland taken from a male mouse and found that it was just as potent as the snake venom protein in inducing nerve growth in cultures." (Cohen, 2008, p. 33794)

Nerve growth factor (or NGF) was formally named in 1954 (Finger, 2013, p. 308). Three seminal papers were published in the March issue of *PNAS* in 1960. In the first one, Stan described the isolation of the protein stimulating neuronal growth, the orienting neural processes to specific targets, and the preparation of its antiserum. After 12 days from injection of this factor in newborn mice, a remarkable increase of protein, DNA, and RNA of the dorsal cervical ganglion of the mouse was observed (respectively six, two, and three times greater than that of the control ganglion). At that time, however, "the role of salivary glands with respect to the nerve growth factor [was] not clear"; Rita and her assistant Barbara Booker examined whether this factor was produced elsewhere in the organism and stored in the salivary glands (Cohen, 1960, p. 310). In two papers, Rita and Barbara Booker described the growth-promoting activity of the purified nerve growth factor on various mammalian embryonic ganglia and on sympathetic ganglia of (in vivo) newborn and adult mice (Levi-Montalcini & Booker, 1960a), and the cytological effect of a specific antiserum, which lead to the destruction of the developing sympathetic ganglia (Levi-Montalcini & Booker, 1960b). This phenomenon, subsequently called "immunosympathectomy," gained interest in the 1960s, convincing the skeptics of the biological importance of NGF (Iversen, 2013).

In December 1958, Rita received distressing news, which resonated "like the tolling of a funeral bell": Due to budget restrictions, Hamburger could no longer pay a professor of biochemistry in a zoology department. Rita (who had been appointed Associate Professor in 1956) was promoted to full Professor, but Stan had to go. At the beginning of what Rita herself called the NGF saga, she feared that the research would inevitably be slowed down or even interrupted. Cohen's contribution was fundamental, because he had continued to investigate the biochemical properties of NGF, discovering other effects. Before leaving St. Louis, Stan observed how mice injected with crude (not yet entirely purified) extract of salivary male mouse glands opened their eyes and grew teeth earlier. While at Vanderbilt University in Nashville, Cohen discovered the molecule called EGF (Epidermal Growth Factor), which had a proliferative effect on connective tissue.

Now it was time to discover the structure of that substance and its action mechanism. Rita was aware of the importance of the contribution of a biochemist. As she was no longer able to count on Cohen's collaboration, she was lucky enough to benefit from the help of a young Italian pathologist, Piero Angeletti, from the Washington University Medical School. Angeletti, defined as "a prominent figure in early discoveries" (Levi-Montalcini, 1997, viii), significantly contributed to the research on NGF purification and analysis of its spectrum of activity in the peripheral nervous system (Bradshaw et al., 2017).

BACK TO ITALY
"Heimat" and the Feeling of Family

In 1986, when Rita and Stan Cohen were awarded the Albert Lasker Medical Research Award, she stated that winning the award was particularly gratifying, because for many years "there was doubt that I was—as I really was—responsible for the discovery" (interview by Anthony Liversidge, in *Omni*, March 1988, p. 72). For a long time, Rita feared the scientific community lacked interest in NGF:

> During the 1960-70 decades, the field of NGF was a sort of private hunting ground. Despite the interest aroused by the two articles Stan Cohen and I published in the *PNAS* in 1960, few scientists ventured down our same path, the results being so perplexing and hard to reconcile with prevailing theory. (Levi-Montalcini, 1988, p. 196)

She also felt that her name was not mentioned: "People repeated my experiment and didn't mention my name! I am not a person to be bitter but it was astonishing to find it completely cancelled" (*Omni*, p. 72). Therefore, together with Cohen and Booker, she developed a series of proofs to illustrate the importance of NGF in symposia, conferences, and meetings. Lloyd Green, who met Rita when he was a student, recalled that at the end of each speech, she was always the first to raise her hand, not to ask questions, but to tell the long story of NGF (Abbott, 2009, p. 567).

At the same time, her desire to be reunited with her mother and Paola became more intense. Rita told Viktor of her wish, which happened to occur contemporarily with the project to establish research unity on NGF in Italy. Viktor was understanding: Rita was to complete the semester of the neurobiology course in St. Louis and, during the time she was in Italy (three months), Angeletti would head the laboratory.

For a while, Rita commuted between Rome and Turin (as well as Rome and St. Louis) until the death of her mother. Paola and Rita settled in Rome, in a beautiful house decorated with Paola's paintings and portraits and full of plants and flowers. Problems were arising due to Italian bureaucracy. Nevertheless, in 1961 her project was welcomed by the Italian Institute of Health and by the National Research Council (CNR) and a space was found to set up the laboratory on the premises of the biochemistry department of the Institute of Health.

The Italian adventure began and, with it, her "life commuting between two continents." In addition to Angeletti, Rita could count on Ruth Hogue Angeletti, Rita's only PhD student and postdoctoral fellow, and Ralph Bradshaw, a young Washington University biochemist, who identified the precise sequence of NGF's (118) amino acids (Hogue-Angeletti & Bradshaw, 1971). Twelve years later, a team of researchers in the United States identified the DNA coding for NGF (Scott et al., 1983). Other essential collaborators were Pietro Calissano, Enrico Alleva, Luigi Aloe, and afterward, Antonino Cattaneo with a team of young postgraduates, who wanted to join Rita despite the modest and precarious salary. Calissano's investigations contributed to elucidating the NGF's mechanism of action at the molecular level. This was complicated by the nature of the nerve cells. When cultivated in vitro, they are in their final differentiative stage; in the absence of NGF, they die, making it impossible to conduct parallel research in the absence of this factor.

In 1969, Vincenzo Caglioti decided to transform the small Center of Neurobiology into an official CNR organ: the "Institute of Cell Biology." In 1986, Rita founded the Institute of Neurobiology. In her autobiography, however, she complained that in the early 1980s the CNR demonstrated a lack of interest in neurobiology, instead privileging molecular biology. Rita had to face several obstacles: the (quantitatively) inferior scientific production in Italy; the desire for autonomy and the tendency of Italian researchers not to work as a team; and the chronic lack of funding. But she refused to give up. Indeed, in 2001 she proposed to found the European Brain Research Institute (EBRI) and in 2004 the European Centre for Brain Research (CERC). In the first decade of the 2000s, EBRI showed significant losses. The Turin neurophysiologist Piergiorgio Strata was called upon to improve the situation, and Rita was confident in him. But Strata resigned almost immediately. By 2008 the funding was halved compared to previous years. Nevertheless, Rita was an optimist: research had to continue. Ruth Angeletti recalled that Rita was tireless: she called her collaborators early in the morning and discussions continued until night. Rita found the beauty in the nervous system.

Nobel Prize, Joys and Sorrows

Rita confessed that in the 1960s, because of her disappointment, she decided "not to do any work on NGF," and started a new research line on the development of the peripheral and central nervous system of the *Periplaneta Americana* cockroaches, eventually identifying a molecule promoting neurite growth. This study produced a dozen articles on the mechanism of nervous interaction in these insects.

"But in 1972 I decided I could not give up my child, the NGF." The Nobel Prize and the Lasker award "recognized the truth even more." In 1986, the Nobel Assembly of the Karolinska Institute awarded the Nobel Prize in Physiology or Medicine jointly to Rita and Stan "for their discoveries of 'growth factors'." Their discoveries demonstrated "how a skilled observer can create a concept out of apparent chaos." Stan and Rita opened new fields of widespread importance to basic science. As a direct consequence, we may increase our understanding of many disease states such as developmental malformations, degenerative changes in senile dementia, delayed wound healing, and tumor diseases. The characterization of these growth factors is therefore expected, in the near future, to result in the development of new therapeutic agents and improved treatment in various clinical diseases.

Before and after winning the Nobel Prize, Rita won "plenty of innumerable awards": Justice was done. In 1987, she was awarded the National Medal of Science with the following citation presented by then President Ronald Reagan:

> For a major breakthrough in neurobiology by her discovery of the Nerve Growth Factor and its effect on the growth of the sympathetic nervous system which set the stage for worldwide studies of the molecules involved in normal and malignant growth.

Even before receiving the Nobel Prize, Rita was a member of many national and foreign academies and scientific societies, including the American Academy of Arts and Sciences (1966), the United States National Academy of Sciences (the 10th woman elected, 1968) the Pontifical Academy of Science (the first woman to be admitted, 1974), the Accademia dei Lincei (1990). She received the Max Weinstein Prize from the United Cerebral Palsy Association (1963), the Antonio Feltrinelli Prize (1969), the William Thomson Wakeman Research Award of the National Paraplegic Foundation (1974), the Lewis S. Rosenstiel Award for Distinguished Work in Basic Medical Research of Brandeis University (1982), the Louisa Gross Horwitz Prize from Columbia University (1983), the Ralph W. Gerard Prize in Neuroscience (1985), and the Albert Lasker Basic Medical Research Award (1986).

Some historians observed that, as the years passed, her "roller coaster" eased up a little. "She buried the hatched with literally everybody in the field," Ralph Bradshaw remarked (McGrayne, 1993, p. 220) recognizing that "Rita had to endure a great deal of scepticism in the early days and there were times when she was justifiably defensive" (Abbott, 2009, p. 567). In her obituary in *Nature*, he observed that

> Rita has been described as ambitious, autocratic, generous, possessive, aristocratic, demanding, persevering, insightful and totally dedicated to her work. All are accurate. She had disagreements with many scientists who worked on NGF. However, as the importance of her discoveries became increasingly appreciated, she mellowed in her outlook (if not her drive) and seemed to accept the mantle of matriarch that was truly her due. (Bradshaw, 2013)

Awards and honors launched Rita as a media personality. She participated in debates, meetings, conferences, and the initial skepticism of the scientific community was overcome. According to Michel Goedert, scientists at the time were mostly familiar with hormones. The protein was not released into the blood, but acted to promote cell growth (Watts, 2013).

But it was not all fun and games. No matter that Rita dedicated her Nobel Prize to Hamburger, "who promoted and took part in this research, and to whom I am forever indebted for his invaluable suggestions and generosity. Without him, the Nerve Growth Factor would never have come to our attention," as she remarked in her Nobel Lecture (Levi-Montalcini, 1986). In the scientific community, some neuroscientists were convinced that the Nobel Committee should also have honored Hamburger, who was 88 years old. In the "Perspectives" of *Trends in Neurosciences*, Dale Purves and Joshua Sanes of the Washington University Medical School objected that "whereas biologists of all denominations are delighted by the award to Levi-Montalcini and Cohen, many neuroscientists are puzzled by the omission of Viktor Hamburger from the prize," claiming that this "exclusion [tended] to obscure a line of research that now spans more than 50 years" (Purves & Sanes, 1987, p. 231). This opinion must have been widely shared, because in 2001, W. Maxwell Cowan commented that "by not including Viktor Hamburger, the Nobel committee had failed to appreciate the significance of his earlier contributions that had paved the way to the discovery of NGF" (Cowan, 2001, pp. 551–552). As reported in *The New York Times* on the 14th of October 1986, Jean Lauder of the University of North Carolina—at the time President of the International Society of Developmental Neuroscience—said that she and others were considering writing to *Science* and *Nature* to express their view that Hamburger should have shared the Nobel Prize.

The interview mentioned above with *Omni* had an adverse effect: perhaps to defend the Nobel Committee for its decision, Rita sustained her "priority," declaring that "Viktor Hamburger was not there when I made the discovery [. . .] He was in Boston and I was in Rio de Janeiro all by myself when I discovered how to elucidate the way NGF works. So I believe I really am the discoverer of NGF." Disappointment with her failure to recognize Viktor's role in the NGF discovery had an impact on the reception of *In Praise of Imperfection*. In a review for *Science*, Purves observed that the latter half of the book, covering Rita's career in the United States, was "less satisfying" (Purves, 1988, p. 1366), because crucial insights "were depicted as a series of revelations." The account of her life outlined a sweetened vision of science and scientific progress: Readers could scarcely appreciate the doubts and conflicts behind scientific advancement. The contributions by Levi, Hamburger, and Angeletti were deliberately left in the background. The personal side of this story was judged "inadequate," and Purves highlighted Rita's "aggressive spirit" and "fierce competitor" attitude, elements which were not revealed in her autobiography. Sarcastically, he concluded that this gap would be filled by the numerous biographers who would have praised Levi-Montalcini.

Hamburger, who had a completely different style and personality from Rita and was awarded the National Medal in Science in 1989, only commented that he did not resent the decision of the Nobel Committee, but that Rita had no respect for his science. When Rita returned to St. Louis in 1991, Viktor (91 years old at the time) did not join the dinner with her (McGrayne, 1993, p. 221).

Another "shameful outrage" against Rita (see *Independent*, 16th of February 1994) was represented by the malevolent assumption that the Italian pharmaceutical company Fidia of Abano Terme (Padua) had spent part of 14bn lire to influence the Nobel Committee. The Nobel Assembly rejected the charges.

But in the end, these shadows were passing, and Rita's image was not affected. In 2001 she was nominated senator-for-life by Italian President Carlo Azeglio Ciampi, in recognition of her scientific and social efforts. This position enabled her to participate in parliamentary debates. In the Senate, she was keen to ensure that all laws passed had effects on science, influencing many key policy questions. Under the Prodi government (2006–2008), she was continually present in Senate sessions, always voting in favor of the Government, and in some cases her vote was crucial to avoid its fall. Celebrating her 100th birthday, *Nature* described the story of her decisive vote in 2006. Rita threatened not to give her vote, if they did not agree to eliminate that section of the budget that cut funds to science. "She won" (Abbott, 2009, p. 565). In Italy she was President of the Institute of the *Italian Encyclopaedia* founded by Giovanni Treccani (1993–1998) and Honorary President of the National Committee for Bioethics. In 2010, the Minister of Education, University and Research launched the "Progetto Montalcini" for the return of young researchers to Italy. In 1995, she was elected Foreign Member of the Royal Society and in 2009 she received the Wendell Krieg Lifetime Achievement Award established by the Cajal Club. In 1999, she became FAO Goodwill Ambassador and, over time, held many honorary degrees including those from Uppsala University, Weizmann Institute (Israel), Saint Mary University (London), Constantinian University (United States), University of Trieste, Polytechnic University of Turin, Complutense University of Madrid, McGill University. She was conferred with the title of Grand Officer of the Order of the Legion of Honour (France) and of Lady of the Grand Cross of the Order of Isabel the Catholic. The asteroid 9722 Levi-Montalcini, discovered in 1981, was named in her honor.

In April 2009, her closest collaborators dedicated a book of "unpublished portraits" to her (Alleva et al., 2009). Colleagues and pupils unanimously described her intellectual curiosity, her contagious enthusiasm, her fight against discrimination, her *ante-litteram* feminism, her constant work to affirm young neuroscientists, her capacity to be a role model for young female researchers, and her commitment in support of the Foundation for Africa. In 1992, influenced by Albert Schweitzer, Rita and her sister Paola established, in memory of their father, the "Rita Levi-Montalcini Foundation" to help young African women find scholarships "to improve their chances of becoming scientists" (quoted in Abbott, 2009, p. 567). In addition to her commitment to education, Rita became interested in the issue of ageing, and saw an antidote against the decline of the capabilities of the aging brain and intellectual activity (Bentivoglio, 2013).

Luigi Aloe remembered that she was not only a woman of remarkable culture, but also a very fashionable woman, and a real force of nature in the laboratory, echoing an opinion that Viktor had expressed: "She sees things that others cannot see." She had remarkable observational skills and did not love statistical analysis, preferring "experiments with a yes or no answer" (Chao & Calissano, 2013, p. 385). Calissano emphasized the role played by her imagination, which was a determining factor in her experiments. Calissano also reported that there was a plaque with Einstein's famous quote, "imagination is more important than knowledge," in the cell-culture room in the Centre of Neurobiology in Rome. Rita used to say that her scientific attitude was a mix of intuition and imagination, and not merely one of complex reasoning. She applied the same intuition to recruitment at the Centre of Neurobiology: Dismissing candidates' CVs, she had a peculiar, "artistic" sensibility that she used to find the most promising young talents devoted to research. Rita also admired the figure of Martin Luther King, Jr. When he was assassinated in 1968, she took part in a march in his honor in St. Louis. A large poster of the American civil rights leader dominated her office, above the quote: "A man who is not ready to die for his ideas is not fit to live."

Some Feminine Curiosity and Epilogue

Photos and interviews from the last few years of Rita's life always portray an old and beautiful woman with a sweet expression and a gentle smile. Rita was always very elegant, impeccably combed and dressed. The style of her clothes was unmistakable: They were creations by Roberto Capucci. For the Nobel Prize Ceremony, Capucci offered Rita a velvet dress in three colors: three very dark tones of green, red, and purple with a small tail. At first, she was somewhat perplexed, but because she would be the only woman among all men in tails, Rita accepted the proposal. She had a very thin physique. There were three fixed points to follow: She liked narrow waists, puffed sleeves, and high 19th-century necks. The puffed sleeves served to accentuate her shoulders, which were minute. The clothes had to be *longuette*, and she always wore heeled shoes. Rita loved silks, such as georgette, but also very light wools and *plissés*. As for the colors, she preferred black, all shades of gray, but also the darker tones of other colors. Even in old age "with her high heels and the swing of her tailored coat, she still looks as though she stepped off the pages of a fashion magazine" (Abbott, 2009, p. 567).

Her beautiful jewelry often turned the heads of many other women. In 1982, Maria Grazia Spillantini, Professor of Molecular Neurology in the Department of Clinical Neurosciences at the University of Cambridge, met Rita for a fellowship, establishing a collaboration that would last 30 years. From a female's perspective, she observed: "Although she was passionate about science she was also very feminine. She dressed very elegantly and had beautiful jewellery. She designed some of it herself" (Watts, 2013). The brooch that almost always appears in photographs of her (also at the Nobel Prize award ceremony in 1986) was special: created by her brother, it represented a sort of talisman, the symbol of a family bond, and a sign of a strong taste. On her right wrist, Rita wore a bracelet she designed, decorated with the lily of Florence, like a tiny cameo. Another bracelet was in the style of ancient Egypt, other jewels were copies of Renaissance jewels, and her pearl necklace belonged to her mother.

She had a gracious, grateful, but "very assertive" personality. Although the concept of "apoptosis" was introduced in 1972, she asserted that she had discovered cell death many years earlier: "I discovered apoptosis 30 years before it was discovered, because I saw also cells that die. What is the reason? And then in 1972 it was given the name of apoptosis." She was referring to a description of a spontaneous form of neuronal death in the chick embryo observed with Levi in 1940s (Chao, 2010, p. 8; Aloe, 2013, p. 140).

In the chapters dedicated to Rita within the *Nobel Prize Women in Science* (McGrayne, 1993; see also Yount, 2009), there are several anecdotes on her determined character. Particularly entertaining is the story of how she flew in the copilot's seat to attend a conference in Paris, after noticing she was not booked on the flight. Having lost her luggage during another flight, at a conference at Harvard University she refused to wear her rumpled traveling clothes and wore the only available clean dress: an evening gown. Robert Provine, one of Rita and Viktor's pupils, stressed her theatrical attitude—one that was not limited merely to her clothing and style. He recounts how her Comparative Neuroanatomy lecture courses were very well-attended and her regal entrance to the seminar hall was preceded by a group of assistants and technicians who would set up her projector and load her slides for her. (Provine, 2001, p. 146; Rodríguez de Romo, 2007, pp. 283–285). She became famous for her sophisticated dinner parties organized with typical Piedmontese dishes: truffles, chicken liver paté, *filet en chemise*, ice cream, and so on.

Rita made no attempt to hide her proud character even when she was appointed to the Pontifical Academy by Pope Paul VI. The American neuroscientist Thomas A. Woolsey recalled that, in the presence of the Pope, instead of kneeling and kissing his hand, she "simply stood and shook the Pope's hand" (Aloe & Chaldakov, 2013b, p. 6). The most lucid, frill-free account of her fantastic adventure she offered herself in an interview with the newspaper, *La Repubblica* on her 99th birthday. Among other things, she recognized she had renounced marriage for science, but not love. She fell in love and was happy. But her only child was the NGF. Rita was "extremely possessive of NGF. She viewed it as her private property. It became her child" (McGrayne, 1993, p. 219; Aloe, 2011, p. 178).

She dared to affirm:

> Without Mussolini and Hitler today I would only be an old lady one step away from her centenary. Thanks to those two, instead, I arrived in Stockholm. I never felt persecuted. I lived my being Jewish in a secular way, without pride and without humility. I do not go to synagogue or church. I do not boast the historical fact of

belonging to a human race that has suffered a lot as some kind of medal, nor have I ever tried to derive moral advantages or reparations. Being Jewish may not be pleasant, it's not comfortable, but it has created an additional intellectual impulse in us. How can we say that Albert Einstein was of inferior race? We should also abolish the concept of race in our minds. There are racists, not races. And I'm only interested in people. ("La Repubblica", December 31st, 2012)

During this interview, Rita stated she went to the laboratory every day to follow microscopic research with her team members precisely as she did 50 years before in America, and that her brain worked even better than when she was young. "I have lost a little sight, and a lot of hearing. In conferences I have trouble seeing the slides and hearing well. But I think more now than I did when I was 20. One's body does what it wants, but I am not my body; I am its mind." She was the longest-living Nobel laureate. Rita used to say that caloric restriction and little sleep contributed to her healthiness, but she declared herself indifferent to health and death. Aged 102 years, she was one of the authors of an article describing how NGF regulates axial rotation in early stages of chick embryo development (Manca et al., 2012).

Her sister Paola passed away in September 2000, and Rita wrote for her the book *The universo inquieto* (2001). Rita died on the 30th of December 2012 in her home in Via di Villa Massimo in Rome, aged 103. When her body was laid in the Senate building, thousands of people went to pay a final tribute to her, and the world's most influential media covered her death. She is buried at the Cimitero Monumentale in Turin, her hometown. In the obituary in *Nature*, Bradshaw commented: "Had her extraordinary life been scripted by Hollywood, it would had been rejected as too improbable" (Bradshaw, 2013, p. 306).

During the 2000s, Hamburger's prediction of "many new trials" in neuroembryology (as Rita Levi-Montalcini had reported in her Nobel Lecture) came true; furthermore, the prophecies of the utilization of the NGF in brain and immunosystem disorders (Levi-Montalcini et al., 1990) have increasingly been confirmed (Zeliadt, 2013, p. 4876). Since 1975, when Aloe and Rita made a seminal experiment that demonstrated that NGF acted on non-neuronal cells, evidence has been accumulated that its influence is "wider than the sky" acting also on immune, epithelial, pancreatic, adipose tissue cells, fibroblasts, and cardiomyocytes. NGF and its receptors likely act against cell degeneration in the nervous system, visual system, and cutaneous and myocardial tissues. (A review of the potential therapeutic role of NGF and brain-derived neurotrophic factor [BDNF] is in Aloe & Chaldakov, 2013a.)

From the beginning of the discovery of NGF, Rita was convinced that the overproduction of NGF could be correlated with certain cancers, while reduced protein production could be associated with other neurological disorders (Finger, 2013, p. 309). For the potential clinical use of NGF and the translational research in Alzheimer's and Huntington's diseases (Tuszynski et al., 2005; Nagahara et al., 2009; Zuccato & Cattaneo, 2007, 2009; Mitra et al., 2018) and other neuropathies (Martinowich et al., 2007), refer also to the review literature (Aloe et al., 2012, 2015; Manni et al., 2013; Aloe & Rocco, 2015; Rocco et al., 2018). Rita's research "was not directly concerned with clinical applications per se" (Chao & Calissano, 2013, p. 387), and although "clinically NGF has not yet proved as valuable as originally hoped" (Watts, 2013), this lack of results must not obscure the value of the pioneering work of Levi-Montalcini (Giudice, 2000, p. 565). For the first time, Rita revealed that nervous growth is *chemically* guided. Through her discovery, she cleared the ground of all hypotheses of both random phenomena or processes guided by less determined forces. Adopting a *holistic* approach in neurobiology, she thought that NGF had an "organismic role":

"It is a universal molecule which is very important for vital roles, the vital role of NGF, which is not only neurogenetic [. . .] NGF is not an organizer. If you take away the organizer, you have no organism to form. If you take [it] away by interjecting mouse or if you take it away by antibody to NGF, the embryo is formed but is very badly formed, and it's doomed to die because there's not a capacity of proliferation, so it will slowly die, not like it will be no formation of the embryo. The embryo is very poorly built." (Chao, 2010, p. 10)

Her results anticipated the demonstration of the role of neurotrophic factors not only in the nervous system, but also in immune and endocrine systems (Tometten et al., 2005; Skaper, 2017) and at the basis of aggressive behavior (Aloe et al., 1986; Alleva et al., 1993; Bigi et al., 1992), memory (Wang et al., 2012; Kopec & Carew, 2013), learning and neuronal plasticity (Conner et al., 2009; Biane et al., 2014), pain (Mizumura & Murase, 2015; Chang et al., 2016; Denk et al., 2017; Lane & Corr, 2017) and fertility (Lougheed, 2012; Palumbo et al., 2013).

Rita was convinced that curiosity, total dedication, and a tendency to underestimate difficulties in the research were more important than intelligence. Without a pre-established plan and following her private inclination and luck, she reached the goal of that imperfection which, more than perfection, she believed belonged to human nature.

REFERENCES

Abbott A (2009) One hundred years of Rita. *Nature*, 458: 564–567.

Alleva E, Aloe L, & Bigi S (1993) An updated role for Nerve Growth Factor in neurobehavioural regulation of adult vertebrates. *Review in the Neurosciences*, 4: 41–62.

Alleva E, De Castro P, & Taranto M (a cura di) (2009) *CuriosaMente: Ritratti inediti di Rita Levi-Montalcini*. Roma: Istituto Superiore di Sanità.

Aloe L (2011) Rita Levi-Montalcini and the discovery of NGF, the first nerve cell growth factor. *Archives Italiennes de Biologie*, 149: 175–181.

Aloe L (2013) In Memoriam Rita Levi-Montalcini (1909–2012). *Growth Factors*, 31 (4): 139–140.

Aloe L, Alleva E, Böhm A, & Levi-Montalcini R (1986) Aggressive behavior induces release of nerve growth factor from mouse salivary gland into the bloodstream. *Neurobiology*, 83: 6184–6187.

Aloe L, & Chaldakov G N (2013a) Homage to Rita Levi-Montalcini, the queen of modern neuroscience. *Cell Biology International*, 37: 761–765.

Aloe L, & Chaldakov G N (2013b) The multiple lives of the nerve growth factor: Tribute to Rita Levi-Montalcini. *Balkan Medical Journal*, 30: 4–7.

Aloe L, Rocco M L, Bianchi P, & Manni L (2012) Nerve growth factor: From the early discoveries to the potential clinical use. *Journal of Translational Medicine*, 10: 239.
Aloe L, Rocco M L, Balzamino B O, & Micera A (2015) Nerve growth factor: A focus on neuroscience and therapy. *Current Neuropharmacology*, 13 (3): 294–303.
Aloe L, & Rocco M L (2015) NGF and therapeutic prospective. What have we learned from the NGF transgenic models? *Ann Ist Super Sanità*, 51 (1): 5–10.
Angeletti R H, & Bradshaw R A (1971) Nerve growth factor from mouse submaxillary gland: Amino acid sequence. *Proceedings of the National Academy of Sciences of the United States of America*, 68: 2417–2420.
Bentivoglio M (2013) Looking at the future with Rita. *Neuroscience* 252: 438–442.
Bentivoglio M, Vercelli A, & Filogamo G (2006) Giuseppe Levi: Mentor of three Nobel laureates. *Journal of History of Neurosciences*, 15: 358–368.
Biane J, Conner J M, & Tuszynski M H (2014) Nerve growth factor is primarily produced by GABAergic neurons of the adult rat cortex. *Frontiers in Cellular Neuroscience*, 8: 220.
Bigi S, Mastripieri D, Aloe L, & Alleva E (1992) NGF decreases isolation-induced aggressive behavior, while increasing adrenal volume, in adult male mice. *Physiology & Behavior*, 51: 337–343.
Bradshaw R A (2013) Rita Levi-Montalcini (1909–2012) Nobel prizewinning neurobiologist and eminent advocate for science. *Nature*, 493: 306.
Bradshaw R A, Mobley W, & Rush R A (2017) Nerve growth factor and related substances: A brief history and an introduction to the International NGF Meeting Series. *International Journal of Molecular Sciences*, 18: 1143.
Bueker E D (1948) Implantation of tumors in the hind limb field of the embryonic chick and the developmental response of the lumbosacral nervous system. *The Anatomical Record*, 102: 369–389.
Chang D S, Hsu E, Hottinger D G, & Cohen S P (2016) Anti-nerve growth factor in pain management: Current evidence. *Journal of Pain Research*, 9: 373–383.
Chao M V (2010) A Conversation with Rita Levi-Montalcini. *Annual Review Physiology*, 72: 1–13.
Chao M V, & Calissano P (2013) Rita Levi-Montalcini: In memoriam. *Neuron*, 77: 385–387.
Cohen S (1960) Purification of a nerve growth-promoting protein from the mouse salivary gland and its neuro-cytotoxic antiserum. *Proceedings of the National Academy of Sciences of the United States of America*, 46: 302–311.
Cohen S (1962) Isolation of a mouse submaxillary gland protein accelerating incisor eruption and eyelid opening in the newborn animal. *Journal of Biological Chemistry*, 237: 1535–1562.
Cohen S (2008) Origins of growth factors: NGF and EGF. *Journal of Biological Chemistry*, 283: 33793–33797.
Cohen S, & Levi-Montalcini R (1956) A nerve growth-stimulating factor isolated from snake venom. *Proceedings of the National Academy of Sciences of the United States of America*, 42: 571–574.
Cohen S, Levi-Montalcini R, & Hamburger V (1954) A nerve growth-stimulating factor isolated from sarcom as 37 and 180. *Proceedings of the National Academy of Sciences of the United States of America*, 40: 1014–1018.
Conner J M, Franks K M, Titterness A K, Russell K, Merrill DA, Christie B R, Sejnowski T J, & Tuszynski M H (2009) NGF is essential for hippocampal plasticity and learning. *Journal of Neuroscience*, 29: 10883–10889.
Cowan W M (2001) Viktor Hamburger and Rita Levi-Montalcini: The path to the discovery of nerve growth factor. *Annual Review of Neuroscience*, 24: 551–600.
Denk F, Bennett D L, & McMahon S B (2017) Nerve growth factor and pain mechanisms. *Annual Review of Neuroscience*, 40: 307–325.
Finger S (2013) Obituary. Rita Levi-Montalcini (1908–2012). *Journal of the History of Neurosciences*, 22: 307–309.

Giudice G (2000) From a home-made laboratory to the Nobel Prize. An interview with Rita Levi-Montalcini. *International Journal of Developmental Biology*, 44: 563–566.
Grignolio A (2018) Nota bibliografica su Giuseppe Levi. *Medicina nei secoli. Arte e Scienza*, 30: 423–446.
Hamburger V (1992) History of the discovery of neuronal death in embryos. *Journal of Neurobiology*, 23:1116–1123.
Hamburger V (1993) The history of the discovery of the nerve growth factor. *Journal of Neurobiology*, 24: 893–897.
Hamburger V, & Levi-Montalcini R (1949) Proliferation, differentiation and degeneration in the spinal ganglia of the chick embryo under normal and experimental conditions. *Journal of Experimental Zoölogy*, 111: 457–502.
Hollyday M (1989) Review of *In Praise of Imperfection. The Quarterly Review in Biology*, 64: 183–184.
Iversen L L (2013) Rita Levi-Montalcini: Neuroscientist par excellence. *Proceedings of the National Academy of Sciences of the United States of America*, 110: 4862–4863.
Kopec A M, & Carew T J (2013) Growth factor signaling and memory formation: Temporal and spatial integration of a molecular network. *Learning & Memory*, 20: 531–539.
Lane N E, & Corr M (2017) Osteoarthritis in 2016: Anti-NGF treatments for pain—Two steps forward, one step back? *Nature Reviews Rheumatology*, 13: 76–78.
Levi-Montalcini R (1986) Nobel lecture: The nerve growth factor: Thirty-five years later. https://www.nobelprize.org/uploads/2018/06/levi-montalcini-lecture.pdf.
Levi-Montalcini R (1987) *Elogio dell'imperfezione*. Milano: Garzanti. Translated by L. Attardi, *In Praise of Imperfection*. New York: Basic Books, 1988.
Levi-Montalcini R (1992) NGF: An uncharted route. In F G Worden, J P Swazey, & A Adelman (Eds.), *The Neurosciences: Paths of Discovery*, pp. 245–265. Boston: Berkhäuser.
Levi-Montalcini R (1993) *Il tuo futuro*. Milano: Garzanti.
Levi-Montalcini R (1996) *Senz'olio contro vento*. Milano: Baldini & Castoldi.
Levi-Montalcini R (1998) *L'asso nella manica a brandelli*. Milano: Baldini & Castoldi.
Levi-Montalcini R (1999) *La galassia mente*. Milano: Baldini & Castoldi.
Levi-Montalcini R (2000) *Il cantico di una vita*. Milano: Cortina.
Levi-Montalcini R (2001) *Un universo inquieto. Vita e opere di Paola Levi Montalcini*. Milano: Baldini & Castoldi.
Levi-Montalcini R (2002) Carlos Chaga Filho: Scientist and humanist. In: The challenge of sciences. A tribute to Carlos Chaga. Vatican City: Pontifical Academy of Sciences. *Scripta Varia*, 103, 118–124.
Levi-Montalcini R (Ed.) (1997) *The Saga of the Nerve Growth Factor: Preliminary Studies, Discovery, Further Development*. Singapore: World Scientific Publishing.
Levi-Montalcini R, Aloe L, & Alleva E (1990) A role for nerve growth factor in nervous, endocrine and immune systems. *Progress in Neuroendocrineimmunology*, 3: 1–10.
Levi-Montalcini R, & Booker B (1960a) Excessive growth of the sympathetic ganglia evoked by a protein isolated from mouse salivary glands. *Proceedings of the National Academy of Sciences of the United States of America*, 46: 373–384.
Levi-Montalcini R, & Booker B (1960b) Destruction of the sympathetic ganglia in mammals by an antiserum to a nerve-growth protein. *Proceedings of the National Academy of Sciences of the United States of America*, 46: 384–391.
Levi-Montalcini R, & Hamburger V (1951) Selective growth stimulating effects of mouse sarcoma on the sensory and sympathetic nervous system of the chick embryo. *Journal of Experimental Zoölogy*, 116: 321–361.
Levi-Montalcini R, & Levi G (1942) Les conséquences de la destruction d'un territoire d'innervation périphérique sur le développement des centres nerveus correspondants dans l'embryon de poulet. *Archives de Biologie*, 53: 537–545.

Levi-Montalcini R, & Levi G (1943) Recherches quantitatives sur la marche du processus de différenciation des neurons dans les ganglions spinaux de l'embryon de Poulet. *Archives de Biologie*, 54: 189–206.
Levi-Montalcini R, & Levi G (1944) Correlazioni nello sviluppo tra varie parti del sistema nervoso. I. Conseguenze della demolizione dell'abbozzo di un arto sui centri nervosi nell'embrione di pollo. *Pontificiae Academiae Scientiarum Commentarii*, 8: 527–575.
Levi-Montalcini R, Meyer H, & Hamburger V (1954) In vitro experiments on the effects of mouse sarcomas 180 and 37 on the spinal and sympathetic ganglia of the chick embryo. *Cancer Research*, 14: 49–57.
Lillie F (1909) *The Development of the Chick: An Introduction to the Chick*. New York: Holt.
Liversidge A (1988) Interview: Rita Levi-Montalcini. *Omni* (March), 70–74 and 102–105.
Lougheed K (2012) Nerve-growth protein linked to ovulation. *Nature News* https://www.nature.com/news/nerve-growth-protein-linked-to-ovulation-1.11239#auth-1.
Manca A, Capsoni S, Di Luzio A, Vignone D, Malerba F, Paoletti F, Brandi R, Arisi I, Cattaneo A, & Levi-Montalcini R (2012) Nerve growth factor regulates axial rotation during early stages of chick embryo development. *Proceedings of the National Academy of Sciences of the United States of America*, 109: 2009–2014.
Manni L, Rocco ML, Bianchi P, Soligo M, Guaragna M, Paparo Barbaro S, & Aloe L (2013) Nerve growth factor: Basic studies and possible therapeutic applications. *Growth Factors*, 31: 4.
Martinowich K, Manji H, & Lu B (2007) New insights into BDNF function in depression and anxiety. *Nature Neuroscience*, 10: 1089–1093.
McGrayne S B (1993) *Nobel Prize Women in Science. Their Lives, Struggles and Momentous Discoveries*. New York: Birch Lane.
Mitra S, Behbahani H, & Eriksdotter M (2019) Innovative therapy for Alzheimer's disease—With focus on biodelivery of NGF. *Frontiers in Neuroscience*, 13: 38.
Mizumura K, & Murase S (2015) Role of nerve growth factor in pain. *Handbook of Experimental Pharmacology*, 227: 57–77.
Nagahara A H, Merrill D A, Coppola G, Tsukada, Schroeder B E, Shaked G M, Wang L, Blesch A, Kim A, Conner J M, Rockenstein E, Chao M V, Koo E H, Geschwind D, Masliah E, Chiba A A, & Tuszynski M H (2009) Neuroprotective effects of brain-derived neurotrophic factor in rodent and primate models of Alzheimer's disease. *Nature Medicine*, 15: 331–337.
Palumbo M A, Giuffrida E, Gulino F A, Leonardi E, Cantarella G, & Bernardini R (2013) Nerve growth factor (NGF) levels in follicular fluid of infertile patients undergoing in vitro fertilization (IVF) cycle. *Gynecological Endocrinology*, 29: 1002–1004.
Piazza A (2018) Portrait of Giuseppe Levi. Medicina nei secoli. *Arte e Scienza*, 30: 15–30.
Provine R R (2001) In the Trenches with Viktor Hamburger and Rita Levi-Montalcini (1965–1974): A Student's Perspective. *International Journal of Developmental Neuroscience*, 19: 143–149.
Purves D (1988) Struggles and discovery: In praise of imperfection. *Science*, 241: 1366.
Purves D, & Sanes J (1987) The 1986 Nobel Prize in physiology or medicine. *Trends in Neuroscience*, 10: 231–235.
Ribatti D (2018) *Il maestro dei Nobel. Giuseppe Levi, anatomista e istologo*. Roma: Carocci.
Rocco M L, Soligo M, Manni L, & Aloe L (2018) Nerve growth factor: Early studies and recent clinical trials. *Current Neuropharmacology*, 16 (10): 1455–1465.
Rodríguez de Romo A C (2007) Chance, creativity, and the discovery of the nerve growth factor. *Journal of the History of the Neurosciences*, 16: 268–287.
Sandrone S (2013) Rita Levi-Montalcini (1909–2012). *Journal of Neurology*, 260: 240–241.
Scott J, Selby M, Urdea M, Quiroga M, Bell G I, & Rutter W J (1983) Isolation and nucleotide sequence of a cDNA encoding the precursor of mouse nerve growth factor. *Nature* 302: 538–540.
Shorey M L (1909) The effect of the destruction of peripheral areas on the differentiation of the neuroblasts. *Journal of Experimental Zoölogy*, 8: 25–63.

Shorey M L (1911) Study of the differentiation of neuroblasts in artificial culture media. *Journal of Experimental Zoölogy*, 10: 85–93.
Skaper S D (2017) Nerve growth factor: A neuroimmune crosstalk mediator for all seasons. *Immunology*, 151: 1–15.
Spemann H, & Mangold H (1924) Induction of embryonic primordia by implantation of organizers from a different species. *Archiv für Mikroskopische Anatomie und Entwicklungsmechanik*, 100: 599–563.
Strata P (2018) Rita Levi-Montalcini and her major contribution to neurobiology. *Rendiconti Lincei. Scienze Fisiche e Naturali*, 29: 737–753.
Tometten M, Blois S, & Arck P C (2005) Nerve growth factor in reproductive biology: Link between the immune, endocrine and nervous system? *Chemical Immunology and Allergy*, 89: 135–148.
Tuszynski M H, Thal L, Pay M, Salmon D P, Sang U H, Bakay R, Patel P, Blesch A, Vahlsing H L, Ho G, Tong G, Potkin S G, Fallon J, Hansen L, Mufson E J, Kordower J H, Gall C, Conner J (2005) A phase 1 clinical trial of nerve growth factor gene therapy for Alzheimer disease. *Nature Medicine*, 11: 551–555.
Vetrano M (2018) https://rivistasavej.it/luniverso-inquieto-di-paola-levi-montalcini-5ad5f4fcee86
Visintini F, & Levi-Montalcini R (1939) Relazione tra differenziazione strutturale e funzionale dei centri e delle vie nervose nell'embrione di pollo. *Archives Suisses de Neurologie et de Psychiatrie*, 43: 1–45.
Wang S H, Liao X-M, Liu D, Hu J, Yin Y-Y, Wang J-Z, & Zhu L-Q (2012) NGF promotes long-term memory formation by activating poly(ADP-ribose) polymerase-1. *Neuropharmacology*, 63: 1085–1092.
Watts G (2013) Obituary. Rita Levi-Montalcini. *Lancet*, 381: 288.
Willier B H (1957) Frank Lillie. *Biographical Memoirs 30*, pp. 77–236. Washington, DC: National Academy of Sciences.
Yount L (2009) *Rita Levi-Montalcini: Discoverer of Nerve Growth Factor*. New York: Chelsea House.
Zeliadt N (2013) Rita Levi-Montalcini: NGF, the prototypical growth factor. *Proceedings of the National Academy of Sciences of the United States of America*, 110: 4873–4876.
Zuccato C, & Cattaneo E (2007) Role of brain-derived neurotrophic factor in Huntington's disease. *Progress in Neurobiology*, 8: 294–330.
Zuccato C, & Cattaneo E (2009) Brain-derived neurotrophic factor in neurodegenerative diseases. *Nature Review Neurology*, 5: 311–322.

INDEX

Page numbers followed by *f* indicate figures.